A Practical Guide to Mechanical Ventilation

A Practical Guide to Mechanical Ventilation

Edited by Jonathon D. Truwit and Scott K. Epstein

WILEY-BLACKWELL

A John Wiley & Sons, Ltd., Publication

This edition first published 2011, © 2011 by John Wiley & Sons, Ltd

Wiley-Blackwell is an imprint of John Wiley & Sons, formed by the merger of Wiley's global Scientific, Technical and Medical business with Blackwell Publishing.

Registered office: John Wiley & Sons Ltd, The Atrium, Southern Gate, Chichester, West Sussex, PO19 8SQ, UK

Editorial Offices:
9600 Garsington Road, Oxford, OX4 2DQ, UK
The Atrium, Southern Gate, Chichester, West Sussex, PO19 8SQ, UK
111 River Street, Hoboken, NJ 07030-5774, USA

For details of our global editorial offices, for customer services and for information about how to apply for permission to reuse the copyright material in this book please see our website at www.wiley.com/wiley-blackwell

Library of Congress Cataloguing-in-Publication Data

A practical guide to mechanical ventilation / edited by Jonathon D. Truwit and Scott K. Epstein.
      p. ; cm.
   Includes index.
   ISBN 978-0-470-05807-7 (pbk.)
   1. Artificial respiration–Handbooks, manuals, etc.   I. Truwit, Jonathon D.   II. Epstein, Scott K.
[DNLM: 1. Respiration, Artificial–methods.   2. Respiratory Tract Diseases–therapy.   3. Ventilator Weaning–methods.   4. Ventilators, Mechanical. WF 145]
   RC87.9.P69 2011
   615.8'36–dc22

2010037010

A catalogue record for this book is available from the British Library.

This book is published in the following electronic formats: ePDFs: 978-0-470-97659-3; Wiley Online Library: 978-0-470-97660-9; ePub: 978-0-470-97664-7

Set in 10.5 on 12.5 pt Times by Toppan Best-set Premedia Limited
Printed and bound in Singapore by Fabulous Printers Pte Ltd

First Impression 2011

Contents

Contributors

Mark R. Bowling, MD
Assistant professor of medicine
Division of Pulmonary, Critical Care,
    and Sleep Medicine
University of Mississippi
Jackson, MS, USA

David L. Bowton, MD
Section Head, Critical Care
    Anesthesia
Professor, Critical Care
    Anesthesia
Wake Forest University
Winston-Salem, NC, USA

Jeremy S. Breit, MD
Fellow, Pulmonary, Critical Care,
    Allergy and Immunology
Wake Forest University
Winston-Salem, NC, USA

Kyle B. Enfield, MD, MPH
Assistant Professor of
    Medicine
Pulmonary and Critical Care
    Medicine
University of Virginia
Charlottesville, VA, USA

Scott K. Epstein, MD, FCCP
Dean for Educational Affairs
Professor of Medicine
Tufts University School of Medicine,
    Boston, MA, USA

Daniel C. Grinnan, MD
Assistant Professor of Medicine
Division of Pulmonary and Critical
    Care Medicine
Virginia Commonwealth University
Richmond, VA, USA

Edward F. Haponik, MD
Professor, Pulmonary, Critical Care,
    Allergy, and Immunologic Medicine
Wake Forest University
Winston-Salem, NC, USA

Robert Duncan Hite, MD, FCCP,
    FACP
Professor and Chief,
Section on Pulmonary, Critical Care,
    Allergy and Immunology
Co-Chair, WFUBMC Critical Care
    Services
Wake Forest University
Winston-Salem, NC, USA

Drew A. MacGregor, MD
Professor, Critical Care Anesthesia,
   Pulmonary, Critical Care, Allergy,
   and Immunology,
Wake Forest University
Winston-Salem, NC, USA

Rodolfo M. Pascual, MD
Assistant Professor
Pulmonary, Critical Care, Allergy and
   Immunology
Wake Forest University
Winston-Salem, NC, USA

Scott van Poppel, MD
Fellow in Anesthesiology
Critical Care Division
Wake Forest University
Winston-Salem, NC, USA

Maged A. Tanios, MD, MPH
Director, Intensive Care Unit
St. Mary Medical Center
Long Beach, California
Associate Clinical Professor of
   Medicine
University of California,
Irvine, CA, USA

Jonathon D. Truwit, MD, MBA
E. Cato Drash Professor of Medicine
Chief, Pulmonary and Critical Care
   Medicine
Senior Associate Dean for Clinical
   Affairs
Chief Medical Officer
Box 800793
University of Virginia,
Charlottesville, VA, USA

Ali S. Wahla
Consultant Pulmonologist & Critical
   Care Physician
Shaukat Khanum Memorial Cancer
   Hospital and Research Center,
   Lahore, Pakistan

Marjolein de Wit, MD, MS
Assistant Professor of Medicine
Division of Pulmonary and Critical
   Care Medicine
Virginia Commonwealth University
Richmond, VA, USA

Part I
Noninvasive ventilation

1.1 Introduction to noninvasive ventilation

Daniel C. Grinnan[1] and Jonathon D. Truwit[2]

[1] *Division of Pulmonary and Critical Care Medicine, Virginia Commonwealth University, Richmond, VA, USA*
[2] *Division of Pulmonary and Critical Care Medicine, University of Virginia, Charlottesville, VA, USA*

1.1.1 Case presentation

You are called by a 45-year-old male with amyotrophic lateral sclerosis after recently starting him on nocturnal noninvasive ventilation by a nasal mask. He stated that his symptoms of morning headache and daytime fatigue have improved slightly. However, he can only wear the nasal mask for a few hours at a time. He has an air leak from the mask which leads to dryness of his eyes. He also states that his sinuses feel "stopped up" at the end of each use. In response to this, he has tightened the straps of the nasal mask. This helped decrease the air leak, but now he has developed soreness at the bridge of his nose, and he fears that the skin will break down. What should be done to help him?

1.1.2 Introduction

Over the past twenty years, evidence for the use of noninvasive ventilation (NIV) in acute and chronic respiratory failure has led to its widespread use. In fact, for several conditions, including acute chronic obstructive pulmonary disease (COPD) exacerbations, NIV is part of the recommended patient management. However, a

A Practical Guide to Mechanical Ventilation, First Edition.
Edited by Jonathon D. Truwit and Scott K. Epstein.
© 2011 John Wiley & Sons, Ltd. Published 2011 by John Wiley & Sons, Ltd.

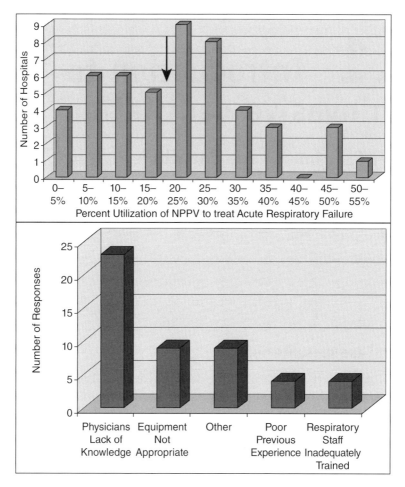

Figure 1.1.1 (Top) The use of NIV in the setting of acute respiratory failure varies widely between hospitals, with a median use of 20%. (Bottom) The most common reason for a failure to initiate NIV in the setting of acute respiratory failure is a lack of knowledge by the physician. (Reproduced with permission [1].)

survey by Maheshwari and colleagues [1] showed that NIV is underutilized in the setting of acute respiratory failure in the United States. The reason most often cited for this underutilization was "physicians lack of knowledge." (Figure 1.1.1) Surveys in the United Kingdom [2] and in Europe [3] also found that NIV was underutilized, if hospitals offered it at all. Therefore, it is hoped to increase practitioner awareness regarding the use of NIV. In this chapter, the history of NIV and the basic equipment that is used when using NIV are reviewed.

1.1.3 History

Noninvasive positive pressure ventilation was first used in the 1930s when Barach used continuous positive airway pressure to successfully treat acute pulmonary edema [4]. In the 1940s, the use of intermittent positive pressure breathing (IPPB) became popular and was continued through the early 1980s [5]. IPPB was usually delivered via a mouthpiece and was used to assist with the delivery of nebulized medications for patients with obstructive lung disease. As such, it was used to deliver positive pressure breaths for only about an hour a day, broken into 3–4 intervals. A prospective, randomized, controlled trial sponsored by the National Institutes of Health (NIH) did not show any benefit to using IPPB over nebulized treatments alone in patients with COPD (IPPB trial group). Thereafter, its use slowly declined. Of note, the relatively short course of daily IPPB likely contributed to the poor study results [5]. The use of nocturnal NIV dates back to the 1960s, when patients with neuromuscular disease used either simple mouthpieces or oronasal masks as their interface [5]. While popular at certain centers, the general difficulty using these interfaces prevented widespread use at that time. The use of NIV did not become widespread until the mid-1980s, when the nasal mask was proven an effective means of delivering NIV to patients with obstructive sleep apnea while enhancing comfort and adherence [6]. Since that time, the use of NIV has gained acceptance as a treatment for both acute and chronic respiratory failure in a variety of conditions.

As noninvasive positive pressure ventilation has gained increasing acceptance, the use of noninvasive negative pressure ventilation has declined. The iron lung was invented by Philip Drinker in 1928, improved by JH Emerson in 1931, and was commonly used to treat respiratory failure from acute poliomyelitis through the 1950s [5]. The polio epidemic also led to the creation of the rocking bed, which used gravity to create diaphragmatic movement and create tidal volumes. In addition, the pneumobelt was created around this time. The pneumobelt is strapped around the abdomen, and a rubber bladder inflates to compress the abdomen and assist with diaphragmatic movement. While all of these methods have been used in recent years, they are no longer readily available in most hospitals or from supply companies. Because of its simple design, portability, and relative comfort to the patient, noninvasive positive pressure equipment has largely replaced the iron lung, the rocking bed, and the pneumobelt. Therefore, in the remainder of this text, the discussion of noninvasive ventilation (NIV) will be limited to the use of noninvasive positive pressure ventilation.

1.1.4 Different modes of noninvasive ventilation

1.1.4.1 Selecting a mode

Noninvasive ventilators, like intensive care mechanical ventilators, are controlled by either setting the volume desired for each breath (volume mode) or by setting a pressure that will be delivered to the airway to assist with breathing (pressure mode). Changes in volume and pressure are directly proportional and are linked by lung and chest wall compliance ($C = \Delta V/\Delta P$). When a volume mode is used, the tidal volume provided by the ventilator will be fixed. If the compliance of the lungs is very low, then a high amount of pressure will be needed to deliver that volume. If there is a leak in the system, then the actual tidal volume delivered to the lungs may be lower than prescribed, as the machine cannot know how much air is delivered to the patient and how much is lost. Alternatively, if a pressure mode is used, the pressure will be fixed and the tidal volume will vary with compliance. The same pressure may generate adequate volumes in a patient with highly compliant lungs but would generate inadequate tidal volumes in a patient with poor chest wall compliance. If there is a leak in the system while in pressure mode, the machine will compensate for the leak until the set pressure is reached, so the patient may receive the same tidal volume regardless of whether or not a leak is present.

NIV also offers the options of being spontaneous, controlled, or a combination (assist-control or spontaneous times mode). If the ventilator is on a spontaneous mode, it will react to a preset patient trigger and will then support the breath. If the patient is apneic, then the ventilator will not deliver any breaths. Alternatively, if the patient is on a controlled mode, then the ventilator will initiate a breath at a time specified by the operator, not the patient. If the patient initiates a breath between ventilator breaths, the ventilator will not support that breath. With combined modes, a respiratory rate is usually set below the patient's spontaneous respiratory rate. If the patient's respiratory rate drops below the specified rate, the ventilator will initiate breaths at this specified rate. If the patient is breathing above the set rate, then each breath will be initiated by the patient and supported by the ventilator.

It is also important to specify whether or not a pressure gradient is applied between inspiration and expiration. Two popular modes of noninvasive ventilation, continuous positive airway pressure (NIV-CPAP) and pressure support (NIV-PS), are pressure modes. However, NIV-CPAP gives a continuous pressure throughout the respiratory cycle. NIV-PS gives additional support during inspiration and a continuous (but lower) pressure during expiration. In the NIV-PS mode, with a BiPAP machine, the inspiratory support is termed the IPAP (inspiratory positive airway pressure), while the expiratory support is termed the EPAP (expiratory positive airway pressure), and the difference between IPAP and EPAP is the amount of pressure support provided. Airway pressures can be regulated by a mechanical ventilator in the PS mode or a BiPAP machine.

With the exception of patients with central sleep apnea, NIV is usually started with a spontaneous mode of breathing. This allows the patient to control the respiratory rate, inspiratory time, and expiratory time. In pressure modes such as NIV-CPAP and NIV-PS, flow (Q) will depend on the set pressures, the patient's respiratory drive, the airway resistance, and the presence or absence of a leak. This can be understood through the equation $Q = \Delta P/R$, where ΔP is the pressure gradient between airway and alveoli as developed by the patient (negative pleural pressure) and ventilator (positive airway pressure) and R is airway resistance.

1.1.4.2 Ventilator triggering

In spontaneously triggered breaths, the ventilator can be triggered by either a change in pressure or by a change in flow. Some ventilators have a preset trigger, while some allow the sensitivity of the trigger to be changed by the operator. If the sensitivity of a ventilator requires a large drop in pressure or change in flow at the airway, then significant effort will be expended by the patient prior to ventilator support, thus increasing the patient's work of breathing. At the other extreme, if the ventilator trigger sensor is responsive to very small changes in pressure or flow then frequent triggering of the ventilator by air leaks and attendant breath stacking may result. Because flow triggering is more sensitive than pressure triggering, it reduces the work of breathing in spontaneous modes and has become the standard method of triggering on newer ventilator models [7, 8].

1.1.4.3 Ventilator cycling

In addition to selecting the proper mode and inspiratory trigger sensitivity, the cycling between inspiration and expiration should be assessed when starting NIV. The trigger for stopping ventilator assistance during inspiration can be either a decrease in flow to a percentage of the maximal flow rate (usually 25% of the maximal rate) or a set flow rate [9]. Some ventilators allow adjustment of this trigger, while others are preset. If the flow rate for breath delivery cessation is too high then the breath will be stopped early. Too low an inspiratory flow rate cut off will result in prolongation of the inspiratory time and increased expiratory work of breathing. This later scenario can be problematic in patients with COPD, who rely of a prolonged expiratory time to prevent auto-PEEP (positive end-expiratory pressure). Therefore, in COPD, a high flow threshold (25–40% of the maximal pressure) should be selected [9].

1.1.4.4 Proportional assist ventilation (PAV)

PAV is a newer mode of ventilation that attempts to assist each breath in proportion to the effort that the patient is able to make. It utilizes an in-line pneumotachograph to continuously track a patient's inspiratory flow. The ventilator can make quick adjustments to the patient's respiratory effort. Therefore, the operator is able to control the proportion of ventilation that is assisted to better closely meet the patient's needs [5]. While small studies have indicated that PAV is more comfortable than NIV-PS [10], this has not yet translated into clinical outcomes. Of the few small studies that have compared PAV with NIV-PS, no significant improvements in hypercapnia [11] or inspiratory muscle unloading [12] were found with PAV.

1.1.4.5 Ventilator type

In the setting of acute respiratory failure, management with NIV requires close monitoring and usually requires care in an intensive care unit or a "step-down" unit.

Portable ventilators were initially designed for home use in patients with chronic respiratory failure. As the applicability of NIV expanded to include certain patient populations with acute respiratory failure, it was recognized that these portable ventilators had shortcomings in the acute setting. These early generation portable ventilators had limited pressure generating capacities (25–35 cm H_2O), lacked oxygen blenders to deliver a high fraction of inspired oxygen (FiO_2), lacked waveform display to assist with ventilator management, and did not have the alarms of an intensive care ventilator [5]. In addition, portable ventilators often have one circuit for both inspiratory and expiratory gases. When the flow through the system is slow, there is a potential for rebreathing carbon dioxide, which can increase the time required to correct hypercapnia [13]. Therefore, intensive care ventilators became the standard for delivering NIV in patients with acute respiratory failure. In 2001, a French survey found that intensive care ventilators were used for NIV in 76% of the cases involving acute respiratory failure [3].

More recent portable ventilators have corrected many of these problems. Current portable ventilators have oxygen blenders and can deliver high FiO_2, they can deliver higher pressures, have improved alarms, and several have waveform analysis. Also, while many still use a single circuit for inspiratory and expiratory gases, setting the EPAP at 4 cm H_2O or greater generally prevents rebreathing [9]. In addition, a small leak (which is usually present in NIV) helps to avoid rebreathing. Portable ventilators have been shown to compensate for leaks better than intensive care ventilators, allowing for improved patient triggering and decreased dysynchrony [14]. However, intensive care ventilators still deliver more accurate FiO_2, have better alarms (which are not always needed with NIV), and have separate tubing for inspiratory and expiratory gases to allow for less opportunity of rebreathing exhaled gas [15]. Therefore, selection must take the patient into consideration. The clinician must also be aware of interventions for potential problems when applying NIV (Table 1.1.1). If the patient is very hypoxemic, an intensive care ventilator may still be preferred to allow more accurate FiO_2. However, in most other settings, newer portable ventilators may improve synchrony and comfort.

1.1.5   Interface

Interfaces are the devices that connect a ventilator circuit to the face. The type of interface used to deliver NIV can have a large influence on patient comfort, adherence with NIV, and efficacy of NIV. The traditional interfaces used to administer NIV are the nasal mask and the orofacial mask (Figure 1.1.2). In the acute setting, either the nasal or the oronasal mask can deliver NIV from either a portable ventilator or a critical care ventilator. Another option is the nasal pillows device. Patients with chronic respiratory failure requiring long-term NIV during the day (in addition to the night) may use the simple mouthpiece or the mouthpiece with lip seal. Recently, the helmet device has been used, although its use is mostly confined to research purposes at present. The choice of which interface to use for a patient requires knowledge of the advantages and disadvantages of each.

Table 1.1.1 Common problems in NIV, problems that may lead to their occurrence, and how to correct the problem.

Problem	Potential cause	Corrective measure
1. Inspiratory trigger failure	Air leak	Adjust mask or change type
	Autocycling	Adjust trigger sensitivity
	Increased work of breathing	Adjust trigger sensitivity or change to a flow trigger if pressure trigger used
2. Inadequate pressurization	Pressure rise time too long	Reduction of pressure rise time
	Pressure support too low	Increase inspiratory pressure
3. Failure to cycle into expiration	Air leak leading to "inspiratory hang up"	Adjust mask or consider switch from nasal to face mask
	High end-inspiratory flow	Increase end-inspiratory flow threshold and set time limit for inspiration
4. CO_2 rebreathing	Single circuit with no true exhalation valve	Use two lines and use non-rebreathe valve
	High respiratory rate	Lower respiratory rate
	No PEEP	Add PEEP to wash out (lavage) mask
	Large mask dead space	Reduce dead space with padding

Reproduced with permission [9].

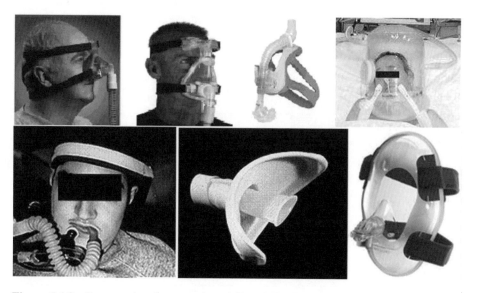

Figure 1.1.2 Common interfaces used to deliver NIV. Top far left: Nasal mask. Top left: Oronasal mask. Top right: Nasal pillows. Top far right: Helmet system. Bottom left: Simple mouthpiece. Bottom right: Mouthpiece with lip seal.

1.1.5.1 Nasal mask and oronasal mask

The nasal mask was the first method for delivering NIV. A comparison between advantages and disadvantages of oronasal and nasal masks is outlined in Table 1.1.2. The nasal mask permits easier expectoration of secretions, liquid consumption and has less respiratory dead space than the oronasal mask. Furthermore, the nasal mask is less claustrophobic than the oronasal mask and patients can talk much easier with a nasal interface. The orofacial mask is more likely to be associated with skin ulceration during prolonged use [16]. However, the nasal mask is very difficult to use in patients with acute respiratory failure (ARF). Patients in ARF are mouth breathers, and this creates a large leak when attempting NIV with a nasal mask. Chin straps and other devices created to decrease the amount of mouth breathing are relatively contraindicated, as the patient is often dependent on this additional ventilation.

Growing evidence supports the common clinical practice of using oronasal interface over a nasal mask in patients with ARF. The oronasal mask provides more rapid improvement in hypercapnia and minute ventilation [17, 18]. Recently, a prospective, randomized, controlled trial compared the utility of the oronasal mask with the nasal mask in patients with ARF [19]. While no difference in rates of intubation or death were noted, most patients (75%) in the nasal mask group were changed to an oronasal mask within six hours due to mouth breathing and the resultant air leak. This study supports the use of the oronasal mask as the standard interface in patients with ARF. However, the duration of continuous oronasal mask use should be limited to decrease the rate of skin ulceration and the time a patient has without oral nutrition. As patients improve, intermittent oronasal mask use or a transition to a nasal mask to enhance comfort and compliance should be considered.

Table 1.1.2 A comparison of the advantages and disadvantages of nasal and oronasal masks.

Clinical aspect	Oronasal mask	Nasal mask
Mouth leak and mouth breathing	+	−
Influence of dental status	+	−
Airway pressure	+	−
Dead space	−	+
Communication	−	+
Eating, drinking	−	+
Expectoration	−	+
Risk of aspiration	−	+
Risk of aerophagia	−	+
Claustrophobia	−	+
Comfort	−	+

A plus indicates superiority of one interface over the other with respect to that clinical aspect.
Reproduced with permission [9].

In the setting of chronic respiratory failure, the oronasal mask is infrequently used. The nasal mask is the preferred interface with nocturnal NIV. The majority of studies in patients using nocturnal NIV have used the nasal mask as the interface, and it is generally well tolerated. However, nasal masks are prone to air leaks. If the mask–face seal pressure is >2 cm H_2O, then a leak is generally avoided [20]. While ventilators made for NIV generally compensate for air leaks and maintain pressure and allow effective triggering, air leaks can still affect the patient's comfort. Air leaks cause a decrease in the absolute humidity of the system, increase patient–ventilator asynchrony, lead to decreased FiO_2, and can lead to irritation of the eyes and dry mouth [14].

Often, the presence of a leak is a sign that the nasal mask is not sized or fitted properly. Nasal masks that are too large often require excessive tightening to prevent air leaks. If one or two fingers cannot be placed inside the straps (usually Velcro), they are probably too tight [21]. Over time, if the mask remains too tight (greater than skin capillary pressure), skin breakdown can occur on the bridge of the nose, sometimes leading to ulceration. In certain populations, such as the immunocompromised, this can be particularly concerning. There are several ways to prevent skin breakdown in patients using nasal masks. Firstly, maintain the lowest mask–face seal pressure that avoids significant leak. Because this pressure is not routinely measured in clinical practice, an experienced practitioner should frequently monitor the mask fit and assess for signs of skin breakdown. Wound care tools (gauze or duoderm) can create padding to prevent injury, but the interface should also be addressed if it is uncomfortable. If the mask has been sized improperly, the correct mask should be supplied immediately. Also, a forehead spacer (Figure 1.1.3) can be used to relieve pressure from the bridge of the nose. Once skin breakdown has developed, the interface should be changed if at all possible. For example, transition from a nasal mask to a full face mask or nasal pillows system may relieve areas with skin breakdown.

When using NIV to treat chronic respiratory failure, humidification has the benefits of decreasing the work of breathing while providing comfort and increasing

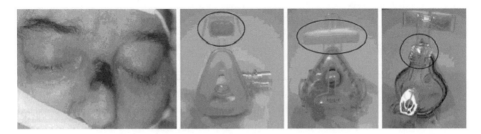

Figure 1.1.3   On the far left, a patient with skin breakdown from a nasal mask. The next three pictures show different forehead spacers that can be used to relieve pressure from the bridge of the nose and prevent skin breakdown.

adherence with NIV [22]. The circuit of the ventilator can be changed to provide heated humidity in certain patients who continue to be "mouth breathers" and are unable to effectively humidify the gases while in their upper airway. However, heated humidifiers should not be routinely used, as most patients do well without their use and they are expensive. A chin strap can be used to prevent mouth breathing in patients using nasal masks. The chin strap can be effective in reducing air leak and hypercapnia in selective patients, although it is not always effective [23].

1.1.5.2   Nasal pillows

Nasal pillows are an alternative to nasal masks for the chronic use of nocturnal NIV. Nasal pillows are two soft plastic plugs that fit into the nares and seal with the help of positive pressure [15]. In patients with obstructive sleep apnea, nasal pillows provided less air leak and better sleep quality compared with the nasal mask [24]. Nasal pillows can also be used for NIV in patients with claustrophobia, who may find this interface less confining compared with nasal masks, oronasal masks, or the helmet. While there is little research comparing nasal pillows to nasal masks in populations other than sleep apnea, they are readily available in clinical practice and commonly used to deliver chronic NIV.

1.1.5.3   Full face mask

Development of a new interface has caused difficulty with current nomenclature. Previously, the oronasal mask had also been called the full face mask. However, with the development of an interface that covers the entire face (Figure 1.1.1), the term full face mask now refers to this interface. The oronasal mask should therefore only be called by this name. The full face mask was developed to decrease skin breakdown, air leaks, and the sense of claustrophobia created in some who use the nasal or oronasal masks [20]. It has been used in patients with acute respiratory failure who could not tolerate oronasal or nasal interfaces. The full face mask was found to significantly improve gas exchange and often prevent intubation in this population [25, 26]. Therefore, if available, it should be considered in those who are candidates for NIV but cannot use an oronasal or nasal mask.

1.1.5.4   Helmet

The helmet has been created as an alternative interface to deliver NIV. It is comprised of a plastic helmet attached to a soft collar (Figure 1.1.1) which fits around the neck. It has been proposed primarily to treat acute respiratory failure as an alternative to the oronasal mask. Because the helmet does not contact the head, it has the advantage of providing increased comfort and longer use compared with the oronasal mask [27]. However, the helmet's large size yields a large dead space, which has raised concerns regarding the ability of the helmet to correct hypercapnic respiratory failure. In fact, when compared with the oronasal mask in patients with acute respiratory failure, the helmet has a smaller reduction in carbon dioxide levels compared with the oronasal mask, and this may have contributed to NIV failure [28]. Patients using the helmet also have a longer delay to trigger inspiration compared with the face mask, but this can be offset by increasing the PEEP and pressure support [29]. While the helmet is tolerated well in patients with acute respiratory failure, the patient and the ventilator settings require careful monitoring while it is in use [30]. At present, the helmet is not available for use in the United States.

1.1.6 Case presentation revisited

It was suspected that the initial nasal mask was too large. Large masks often create air leaks that irritate the conjunctiva. When attempts are made to decrease the air leak by tightening the straps, the extra pressure can cause pressure sores over the nasal bridge. The sensation of feeling "stopped up" could result from the leak as well. When leaks are large, the absolute humidity in the system is decreased, which can lead to dry nasal secretions and sinus pressure. This sensation could also be from the transmission of positive pressure to the sinuses, which can frequently cause sinus pain.

The oxygen supply company was contacted, and it was requested that the patient be fitted with a smaller mask. Gauze padding under the new mask was used for a couple of weeks, so that the nasal bridge would not be irritated. To improve patient tolerance, both airway pressure settings, IPAP and EPAP, were decreased by 3–5 cm H_2O and later returned to original set pressures. In addition, we added a nasal corticosteroid to decrease inflammation and permit easier breathing. With these changes, the patient reported resolution of the initial problems, and was able to wear a nasal mask without difficulty. It would have been acceptable to transition the patient to nasal pillows, as this device would likely have corrected the eye pain and prevented skin breakdown. However, the problems with the sinuses would still require attention.

References

1. Maheshwari, V. *et al.* (2006) Utilization of noninvasive ventilation in acute care hospitals: a regional survey. *Chest*, **129**, 1226–1233.
2. Doherty, M. and Greenstone, M. (1998) Survey of non-invasive ventilation (NIV) in patients with acute exacerbations of chronic obstructive pulmonary disease (COPD) in the UK. *Thorax*, **53**, 863–866.
3. Carlucci, A. *et al.* (2001) Noninvasive versus conventional mechanical ventilation: an epidemiologic survey. *Am. J. Respir. Crit. Care Med.*, **163** (4), 874–880.
4. Barach, A.L. *et al.* (1938) Positive pressure respiration and its application to the treatment of acute pulmonary edema. *Ann. Intern. Med.*, **12**, 754–795.

5. Mehta, S. and Hill, N. (2001) Noninvasive ventilation. *Am. J. Respir. Crit. Care Med.*, **163**, 540–577.

6. Sullivan, C.E., Issa, F.G., Berthon-Jones, M. and Eves, L. (1981) Reversal of obstructive sleep apnea by continuous positive airway pressure applied through the nares. *Lancet*, **1**, 862–865.

7. Aslanian, P. *et al.* (1998) Effects of flow triggering on breathing effort during partial ventilatory support. *Am. J. Respir. Crit. Care Med.*, **157**, 135–143.

8. Nava, S. *et al.* (1997) Physiological effects of flow and pressure triggering during non-invasive mechanical ventilation in patients with chronic obstructive pulmonary disease. *Thorax*, **52**, 249–254.

9. Schonhofer, B. and Sorter-Leger, S. (2002) Equipment needs for noninvasive mechanical ventilation. *Eur. Respir. J.*, **20**, 1029–1036.

10. Mols, G. (2005) 'Simplify your life' does not necessarily work when applying automatic tube compensation and proportional assist ventilation. *Crit. Care Med.*, **33** (9), 2125–2126.

11. Winck, J.C. *et al.* (2004) Tolerance and physiologic effects of nocturnal mask pressure support vs proportional assist ventilation in chronic ventilatory failure. *Chest*, **126** (2), 382–388.

12. Varelmann, D. *et al.* (2005) Proportional assist versus pressure support ventilation in patients with acute respiratory failure: cardiorespiratory responses to artificially increased ventilatory demand. *Crit. Care Med.*, **33** (9), 1968–1975.

13. Ferguson, G.T. and Gilamartin, M. (1995) CO_2 rebreathing during BiPAP ventilatory assistance. *Am. J. Respir. Crit. Care Med.*, **151** (4), 1126–1135.

14. Miyoshi, E. *et al.* (2005) Effects of gas leak on triggering function, humidification, and inspiratory oxygen fraction during noninvasive positive airway pressure ventilation. *Chest*, **128**, 3691–3698.

15. Hess, D. (2006) Noninvasive ventilation in neuromuscular disease: equipment and application. *Respir. Care*, **51** (8), 896–912.

16. Navalesi, P. *et al.* (2000) Physiologic evaluation of noninvasive mechanical ventilation delivered with three types of masks in patients with chronic hypercapnic respiratory failure. *Crit. Care Med.*, **28**, 1785–1790.

17. Pravinkumar, S.E. (2009) A face that matters in distress: interface selection for acute noninvasive ventilation. *Crit. Care Med.*, **37** (1), 344–345.

18. Meduri, G.U. *et al.* (1996) Noninvasive positive pressure ventilation via face mask: first-line intervention in patients with acute hypercapnic and hypoxemic respiratory failure. *Chest*, **109**, 179–193.

19. Girault, C. *et al.* (2009) Interface strategy during noninvasive positive pressure ventilation for hypercapnic acute respiratory failure. *Crit. Care Med.*, **37**, 124–131.

20. Nava, S. *et al.* (2009) Interfaces and humidification for noninvasive mechanical ventilation. *Respir. Care*, **54** (1), 71–82.

21. Meduri, G.U. and Spencer, S.E. (2001) Noninvasive mechanical ventilation in the acute setting. Technical aspects, monitoring and choice of interface. *Eur. Respir. Mon.*, **16**, 106–124.

22. Lellouche, F. *et al.* (2002) Effect of the humidification device on the work of breathing during noninvasive ventilation. *Intensive Care Med.*, **28**, 1582–1589.

23. Gonzalez, J. *et al.* (2003) Air leaks during mechanical ventilation as a cause of persistent hypercapnia in neuromuscular disorders. *Intensive Care Med.*, **29** (4), 596–602.

24. Massie, C.A. *et al.* (2003) Clinical outcomes related to interface type in patients with obstructive sleep apnea/hypopnea syndrome who are using continuous positive airway pressure. *Chest*, **123** (4), 1112–1118.

25. Criner, G. *et al.* (1994) Efficacy of a new full face mask for noninvasive positive pressure ventilation. *Chest*, **106** (4), 1109–1115.
26. Roy, B. *et al.* (2007) Full face mask for noninvasive positive-pressure ventilation in patients with acute respiratory failure. *J. Am. Osteopath.*, **107** (4), 148–156.
27. Tonnelier, J.M. *et al.* (2003) Noninvasive continuous positive airway pressure ventilation using a new helmet interface: a case-control prospective pilot study. *Intensive Care Med.*, **29**, 2077–2080.
28. Antonelli, M. *et al.* (2004) Noninvasive positive pressure ventilation using a helmet in patients with acute exacerbations of chronic obstructive pulmonary disease. *Anesthesiology*, **100**, 16–24.
29. Moerer, O. *et al.* (2006) Influence of two interfaces for noninvasive ventilation compared to invasive ventilation on the mechanical properties and performance of a respiratory system: a lung model study. *Chest*, **129**, 1424–1431.
30. Chiumello, D. (2006) Is the helmet different than the face mask in delivering noninvasive ventilation? *Chest*, **129**, 1402–1403.

1.2 Physiology of noninvasive ventilation

Daniel C. Grinnan[1] and Jonathon D. Truwit[2]

[1] *Division of Pulmonary and Critical Care Medicine, Virginia Commonwealth University, Richmond, VA, USA*
[2] *Division of Pulmonary and Critical Care Medicine, University of Virginia, Charlottesville, VA, USA*

1.2.1 Case presentation

A 55-year-old with post-polio syndrome presents to clinic for further evaluation. He has developed morning headaches and some mild dyspnea. An arterial blood gas reads 7.35/55/70, with SaO_2 of 94%. After a lengthy discussion, he agrees to start nocturnal noninvasive ventilation with pressure support (NIV-PS) with a nasal interface. The discussion raises several questions. How can chronic nocturnal hypercapnia progress to daytime hypercapnia? How long should one try nocturnal NIV before improvement in daytime hypercapnia is seen? What is the best way to follow response to therapy over time?

1.2.2 Introduction

Noninvasive ventilation has several theoretical advantages over endotracheal intubation or tracheotomy, and several studies suggest that gas exchange is very similar to these more invasive methods of mechanical ventilation. In the acute setting, despite a clinician's best attempt, some patients require endotracheal intubation

A Practical Guide to Mechanical Ventilation, First Edition.
Edited by Jonathon D. Truwit and Scott K. Epstein.
© 2011 John Wiley & Sons, Ltd. Published 2011 by John Wiley & Sons, Ltd.

following unsuccessful noninvasive ventilation. In this chapter, the physiology behind the most common problems leading to failure of NIV in patients with acute respiratory failure is discussed, including mask leaks and ventilator asynchrony. When noninvasive ventilation is used chronically, patients often have difficulty tolerating the interface due to upper respiratory tract complaints. The physiology of the upper airway in reference to NIV is also discussed. Additionally, when used chronically, NIV and its pressure settings can be difficult for physicians to titrate. As different diseases have different physiologic explanations for improved gas exchange with NIV, it is important to review this physiology.

1.2.3   Patient–ventilator interaction in acute respiratory failure

There are several problems that can lead to ineffective noninvasive ventilation or intolerance to noninvasive ventilation. In Chapter 1.1 the problem of carbon dioxide rebreathing and mask leaks were discussed. Problems with patient–ventilator inter- action are another common reason for patient discomfort, ineffective noninvasive ventilation, and discontinuation of mechanical ventilation. Inspiratory triggering asynchrony may occur due to ineffective ventilator triggering during patient inspira- tion or due to decreased rate of inspiratory pressure rise during the inspiratory cycle [1, 2]. Expiratory triggering asynchrony can occur if there is ineffective termination of a mechanically delivered breath or if expiratory positive airway pressure is inef- fectively delivered. In cases of asynchrony due to ineffective triggering, there is a phase shift between the patient's neural signaling and the ventilator's response [1]. This leads to increased work of breathing and patient discomfort. An example of patient–ventilator asynchrony is shown in Figure 1.2.1.

While not often used in clinical practice, the pressure time product (PTP) is a common indicator of the work of breathing in clinical research. The pressure time product is the product of the average inspiratory pressure (starting from the onset of effort) and the duration of inspiration: PTP = Pavg × Ti. The PTP was developed to account for energy expenditures during the dynamic and isometric phases of respiration, whereas other measures of work of breathing require a change in the volume (thus accounting for only the dynamic phase) [37]. Therefore, the PTP should more directly measure the total energy (in addition to the total work) of breathing than other means of measuring work of breathing. Thus, the PTP often allows for comparisons of work of breathing with different modes, amounts of leak, and so on. Much of the research on the effect of patient–ventilator interaction on work of breathing has used the PTP.

There are several different factors that can lead to asynchrony in noninvasive ventilation. The presence of a leak, the type of interface, the mode of noninvasive ventilation, and the method of triggering the ventilator to stop inspiration have all been identified as causes for asynchrony.

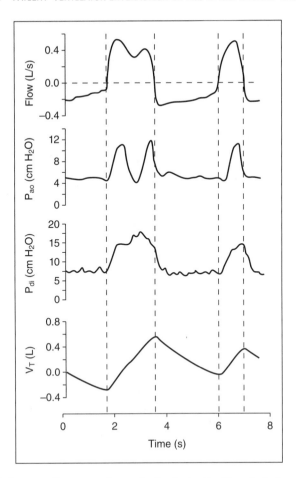

Figure 1.2.1 Patient–ventilator asynchrony. In the first patient breath (between seconds 2 and 4), there is an initial positive airway pressure (Pao), indicating effective noninvasive ventilation. This is preceded by a downward reflection in the Pao, indicating patient effort on top of ventilator effort. This resulted in a transient decrease in airflow and prolonged total inspiratory time compared with the second breath. (Reproduced with permission [7].)

1.2.3.1 Asynchrony and air leak

The presence of a leak is the most common cause of asynchrony [2]. This may present as an inability of the ventilator to trigger inspiration. A leak causes faulty inspiratory triggering by delaying inspiratory triggering, by decreasing ventilator sensitivity, or both. A leak may also prevent effective transition from inspiration to expiration. As the end of inspiration is recognized by the ventilator as inspiratory flow decay to a certain threshold, and a leak can prevent recognition of this decay, a leak can prevent the "cycling off" of inspiration and lead to asynchrony. During inspiration, if a leak prevents adequate transmission of pressure from the ventilator to the airways, then the patient will use significant effort to breathe during attempted inspiration. Such asynchrony is shown in Figure 1.2.1. During expiration, a leak will prevent expiratory positive airway pressure from being transmitted to the airways. Especially in those with obstructive lung disease, this may lead to active respiratory muscle use in during expiration and difficulty triggering inspiration.

1.2.3.2   Ventilator mode and asynchrony

The introductory chapter reviewed the various modes that can be used. In this section, the effect of different modes on asynchrony are discussed.

Because noninvasive ventilation, continuous positive airway pressure (NIV-CPAP) provides continuous ventilatory support, it does not need to distinguish between inspiration and expiration. Therefore, asynchrony does not occur with NIV-CPAP. This is a potential advantage for NIV-CPAP, as NIV-PS should only be used when an operator experienced with the management of asynchrony is available.

Bilevel or noninvasive ventilation with pressure support (NIV-PS) is commonly associated with asynchrony, and this is one of the more common reasons for its discontinuation [3, 4]. NIV-PS is designed to deliver a set amount of inspiratory support with each breath, regardless of the patient's level of participation. Asynchrony may develop from ineffective inspiratory triggering (the ventilator does not sense the patient's breath) or from ineffective expiratory triggering (the ventilator continues to supply a breath after the patient begins to exhale). The expiratory triggering asynchrony is influenced by the degree of air leak; the larger the leak, the more time it will take to reach the desired pressure, and the longer inspiration will last.

An alternate mode to NIV-PS is proportional assist ventilation (PAV), which provides inspiratory support in proportion to the effort of the patient. By coupling ventilation effort to patient effort, it is hoped that asynchrony will be eliminated. Expiratory-triggering asynchrony is virtually eliminated, since the cessation of the patient's intrinsic flow will lead to cessation of ventilator flow [5]. This has translated into improved patient comfort and less patient intolerance compared with pressure support ventilation [6]. While PAV has not provided meaningful clinical improvement compared with pressure support ventilation, its use should be considered in a patient having difficulty with expiratory triggering asynchrony. At this time, PAV is not approved by the Food & Drug Administration (FDA) for use with NIV in the United States, as it does not yet have leak compensation built into the ventilator software [2].

1.2.3.3   Interface and asynchrony

Mask leaks can affect the expiratory trigger during pressure support ventilation. The expiratory trigger can be cycled by time or by flow. In the presence of an air

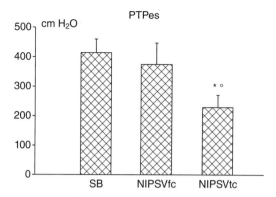

Figure 1.2.2   Time controlled expiratory triggering (NIV-PStc) reduces work of breathing (as assessed by the PTP) compared with flow controlled expiratory breathing (NIV-PSfc). (Reproduced with permission [3].)

leak, the flow cycled trigger develops a progressive phase shift, leading to patient–ventilator asynchrony and increased work of breathing (as determined by the PTP) [3]. By changing patients to a time cycled expiratory trigger, the expiratory triggering asynchrony was reduced and patient discomfort was improved (Figure 1.2.2).

As mentioned in the Chapter 1.1, the helmet is a relatively new interface, designed to decrease skin breakdown and improve comfort compared with mask ventilation. However, the helmet has a large inner volume and a high compliance. These characteristics indicate that a proportion of the inspiratory pressure will be used to pressurize and expand the helmet. This was found to create a phase shift between the start of the patient's inspiratory effort and the ventilator's effort, resulting in a twofold increase in autocycled breaths compared with mask ventilation [7]. This asynchrony translated into a significant increase in the PTP with helmet ventilation compared with mask ventilation (Figure 1.2.3).

In summary, discomfort and failure to decrease the work of breathing are common reasons for the discontinuation of mechanical ventilation in the setting of acute respiratory failure. Patient–ventilator asynchrony plays a significant role in the level of discomfort and can unnecessarily increase the patient's work of breathing. Consideration of the interface, the triggering mechanisms, and the mode may help to improve patient comfort and work of breathing before proceeding with invasive mechanical ventilation.

1.2.4   Upper airway physiology in noninvasive ventilation

With noninvasive ventilation air must traverse the upper airway before arriving in the trachea. If delivered from a nasal mask, for example, air traverses the nasal

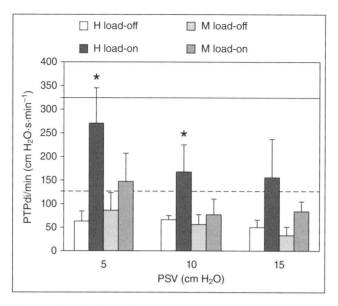

Figure 1.2.3 Increased work of breathing with the helmet interface. When an inspiratory load is applied (to approximate acute respiratory failure), the work of breathing (as assessed by the PTP) is greater with helmet ventilation than mask ventilation at different levels of pressure support (PSV). (Reproduced with permission [7].)

passages, the rhinopharynx, the posterior oropharynx, the larynx, and the glottis with the vocal cords. At each anatomic location, there are considerations that can limit the utility of NIV or can limit a patient's ability to tolerate NIV.

Approximately 40% of patients using chronic nocturnal NIV develop either sore throat, dry nose and throat, or nasal congestion. Not infrequently, these symptoms lead to temporary or permanent discontinuation of NIV. Although the exact mechanism leading to these symptoms remains unknown, it appears that the presence of a leak (either from the mask or from the mouth) is commonly responsible. While commonly used NIV ventilators will maintain adequate pressures despite a leak, the presence of a leak will lead to decreased absolute humidity in the inspired air [8]. In addition, a mouth leak causes unidirectional flow through the nasal passages. Over time, unidirectional flow leads to a marked increase in nasal resistance, which corresponds to the sensation of nasal congestion [9]. The impact of these changes is significant, as only 30% of mouth breathers will be able to tolerate long-term nasal CPAP treatment, compared with 71% of nasal breathers [10].

Several attempts have been made to decrease mouth breathing and increase adherence to nasal CPAP. The use of a chin strap has been advocated to decrease mouth breathing and the arousal index [11]. However, these authors also found that snoring was increased and the respiratory disturbance index was increased with the use of a chin strap. A second approach to decrease mouth breathing is uvulopalatopharyngoplasty (UP3), which has been advocated as a treatment for obstructive sleep apnea. However, there is increasing evidence that patients who have had UP3 are not able to tolerate nasal CPAP therapy as well as those patients who have not had UP3 surgery [12, 13]. Han found that greater resection of the soft palate led to decreased CPAP compliance, while Mortimer found that loss of the soft palatal seal led to increased mouth air leaking. Therefore, it seems that the soft palatal seal is important to prevent mouth breathing and tolerate nasal CPAP. The last approach to decrease mouth breathing is the addition of heated humidification. While it has been shown that heated humidification decreases symptoms of oral and nasal dryness [14], one study found that heated humidification did not decrease nasal resistance [15]. However, this study did not isolate only those patients with mouth leaks, and thus may have included patients not expected to benefit. While heated humidification holds the most promise of the three proposed solutions to mouth leaks, it has not yet been adequately studied.

The glottis may also impact the efficacy of NIV. With increasing minute ventilation delivered through a NIV mask, the vocal cords developed progressive adduction, leading to a narrowed glottis, increased resistance to airflow, and a reduced proportion of tidal volume actually delivered into the lungs. This mechanism may serve as a control against the effects of hyperventilation, although this remains uncertain [16, 17].

When using the NIV-PS mode of ventilation, the practitioner has the option of choosing either a controlled mode or a spontaneous mode of breathing. In one study of normal subjects, the spontaneous mode did not result in increased minute ventilation until the inspiratory positive airway pressure (IPAP) was set at over 20 cm H_2O, causing large numbers of periodic breathing and central apneas. With a controlled mode and a set frequency of 20 breaths/min, greater minute ventilation than with spontaneous mode could be achived despite a lower IPAP [18, 19]. While this data cannot be extrapolated to different disease states, it should be further studied in groups such as those with neuromuscular disease.

In summary, there is a paucity of studies examining the role of the upper airway in noninvasive ventilation. Because endotracheal intubation can often support gas exchange after the failure of noninvasive ventilation, there can be little doubt that the upper airway is important in NIV failures. It appears that the nasal alae, sinuses, pharynx, and glottis may all play a role in the effectiveness of mask ventilation. In addition, it has been learnt that the soft palate is important in controlling mouth leaks, as evidenced by the failure of CPAP following UP3.

1.2.5 The physiology of noninvasive ventilation in hypercapnic respiratory failure

In many disease states, the use of nocturnal NIV has led to improvements in daytime hypercapnia and hypoxemia. There are several different mechanisms that may explain these improvements. Firstly, it is possible that NIV permits chemore-ceptors in the central nervous system to alter their response to carbon dioxide, thus creating more appropriate minute ventilation for the hypercapnia. This implies that the chemoreceptor response to carbon dioxide is impaired. Secondly, it is possible that NIV improves respiratory mechanics. It has been suggested that resting the muscles of respiration during the night may help to refresh the muscles during the day, which would translate to improved maximal inspiratory force in neuromuscu-lar disease and improved dynamic hyperinflation in chronic obstructive pulmonary disease (COPD). Thirdly, it is possible that NIV improves the ventilation/perfusion matching in the lungs, especially in patients with neuromuscular disease. These patients have chest wall restriction and are thus inclined to develop atelectasis. The initiation of positive pressure ventilation may assist with alveolar recruitment, decrease atelectasis, improve ventilation/perfusion matching, and therefore lead to improved oxygenation. Fourthly, in the setting of neuromuscular disease, it is pos-sible that chronic restriction leads to increased alveolar surface forces, which in turn lead to further restriction. NIV may lead to increased alveolar surface area, thus assisting with lung compliance and restriction.

1.2.5.1 Neuromuscular disease

In neuromuscular disease, several small studies have been undertaken to determine which of the above mechanisms may be responsible for improvements in daytime gas exchange with nocturnal NIV. Several investigators have found that static lung compliance is improved following short intervals of NIV in patients with amyotrophic leteral sclerosis (ALS) [20], kyphoscoliosis [21], and muscular dys-trophy or spinal cord injury [22]. Often, the increased compliance is attributed to improved atelectasis [20]. However, one study of 14 patients with neuromuscular disease did not find significant evidence of microatelectasis on high resolution computed tomography (HRCT) [23]. These authors suggested that impaired lung compliance may be secondary to reduced lung elastance from chronically decreased tidal volumes. If the improvement of atelectasis led to the improvement in oxygena-tion in patients with neuromuscular disease, then one would expect to see an increase in the alveolar–arterial oxygen gradient (A–a gradient) with NIV. While large A–a gradients in patients with neuromuscular disease and respiratory failure have been confirmed [24], studies have not revealed that the A–a gradient is decreased with the start of NIV. In fact, two small studies that showed an improve-ment in hypercapnia and hypoxemia failed to show a significant improvement in the A–a gradient [24, 25]. However, the small size of these studies makes their interpretation difficult. Therefore, the role of atelectasis in the improvement of daytime gas exchange following nocturnal NIV has not been adequately investi-gated. Future studies assessing the A–a gradient in a large cohort of patients may be useful.

Some studies have investigated the effect of nocturnal NIV on daytime lung function and muscle strength in neuromuscular disease. These studies have consistently failed to show any significant improvement in FEV1, FVC, or PImax after NIV [24–26]. All of these studies did find significant improvements in gas exchange, making it difficult to attribute the improvements in gas exchange to improvements in muscle strength. However, accurate PImax can be difficult to obtain in patients with neuromuscular disease, especially if they have bulbar symptoms.

Daytime gas exchange from nocturnal NIV is associated with adjustment of the chemoreceptor response to carbon dioxide. In patients with sleep apnea, the ventilatory response to hypercapnia is altered with NIV, and the response to hypercapnia is usually reversed in a two week period [27]. The impaired ventilatory response has been linked to increased sleep fragmentation [28], indicating that the improvement in the hypercapnic response with NIV in sleep apnea is due to restoration of the sleep cycle. Annane and colleagues [24] showed that, in patients with neuromuscular disease, nocturnal NIV improves the ventilatory response to carbon dioxide. They also found a significant correlation between the change in the ventilatory response to carbon dioxide at night and the improvement in daytime hypercapnia. In addition, their subjects had a significant degree of sleep apnea, leading them to believe that correction of apnea led to improved ventilatory response and improved daytime hypercapnia in patients with NMD. Piper evaluated removal of NIV on gas exchange in neuromuscular diseased patients chronically applying NIV [38]. Gas exchange and hypoxic arousal responses before initiation and after withdrawal of NIV were assessed. When NIV was withdrawn after long-term usage, patients had improved gas exchange and improved arousal responses to hypoxemia when compared to pre-initiation NIV assessments. This suggests that central chemoreceptors had been "reset."

In summary, there may be several mechanisms which cause the improvement in daytime gas exchange with nocturnal NIV in neuromuscular disease. While studies do not support that decrements in the work of breathing while on NIV improve gas exchange, it is hard to believe that it does not play a role at all. These patients develop orthopnea, resting shortness of breath, and tachypnea; these are all signs of respiratory muscle fatigue, and this fatigue likely causes hypoventilation. It is also possible that atelectasis and reduced lung elasticity contribute to hypoventilation and hypoxemia; however, there is no definitive evidence of this. Finally, it appears that the ventilatory response to carbon dioxide is altered due to increased sleep fragmentation, and that correcting this sleep fragmentation with NIV contributes to the improvement of gas exchange during the daytime.

1.2.5.2 *Chronic obstructive pulmonary disease (COPD)*

The majority of studies have demonstrated improvements in daytime gas exchange with the use of nocturnal NIV in patients with stable hypercapnic COPD, but not all studies [29–32]. Studies that did not show improvement in gas exchange generally used lower inspiratory pressures than the studies that did show improvement. The mechanism for the improvement in daytime gas exchange with nocturnal NIV has been debated. Unlike patients with neuromuscular disease, available information does not suggest that the resetting of central chemoreceptors is important. Rather, mechanical factors involving respiratory muscle recovery and improvement of dynamic hyperinflation have been proposed.

Several investigators have found that NIV is able to decrease the work that the diaphragm performs in patients with COPD, as evaluated by the pressure time product [30, 33]. By decreasing the work of breathing, the diaphragm would be rested, and respiratory muscle fatigue may be prevented. Therefore, by preventing respiratory muscle fatigue, NIV may improve chronic hypercapnia. However, this theory has a major limitation. Similowski and colleagues [34] showed that patients with stable hypercapnic COPD have intact diaphragm function when compared with normal controls at matched lung volumes. This indicates that patients with hypercapnic COPD do not have diaphragmatic fatigue, and they are not approaching the transdiaphragmatic threshold for fatigue. Therefore, NIV would not be expected to benefit COPD patients by improving diaphragmatic function.

An alternate explanation is that NIV improves dynamic hyperinflation in COPD patients, thereby reducing the residual volume and permitting improved daytime tidal volumes and minute ventilation, which in turn leads to improvement of daytime gas exchange. Some studies have found that the intrinsic positive end-expiratory pressure (PEEP) is reduced after NIV is applied [29, 30]. With the use of high inspiratory pressures, lung function has been altered with nocturnal NIV (residual volume was decreased, and the residual capacity was increased) [29]. In addition, the daytime minute ventilation and tidal volumes have been significantly increased in patients receiving nocturnal NIV with high inspiratory levels [29, 35]. Lastly, a strong correlation between daytime carbon dioxide improvement and reduction in dynamic hyperinflation has been found (Figure 1.2.4) [29]. Therefore, while not conclusively proven, there is reasonable evidence to suggest that improvements in dynamic hyperinflation are responsible for improvements in daytime hypercapnia in stable hypercapnic COPD patients.

Clinical results have not shown a clear indication for the use of NIV in patients with stable hypercapnic COPD. Several studies that have failed to show an improvement in important disease parameters (survival, exacerbations, hospitalizations) with nocturnal NIV use. While daytime hypercapnia can be improved with NIV utilizing high inspiratory pressures, this does not seem to correlate with improved clinical parameters. As recently suggested, perhaps hypercapnia represents a favorable response of the central nervous system, carefully chosen through natural selection to decrease the minute ventilation and dyspnea in people with emphysema [36]. Hypercapnia would represent a useful clinical target if it represented respiratory muscle weakness. However, in the absence of diaphragmatic weakness, altering the lung mechanics to reduce dynamic hyperinflation may or may not be

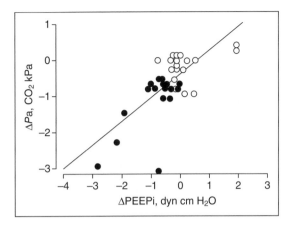

Figure 1.2.4 The correlation between the change in intrinsic PEEP and the change in diurnal carbon dioxide concentration. (Reproduced with permission [29].)

beneficial to the patient. As mentioned above, patients with stable hypercapnia from COPD do not approach the threshold for diaphragmatic fatigue under normal circumstances [34]. Therefore, it is not entirely surprising that improvement in carbon dioxide levels have not correlated with improvement in clinical outcomes.

1.2.6 Summary

While noninvasive ventilation confers several advantages over invasive ventilation, including less sedative use and fewer respiratory infections, it can be difficult to maintain patients with NIV. Understanding the physiology of the ventilator and the respiratory system bring awareness to the complications that can occur with NIV and provide insight into their solutions.

1.2.7 Case presentation revisited

The patient under consideration has developed chronic hypercapnic respiratory failure. As mentioned above, there are several mechanisms that have been proposed to explain the development of daytime hypercapnia. It appears likely that chronic respiratory muscle weakness and hypoventilation eventually lead to daytime hypercapnia in patients with chronic neuromuscular disease. It is interesting that nocturnal NIV use will often improve or reverse the daytime hypercapnia and hypoxemia. In the setting of neuromuscular disease, it appears likely that this reversal is due to the resetting of the central drive to breath. It may take 4–6 weeks for this to take effect, and checking for a response to hypercapnia more often than this may lead to unnecessary ventilator adjustments.

References

1. Sassoon, C. and Foster, G. (2001) Patient ventilator asynchrony. *Curr. Opin. Crit. Care*, **7**, 28–33.
2. Chatburn, R. *et al.* (2009) Which ventilators and modes can be used to deliver noninvasive ventilation. *Respir. Care*, **54** (1), 85–99.
3. Calderini, E. *et al.* (1999) Patient-ventilator asynchrony during noninvasive ventilation: the role of expiratory trigger. *Intensive Care Med.*, **25** (7), 662–667.
4. Younes, M. (1994) Proportional assist ventilation, in Principles and Practices of Mechanical Ventilation (ed. M.J. Tobin), McGraw-Hill, New York, pp. 349–369.
5. Fernandez-Vivas, M. *et al.* (2003) Noninvasive pressure support versus proportional assist ventilation in acute respiratory failure. *Intensive Care Med.*, **29**, 1126–1133.
6. Gay, P.C. *et al.* (2001) Noninvasive proportional assist ventilation for acute respiratory insufficiency: comparison with pressure support ventilation. *Am. J. Respir. Crit. Care Med.*, **164** (9), 1606–1611.
7. Racca, F. *et al.* (2005) Effectiveness of mask and helmet interfaces to deliver noninvasive ventilation in a human model of resistive breathing. *J. Appl. Physiol.*, **99**, 1262–1271.
8. Miyoshi, E. *et al.* (2005) Effect of gas leak on triggering function, humidification, and inspiratory oxygen fraction during noninvasive positive airway pressure ventilation. *Chest*, **128** (5), 3691–3698.
9. Richards, G.N. *et al.* (1996) Mouth leak with nasal continuous positive airway pressure increases nasal airway resistance. *Am. J. Respir. Crit. Care Med.*, **154**, 182–186.
10. Bachour, A. *et al.* (2004) Mouth breathing compromises adherence to nasal CPAP therapy. *Chest*, **126** (4), 1248–1254.
11. Bachour, A. *et al.* (2004) Mouth closing device (chin strap) reduces mouth leak during nasal CPAP. *Sleep Med.*, **5** (3), 261–267.
12. Mortimore, I.L., Bradley, P.A., Murray, J.A.M. and Douglas, N.H. (1996) Uvulopalatopharyngoplasty may compromise nasal CPAP therapy in sleep apnea syndrome. *Am. J. Respir. Crit. Care Med.*, **154**, 1759–1762.
13. Han, F. *et al.* (2006) Influence of UPPP surgery on tolerance to subsequent continuous positive airway pressure in patients with OSAHS. *Sleep Breath*, **10** (1), 37–42.
14. Mador, M.J. *et al.* (2005) Effect of heated humidification on compliance and quality of life in patients with sleep apnea using nasal CPAP. *Chest*, **128** (4), 2151–2158.
15. Duong, M. *et al.* (2005) Use of heated humidification during nasal continuous positive airway pressure titration in obstructive sleep apnea syndrome. *Eur. Respir. J.*, **26** (4), 679–685.
16. Jounieaux, V. *et al.* (1995) Effects of nasal positive-pressure hyperventilation on the glottis in normal awake subjects. *J. Appl. Physiol.*, **79**, 176–185.
17. Jounieaux, V. *et al.* (1995) Effects of nasal positive-pressure hyperventilation on the glottis in normal sleeping subjects. *J. Appl. Physiol.*, **79**, 186–183.
18. Parreira, V.F. *et al.* (1997) Effectiveness of controlled and spontaneous modes in nasal two-level positive pressure ventilation in awake and asleep normal subjects. *Chest*, **112**, 1267–1277.
19. Parriera, V.F. *et al.* (1996) Glottic aperature and effective minute ventilation during nasal two-level positive pressure ventilation in spontaneous mode. *Am. J. Respir. Crit. Care Med.*, **154**, 1857–1863.
20. Lechtzin, N. *et al.* (2006) Supramaximal inflation improves lung compliance in subjects with amyotrophic lateral sclerosis. *Chest*, **129**, 1322–1329.
21. Sinha, R. and Bergofsky, E.H. (1972) Prolonged alteration of lung mechanics in kyphoscoliosis by positive pressure hyperinflation. *Am. Rev. Respir. Dis.*, **106**, 47–57.

22. McCool, F.D. *et al.* (1986) Intermittent positive pressure breathing in patients with respiratory muscle weakness: alterations in total respiratory system compliance. *Chest*, **90**, 546–552.

23. Estenne, M. *et al.* (1993) Lung volume restriction in patients with chronic respiratory muscle weakness: the role of microatelectasis. *Thorax*, **48** (7), 698–701.

24. Annane, D. *et al.* (1999) Mechanisms underlying effects of nocturnal ventilation on daytime blood gases in neuromuscular diseases. *Eur. Respir. J.*, **13**, 157–162.

25. Barbe, F. *et al.* (1996) Long-term effects of nasal intermittent positive-pressure ventilation on pulmonary function and sleep architecture in patients with neuromuscular diseases. *Chest*, **110**, 1179–1183.

26. Aboussouan, L.S. *et al.* (2001) Objective measures of the efficacy of noninvasive positive-pressure ventilation in amyotrophic lateral sclerosis. *Muscle Nerve*, **24**, 403–409.

27. Berthon-Jones, M. *et al.* (1987) Time course of change in ventilatory response to carbon dioxide with long-term of CPAP therapy for obstructive sleep apnea. *Am. Rev. Respir. Dis.*, **135**, 144–147.

28. White, D.P. *et al.* (1983) Sleep deprivation and the control of ventilation. *Am. Rev. Respir. Dis.*, **128**, 984–986.

29. Diaz, O. *et al.* (2002) Effects of noninvasive ventilation on lung hyperinflation in stable hypercapnic COPD. *Eur. Respir. J.*, **20**, 1490–1498.

30. Nava, S. *et al.* (2001) Physiologic evaluation of 4 weeks of nocturnal nasal positive pressure ventilation in stable hypercapnic patients with COPD. *Respiration*, **68** (6), 573–583.

31. Clini, E. *et al.* (2002) The Italian multicenter study on noninvasive ventilation in chronic obstructive lung disease patients. *Eur. Respir. J.*, **20** (3), 529.

32. Casanova, C. *et al.* (2000) Long-term trial of nocturnal nasal positive pressure ventilation in patients with severe COPD. *Chest*, **118**, 1582–1590.

33. Nava, S. *et al.* (1993) Effect of nasal pressure support ventilation and external PEEP on diaphragmatic activity in patients with severe stable COPD. *Chest*, **103**, 143–150.

34. Similowski, T. *et al.* (1991) Contractile properties of the human diaphragm during chronic hyperinflation. *N. Engl. J. Med.*, **325**, 917–923.

35. Windisch, W. *et al.* (2006) Nocturnal noninvasive positive pressure ventilation: physiological effects on spontaneous breathing. *Respir. Physiol. Neurobiol.*, **150**, 251–260.

36. Petty, T.L. (2006) CO_2 can be good for you. *Chest*, **129** (2), 494.

37. Grinnan, D. and Truwit, J.D. (2005) Clinical review: respiratory mechanics in spontaneous and assisted ventilation. *Crit. Care*, **9**, 472–484.

38. Piper, A. (2002) Sleep abnormalities associated with neuromuscular disease:pathophysiology and evaluation. *Semin. Respir. Crit. Care Med.*, **23** (3), 211–219.

1.3 Noninvasive ventilation in acute respiratory failure from COPD

Daniel C. Grinnan[1] and Jonathon D. Truwit[2]

[1] *Division of Pulmonary and Critical Care Medicine, Virginia Commonwealth University, Richmond, VA, USA*
[2] *Division of Pulmonary and Critical Care Medicine, University of Virginia, Charlottesville, VA, USA*

1.3.1 Case presentation

A 74-year-old female with a past medical history of tobacco use, hypertension, and hyperlipidemia presents to the emergency room with a one day history of increased shortness of breath. At baseline, she wears two liters of supplemental oxygen for "COPD," and she has dyspnea after ambulating for five minutes. At present, she is using accessory muscles of respiration and is tachypneic. She is alert but confused and mildly agitated. She has some lower extremity edema, but it is not changed from her previous examination (you saw her last month in the emergency room). Her oxygen saturation is 88% on 4 l nasal canula, and her arterial blood gas reveals pH $= 7.21$, $PaCO_2 = 88 \, mm \, Hg$, and $PaO_2 = 55 \, mm \, Hg$. She has been given albuterol and ipratropium treatments, as well as methylprednisolone, but she had no apparent improvement. At this time, you are asked for advice on several questions:

- Should you continue current therapy, start noninvasive ventilation (NIV), or proceed with mechanical intubation?
- If started on noninvasive ventilation, how (and where) should she be monitored?

A Practical Guide to Mechanical Ventilation, First Edition.
Edited by Jonathon D. Truwit and Scott K. Epstein.
© 2011 John Wiley & Sons, Ltd. Published 2011 by John Wiley & Sons, Ltd.

- If noninvasive ventilation is started, should a nasal mask or a full face mask be used?
- If noninvasive ventilation is started, should continuous positive airway pressure (NIV-CPAP) or pressure support (NIPSV) or Bilevel positive airway pressure (BiPAP) be used?
- If noninvasive ventilation is started, what settings should be chosen and how should these be monitored?

This case is readdressed at the end of the chapter and it is hoped to answer these (and other) questions.

1.3.2   Introduction

Chronic obstructive pulmonary disease (COPD) is characterized by obstruction of expiratory flow and is the fourth leading cause of death among adults older than 65 in the United States [1]. COPD exacerbations are the leading cause of acute ventilatory failure in the United States [2]. The natural course of COPD involves a slow progression of expiratory airflow obstruction, which leads to progressive air trapping and lung hyperinflation, resulting in a flattened diaphragm. As such, the diaphragm has lost the zone of apposition and mechanical advantage. Clinically this can be observed as paradoxical motion of the lower rib cage during inspiration (the Hoover sign). To compensate accessory muscles are recruited, which causes increased energy during inspiration. During acute COPD exacerbations, airflow obstruction is increased, leading to further air trapping (increased residual volume) and the patient adapts by assuming a rapid and shallow breathing pattern. This breathing pattern increases intrinsic positive end-expiratory pressure (PEEP), or auto-PEEP (AP), leading to a further increase in the energy needed to start inspiration and increased work of breathing. This increased work of breathing can overwhelm the capacity of the respiratory muscles and lead to hypoxemic and hypercapnic respiratory failure.

Acute exacerbations of COPD can be caused by worsening airway inflammation (asthmatic bronchitis), infectious bronchitis, or pneumonia, among other causes. Acute COPD exacerbations usually repond to medical treatment over the first several days of admission. However, the respiratory muscles may fatigue during this time. Prior to NIV, invasive ventilation was the standard treatment for severe acute COPD exacerbations and attendant respiratory failure. Over the last 15 years, NIV has been increasingly used to treat acute COPD exacerbations. In this chapter, the data supporting the use of NIV in this patient population is summarized.

1.3.3   Physiology of NIV in acute COPD

Physiologic studies have supported the rationale for NIV use and suggested a pressure support mode (NIV-PS) that should be used in acute COPD exacerbations.

Patients with COPD commonly develop further increases in functional residual capacity, which can be assessed by the measurement of AP, (the mean pressure within communicating alveoli at end-exhalation). As AP is a positive pressure and the initiation of inspiratory airflow requires a negative pressure gradient between the upper airway and the distal airway, considerable energy must be spent to overcome AP. This energy is expended during the isometric phase of respiration in patients with acute COPD exacerbations, as flow will not occur until AP is overcome. CPAP provides positive pressure at the nose and mouth, thus reducing the positive pressure gradient between the upper airway and the distal airway at the end of expiration. Theoretically, this should reduce the energy needed to start a breath and help patients with acute COPD exacerbations. In fact, Appendini et al. [3] found that the inspiratory work load is significantly reduced by placing the PEEP of a NIV machine at a level that is 80–90% of the intrinsic PEEP. When they studied the effect NIV-PS, they found that the pressure time product is significantly reduced in patients with acute respiratory failure (ARF) due to COPD when compared with patients treated with CPAP alone [3]. The pressure time product (PTP) is the product of the average inspiratory pressure and the duration of inspiration (PTP = $P_{avg} \times T_i$) and was developed to assess energy expenditures during the dynamic and isometric phases of respiration [4]. Therefore, physiological studies of lung mechanics in acute COPD exacerbations support the use of NIV-PS.

Because esophageal balloons are not placed in normal clinical practice, measurements like intrinsic PEEP, compliance, and resistance are not directly measured in spontaneously breathing patients receiving noninvasive ventilation. Therefore, the initial settings of NIV-PS in patients with COPD are based on previous experience with similar patients, rather than precise physiologic data. Because NIV-PS can be uncomfortable and lead to heightened anxiety and feelings of claustrophobia, it is important to ease the patient into treatment with NIV-PS. Settings are normally started with an inspiratory positive airway pressure (IPAP) of around 10 cm H_2O and an expiratory positive airway pressure (EPAP) of around 5 cm H_2O with a BiPAP machine or PS level of 5 cm H_2O and PEEP of 5 cm H_2O when using an intensive care mechanical ventilator. Often, patients will regain some control and comfort if they are allowed to hold the mask in place (and are able to do so) [2]. In the setting of acute respiratory failure, mask discomfort is the most common reason for NIV discontinuation and is an important reason for NIV failure [2]. Finding a mask that fits the patient appropriately is extremely important. There is an ongoing debate regarding oronasal masks (full face masks) and nasal masks in acute respiratory failure. We believe that full face masks are the preferred initial mask. Oronasal masks permit mouth breathing and reduce oral air leaks, an important consideration in acutely ill patients who are usually mouth breathers [5]. Kwok and colleagues [5] showed that, in the setting of acute respiratory failure, mask intolerance was greater with nasal masks than with oronasal masks. They also found a trend toward greater success of NIV treatment with oronasal masks (65.7%) than with nasal masks (48.6%), although this trend was not significant. For long-term application of NIV, nasal masks are usually more comfortable than oronasal masks [6]. Therefore, clinicians should consider transitioning from oronasal masks to nasal masks in patients who continue to require NIV over several days.

1.3.4   Clinical data on NIV in acute COPD

Several clinical studies have looked at surrogate end points of clinical improvement with NIV in acute COPD exacerbations. It has been shown that NIV improves hypoxemia and hypercapnia [7, 8], decreases the respiratory rate [7, 8], and decreases the cardiac output while maintaining the central venous saturation [9]. The underlying mechanism for these changes appears to be that NIV-PS increases alveolar ventilation leading to improved clearance of carbon dioxide, which increases alveolar oxygenation. This increase in alveolar oxygenation enables one to maintain oxygen content in the face of a reduced cardiac output while maintaining oxygen content [9].

In addition to the above surrogate end points, NIV has been found to significantly decrease the mortality rate, intubation rate, and length of hospital stay in patients with severe acute COPD exacerbations [7] (Figure 1.3.1).

Recent meta-analyses by Lightowler [10] and Keenan *et al.* [11] confirmed that these important end points were significant. Lightowler found that patients treated with NIV had a 0.41 relative risk of mortality, a 0.42 relative risk of intubation, and a 3.24 day reduction in the length of hospital stay. Similarly, Keenan found a

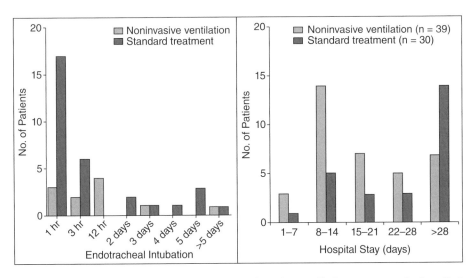

Figure 1.3.1   Bar graphs showing the effect of noninvasive ventilation versus standard medical treatment on (left) time to intubation and (right) length of hospital stay. (Reproduced with permission from [7].)

10% risk reduction in mortality, a 28% risk reduction in rate of intubation, and a 4.57 day reduction in the length of hospital stay. Keenan also performed a subgroup analysis on patients with mild COPD exacerbations (pH > 7.30). In this group, his analysis did not reveal a significant decrease in intubation rate or mortality rate. However, there have only been two small studies on this population, so it is not inappropriate to consider NIV in this population if the work of breathing is increased.

NIV has been well studied in hypercapnic respiratory failure from COPD. It has been shown that NIV-PS improves gas exchange, decreases the rate of intubation, and reduces length of hospital stay compared with conventional treatment [8]. However, there is a significant rate of NIV failure, ranging from 5 to 50% in different series [7, 8, 12]. Determining which patients are likely to fail NIV treatment can lead to the improved initial care and should lead to improved clinical outcomes. Known risk factors for failure of NIV in ARF due to COPD include altered mental status (AMS), high APACHE II score (odds ratio of 5.38 for every five point increase in the APACHE II score) [13], pH, and respiratory rate [14]. In addition, it was recently shown that airway colonization by pathogenic bacteria on admission was a predictor of NIV failure [15]. All patients in that study underwent quantitative culture of either sputum or tracheal aspirate on admission.

As mentioned above, AMS is an independent predictor of NIV failure in patients with acute COPD exacerbations. It is generally assumed that these patients are at an increased risk of aspiration, as they may not be able to protect their airway. Therefore, AMS has long been considered a relative contra-indication to noninvasive ventilation. However, it has been unclear where "the line" should be drawn, since AMS represents a continuum between mild confusion and coma. A recent case control study looked at the rate of NIV failure with progressive levels of AMS (as assessed by the Kelly score) [16]. The Kelly score rates AMS from one to six and describes patients with minimal baseline AMS (Kelly 1), those who are alert and able to follow simple commands (Kelly 2), those who lethargic but arousable and following simple commands (Kelly 3), and those who are stuporous or comatose (Kelly 4–6). In patients with AMS and ARF from COPD, the rate of NIV failure increased from 15% at Kelly score of two, to 25% at Kelly score of three, and to 45% at a Kelly score of greater than three. Compared to matched controls without AMS, only those with Kelly scores greater than three had a significantly higher rate of NIV failure. While this study is not definitive, it suggests that "the line" may be drawn between those who are lethargic but arousable and following basic commands (Kelly 3) and those who are stuporous (Kelly 4). If NIV is attempted in patients who are stuporous, caution and vigilance should be maintained by the clinician.

Recently, efforts have been made to more accurately assess the rate of NIV failure in patients with acute hypercapnic respiratory failure due to COPD. Confalonieri *et al.* [14] recently performed a retrospective analysis on over 1000 patients with ARF and COPD, and their risk stratification system for predicting the likelihood of NIV failure is shown in Figure 1.3.2.

	RR	pH admission < 7.25		pH admission 7.25–7.29		pH admission > 7.25	
		APACHE ≥ 29	APACHE < 29	APACHE ≥ 29	APACHE < 29	APACHE ≥ 29	APACHE < 29
GCS 15	< 30	29	11	18	6	17	6
	30–34	42	18	29	11	27	10
	≥ 35	52	24	37	15	35	14
GCS 12–14	< 30	48	22	33	13	32	12
	30–34	63	34	48	22	46	21
	≥ 35	71	42	57	29	55	27
GCS ≤ 11	< 30	64	35	49	23	47	21
	30–34	76	49	64	35	62	33
	≥ 35	82	59	72	44	70	42

	RR	pH after 2h < 7.25		pH after 2h 7.25–7.29		pH after 2h < 7.25	
		APACHE ≥ 29	APACHE < 29	APACHE ≥ 29	APACHE < 29	APACHE ≥ 29	APACHE < 29
GCS 15	< 30	72	35	27	7	11	3
	30–34	88	59	49	17	25	7
	≥ 35	93	73	64	27	38	11
GCS 12–14	< 30	84	51	41	13	19	5
	30–34	93	74	65	28	39	12
	≥ 35	96	84	78	42	54	20
GCS ≤ 11	< 30	93	74	65	28	39	12
	30–34	97	88	83	51	63	26
	≥ 35	99	93	90	66	76	40

Failure Rate Legend	0–24%	25–49%	50–74%	75–100%

Figure 1.3.2   Percent chance of NIV failure based on respiratory rate, APACHE score, pH, and GCS. The top panel shows the risk of failure based on admission characteristics. The bottom panel shows the risk of failure based on characteristics two hours after admission. GCS = Glasgow coma score, RR = respiratory rate. (Modified with permission [14].)

The improvement in hypercapnic acute respiratory failure that is seen in COPD cannot be extrapolated to other etiologies of hypercapnic ARF. A recent study showed that, while only 19% of patients with hypercapnic ARF due to COPD failed NIV, 47% of patients (matched for age and severity of illness) with hypercapnic ARF due to other causes failed NIV [13].

As NIV has become standard treatment in acute exacerbations of NIV, investigators have started to look at NIV in patients with more severe illness. Early reports suggested that outcomes of patients with severe pneumonia and COPD were poor when treated with NIV [17]. However, subsequent studies have shown that NIV can improve mortality compared with conventional treatment in patients with COPD and severe pneumonia [18]. In this prospective, randomized trial, they also found decreased rates of invasive ventilation and decreased length of intensive care unit stay in the NIV group.

Squadrone *et al.* [19] assessed patients in severe ARF from COPD (pH < 7.25, $PaCO_2 > 70\,mm\,Hg$, and RR > 35) who met criteria for invasive mechanical ventilation. They treated these patients with NIV, and compared results with a historical control group treated with invasive ventilation. They found similar rates of hospital mortality and length of hospital stay. However, they found that the rate of infection was decreased in the group treated with NIV compared with the historical control. It must be noted that the rate of NIV failure was very high (62%) in this group. Once again, it must be stressed that the decision to treat patients with severe ARF from COPD must be accompanied by increased vigilance and a willingness to invasively ventilate if improvement is not seen within the first two hours of NIV.

In clinical practice, NIV is often offered to patients with acute exacerbations of COPD who defer intubation. In fact, the use of NIV in patients who deferred intubation (do not resuscitate, DNR) accounts for about 10% of NIV use in the acute setting [20]. Patients with COPD exacerbations who declare as DNR but are provided NIV are likely to survive that hospitalization [21]. A recent study demonstrated that the one year survival in this cohort was 29.7%, and the one year event free survival was 16.2% [22]. Event free survival was characterized by death or repeat exacerbation requiring NIV. This information may assist physicians as well as patients and their families in deciding whether or not to pursue NIV treatment.

Patients with acute exacerbations of COPD requiring NIV are likely to have repeated hospitalizations. Tuggey and colleagues [23] performed a retrospective analysis to determine if outpatient NIV use led to better utilization of health care resources in patients with recurrent admissions requiring NIV. They found that home NIV use led to significantly fewer hospital days and significantly lower health care costs.

1.3.5 Summary

COPD is the leading cause of acute respiratory failure in the United States, and the development of noninvasive ventilation has changed the management of acute COPD exacerbations. NIV can decrease the need for intubation, decrease hospital stay, and even improve mortality in patients with acute COPD exacerbations. However, it is important to be able to determine when a patient has "failed" NIV or is not appropriate for NIV. This determination requires careful attention (usually in an intensive care unit or emergency room) by experienced clinicians. While NIV can be offered to patients who have refused intubation, it should be recognized (by the practitioner and by the patient or his/her family) that the one year survival in this population is poor. Chung *et al.* report five-year outcomes in patients with COPD after first episode of NIV for an acute exacerbation [24]. One year survival was 72% and two and five years were 52% and 26% respectively. Long term mortality was associated with advanced age, reduced BMI and prior home oxygen.

1.3.6 Case revisited

The case at the beginning of the chapter depicts an elderly female with acute hypoxemic and hypercapnic respiratory failure from a COPD exacerbation. After reading this chapter, it is hoped it is understood that ample evidence supports using NIV in this patient population. The degree of hypercapnia (pH = 7.21) does not prohibit NIV, but (as noted in Figure 1.3.2) the chance of NIV failure is significant, so that close observation is essential to ensure that intubation (if necessary) is not delayed. The presence of agitation is not a contra-indication to NIV but again demands close observation to see if treatment is tolerated. Once NIV has been started, it is recommended monitoring the patient at least every hour for signs of clinical improvement. If significant improvement has not been made after a couple of hours, the patient may require invasive ventilation. It is recommend that patients on NIV for acute respiratory failure be monitored in an intensive care unit setting, unless there is significant experience amongst all staff caring for the patients and clear algorithms for transfer to an intensive care unit exist. It is felt that this patient would be best served using a full face mask initially to prevent air leaks and minimize treatment failure. As the patient improves, transition to a nasal mask may improve comfort. While the helmet is intriguing, it is not approved by the Food & Drug Administration for use in the United States, and further research is needed to recommend its use. In this case (COPD), the patient should be treated with NIV-PS. While there is no consensus on initial levels of support, it is recommended starting with an IPAP of 10 cm H_2O and an EPAP of 5 cm H_2O, with a BiPAP machine or PS level of 5 cm H_2O and PEEP of 5 cm H_2O when using an intensive care mechanical ventilator. Inspiratory and end-expiratory pressures are then carefully titrated to the desired clinical effect.

References

1. Carlucci, A. et al. (2001) Noninvasive versus conventional mechanical ventilation: an epidemiologic survey. Am. J. Respir. Crit. Care Med., 163, 874–880.
2. Pierson, D.J. and Hill, N.S. (2005) Acute ventilatory failure, in Murray and Nadel's Textbook of Respiratory Medicine, 4th edn (eds. R.J. Mason, V.C. Broaddus, J.F. Murray and J.A. Nadel), Elsevier Saunders, Philadelphia, pp. 2379–2398.
3. Appendini, L. et al. (1994) Physiologic effects of positive end-expiratory pressure and mask pressure support during exacerbations of chronic obstructive pulmonary disease. Am. J. Respir. Crit. Care Med., 149 (5), 1069–1076.
4. Grinnan, D.C. and Truwit, J.D. (2005) Clinical review: respiratory mechanics in spontaneous and assisted ventilation. Crit. Care, 9, 3516.
5. Kwok, H. et al. (2003) Controlled trial of oronasal versus nasal mask ventilation in the treatment of acute respiratory failure. Crit. Care Med., 31 (2), 468–473.
6. Navalesi, P. et al. (2000) Physiologic evaluation of noninvasive mechanical ventilation delivered with three types of masks in patients with chronic hypercapnic respiratory failure. Crit. Care Med., 28, 1785–1790.

7. Brochard, L. *et al.* (1995) Noninvasive ventilation for acute exacerbations of chronic obstructive pulmonary disease. *N. Engl. J. Med.*, **333** (13), 817–822.
8. Celikel, T. *et al.* (1998) Comparison of noninvasive positive pressure ventilation with standard medical therapy in hypercapnic acute respiratory failure. *Chest*, **114**, 1636–1642.
9. Diaz, O. *et al.* (1997) Effects of noninvasive ventialation on pulmonary gas exchange and hemodynamics during acute hypercapnic exacerbations of chronic obstructive pulmonary disease. *Am. J. Respir. Crit. Care Med.*, **156**, 1840–1845.
10. Lightowler, J. (2003) Noninvasive positive pressure ventilation for the treatment of respiratory failure due to exacerbations of chronic obstructive pulmonary disease. *BMJ*, **326**, 185–189.
11. Keenan, S.P. *et al.* (2003) Which patients with acute exacerbations of chronic obstructive pulmonary disease benefit from noninvasive ventilation? A systematic review of the literature. *Ann. Intern. Med.*, **138**, 861–870.
12. Carratu, P. *et al.* (2005) Early and late failure of noninvasive ventilation in chronic obstructive pulmonary disease with acute exacerbation. *Eur. J. Clin. Invest.*, **35**, 404–409.
13. Phua, J. *et al.* (2005) Noninvasive ventilation in hypercapnic acute respiratory failure due to chronic obstructive pulmonary disease vs. other conditions: effectiveness and predictors of failure. *Intensive Care Med.*, **31**, 533–539.
14. Confalonieri, M. *et al.* (2005) A chart of failure risk of noninvasive ventilation in patients with COPD exacerbation. *Eur. Respir. J.*, **25**, 348–355.
15. Ferrer, M. *et al.* (2005) Microbial airway colonization is associated with noninvasive ventilation failure in exacerbation of chronic obstructive pulmonary disease. *Crit. Care Med.*, **33** (9), 2003–2009.
16. Scala, R. *et al.* (2005) Noninvasive positive pressure ventilation in patients with acute exacerbations of COPD and varying levels of consciousness. *Chest*, **128**, 1657–1666.
17. Ambrosino, N. *et al.* (1995) Noninvasive mechanical ventilation in acute respiratory failure due to chronic obstructive pulmonary disease: correlates for success. *Thorax*, **50**, 755–777.
18. Confalonieri, M. *et al.* (1999) Acute respiratory failure in patients with severe community aquired pneumonia: a prospective randomized evaluation of noninvasive ventilation. *Am. J. Respir. Crit. Care Med.*, **160**, 1585–1591.
19. Squadrone, E. *et al.* (2004) Noninvasive vs invasive ventilation in COPD patients with severe acute respiratory failure deemed to require ventilatory assistance. *Intensive Care Med.*, **30**, 1303–1310.
20. Levy, M. *et al.* (2004) Outcomes of patients with do-not-intubate orders treated with noninvasive ventilation. *Crit. Care Med.*, **32**, 2002–2007.
21. Meduri, G.U. *et al.* (1994) Noninvasive mechanical ventilation via face mask in patients with acute respiratory failure who refused endotracheal intubation. *Crit. Care Med.*, **22**, 1584–1590.
22. Chu, C.-M. *et al.* (2004) Noninvasive ventilation in patients with acute hypercapnic exacerbation of chronic obstructive pulmonary disease who refused endotracheal intubation. *Crit. Care Med.*, **32** (2), 372–377.
23. Tuggey, J.M. *et al.* (2003) Domiciliary non-invasive ventilation for recurrent acidotic exacerbations of COPD: an economic analysis. *Thorax*, **58**, 867–871.
24. Chung, L.P. *et al.* (2010) Five-year outcome in COPD patients after their first episode of acute exacerbation treated with non-invasive ventilation. *Respirology*, **15**, 1084–1091 doi: 10.1111/j.1440-1843.2010.01795.x.

1.4 Noninvasive ventilation in acute CHF

Daniel C. Grinnan[1] and Jonathon D. Truwit[2]

[1] *Division of Pulmonary and Critical Care Medicine, Virginia Commonwealth University, Richmond, VA, USA*
[2] *Division of Pulmonary and Critical Care Medicine, University of Virginia, Charlottesville, VA, USA*

1.4.1 Case presentation

A 62-year-old with a known history of congestive heart failure (CHF) caused by systolic dysfunction and an ejection fraction of 25% presents to the emergency room with acute respiratory distress. The patient does not have a history of tobacco use or known emphysema. Examination reveals tachypnea with accessory muscle use, bibasilar crackles, scattered wheezes, elevated jugular venous pressures, and bilateral lower extremity pulmonary edema. A chest radiograph is consistent with pulmonary edema and small bilateral effusions, and the brain natriuretic peptide (BNP) is 1340 pg/ml. An arterial blood gas is obtained and reads 7.22/68/62 while the patient is receiving two liters oxygen by nasal canula. While administering diuretic medication and afterload reduction, the decision is made to start noninvasive ventilation. You are asked what mode of noninvasive ventilation you would prefer, with which settings you would like to start, and whether or not to admit the patient to the floor, to the "step-down" unit, or to the intensive care unit. How should you respond?

1.4.2 Introduction

Patients with acute congestive heart failure (CHF) commonly present to the emergency room. Heart failure is the leading cause of hospitalization in patients over

A Practical Guide to Mechanical Ventilation, First Edition.
Edited by Jonathon D. Truwit and Scott K. Epstein.
© 2011 John Wiley & Sons, Ltd. Published 2011 by John Wiley & Sons, Ltd.

age 65 in the United States [1]. Patients with CHF experience the progressive downward spiral of left ventricular dysfunction, pulmonary edema, impaired gas exchange, increased work of breathing, increased oxygen consumption by the diaphragm and accessory muscles, increased cardiac demand, and myocardial ischemia. In most cases of acute CHF, proper management can interrupt this spiral and lead to its reversal. Both invasive and noninvasive positive pressure ventilation lead to decreased left ventricular afterload, decreased work of breathing, and decreased intrapulmonary shunt [2]. Because of the inherent advantages of noninvasive ventilation (NIV) over invasive ventilation, NIV is frequently used in acute CHF. In fact, acute CHF is the second leading use of NIV [3]. However, no single trial has shown a significant mortality benefit to using NIV in this population. In addition, as discussed later, it is debated whether continuous positive airway pressure (NIV-CPAP) or pressure support (NIV-PS) is the superior mode of NIV in acute CHF.

1.4.3   Physiology of NIV-CPAP in CHF

NIV-CPAP assists patients with acute CHF through several mechanisms. These mechanisms can be broken down into improvements in respiratory mechanics and improvements in hemodynamics (Figure 1.4.1).

NIV-CPAP improves respiratory mechanics by decreasing atelectasis and by decreasing the hydrostatic forces leading to pulmonary edema. It is common for patients with acute CHF to develop atelectasis. The enlarged left ventricle leaves less space for the left lower lobe in the thoracic cage. In addition, patients are often immobile due to their illness and are placed in a semi-recumbent position. This enhances the probability of developing left lower lobe atelectasis, since much of this lobe lies posterior to the heart. NIV-CPAP increases the positive pressure in

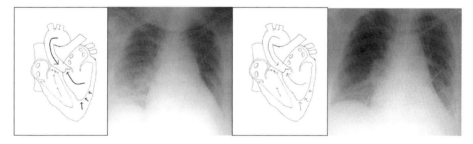

Figure 1.4.1 Congestive heart failure is normally characterized by a state of increased afterload, leading to increased left ventricular wall tension and increased work during systole (far left). Radiographically, this often manifests as interstitial edema (left middle). After NIV-CPAP, the afterload is reduced, leading to decreased left ventricular wall stress and decreased work during systole (right middle). The radiograph on the far right is on the same patient following one hour of NIV-CPAP without diuresis. While left lower lobe atelectasis and cardiomegaly persist, there has been interval improvement in the pattern of interstitial edema.

the alveoli throughout the respiratory cycle, making it more likely that atelectatic alveoli will be "recruited" throughout the respiratory cycle. The increase in the number of functional alveoli improves ventilation/perfusion matching (as the base of the left lower lobe is heavily perfused in the semi-recumbant position).

The Starling equation describes the forces that influence the efflux of fluid across the capillary wall. The equation is defined as: $Jv = LpS [(Pc - Pi) - (\pi c - \pi i)]$, where Jv is the filtration rate, Lp is the conductivity of the capillary membrane, S is the surface area, Pc is the capillary hydrostatic pressure, Pi is the interstitial hydrostatic pressure, πc is the capillary plasma oncotic pressure, and πi is the interstitial plasma oncotic pressure [4]. Because NIV-CPAP increases the pressure in the alveoli and some of this pressure is transferred to the interstitium of the alveoli, the pressure gradient favoring the movement of fluid from the capillaries to the interstitium is reduced, thus reducing the filtration rate.

NIV-CPAP also assists patients with acute CHF by decreasing the load placed on the left ventricle. Left ventricular afterload is the load on the left ventricle during systole, which translates left ventricular wall stress during left ventricular contraction. In acute CHF, the left ventricle usually has increased preload, increased left ventricular end diastolic pressure, increased left ventricular wall stress at end diastole, and increased afterload. This increase in afterload means that increased intraventricular pressure must be created to open the aortic valve and then maintained during the rest of systole [5]. NIV-CPAP decreases the afterload placed on the left ventricle by decreasing the systolic blood pressure [2, 6]. In addition, in patients with decompensated CHF, the increase in intrathoracic pressure from CPAP is partially transmitted to the left ventricle, helping to reduce the left ventricular afterload further [2]. Because the decrease in afterload is not accompanied by a significant decrease in preload in patients with acute CHF [2], their stroke volume and cardiac output are improved [7].

Intuitively, it would be anticipated that noninvasive ventilation with pressure support (NIV-PS) would confer an advantage over NIV-CPAP. By providing a pressure gradient between the inspiratory positive airway pressure (IPAP) and the expiratory positive airway pressure (EPAP), NIV-PS, here with a BiPAP machine, contributes to the work of breathing, thus decreasing patient work of breathing and decreasing respiratory muscle oxygen consumption [8]. This should decrease myocardial demand and improve outcomes in patients with acute CHF. As discussed below, the clinical evidence has yet to confirm that NIV-PS is superior to NIV-CPAP in patients with heart failure.

1.4.4 Does NIV improve clinical outcomes in acute CHF?

Physiological analysis of the effects of NIV in acute CHF have consistently showed significant improvements with NIV. Acute improvements in oxygenation (PaO_2) [9, 10], ventilation (decrease in $PaCO_2$) [9, 10], tachypnea [9], and tachycardia [9] have been shown. Intrapulmonary shunt and work of breathing have also been reduced using NIV in patients with acute cardiogenic pulmonary edema [2]. These physiologic improvements translate into improvements in patient reporting of dyspnea with NIV [10]. As most of the early studies assessing NIV in acute CHF were small studies, they were not powered to detect a difference in mortality. This led to a wave of meta analyses which pooled data from all of these smaller studies to see if a mortality benefit existed with NIV in acute CHF. As with all meta analyses, discrepancies in individual trial design can greatly confound the results and make interpretation difficult. One meta-analysis showed a 43% relative risk reduction in mortality ($p < 0.001$) and a 56% relative risk reduction in need for invasive ventilation ($p < 0.001$) when NIV was compared with conventional treatment alone [11]. (Figure 1.4.2) When NIV-CPAP was compared with conventional treatment in this meta analysis, there was still a significant reduction in mortality ($p = 0.003$) and in the need for invasive ventilation ($p < 0.001$). However, when the existing studies of NIV-PS were compared with conventional treatment alone, the difference

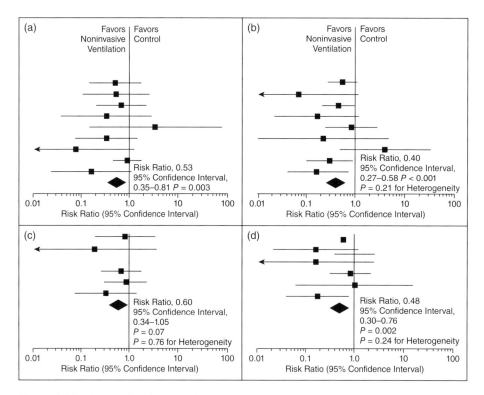

Figure 1.4.2   Forest plots from Masip *et al.* (JAMA) Panel A shows the effect of NIV-CPAP versus conventional treatment on mortality. Panel B shows the effect of NIV-CPAP versus conventional treatment on rate of invasive ventilation. Panels C and D show the effect of NIV-PS versus conventional treatment on mortality rate and rate of invasive ventilation, respectively.

in mortality did not reach statistical significance ($p = 0.07$). A follow up meta-analysis reached similar conclusions [12].

Recently, the 3-CPO trial [10] (a large prospective, randomized, controlled study) compared the efficacy of NIV-CPAP and NIV-PS with conventional treatment. The primary outcomes of the study were mortality and a composite outcome of mortality and rate of intubation. Secondary outcomes included 30-day mortality and various physiological outcomes. While improvements in tachycardia, hypercapnia, and dyspnea were found in those treated with NIV, there was no significant reduction (or trend toward reduction) in mortality among the NIV treated population (Table 1.4.1).

The 3-CPO trial marks the largest prospective, randomized study of NIV in patients with acute CHF exacerbations. Therefore, it is important to look closely at the design and the results before extrapolating the results to clinical practice. It might be assumed that standard therapy (oxygen and medication without NIV) means that patients did not receive NIV under any circumstances. If their assigned treatment did not work and the patient deteriorated, the patient would be intubated. However, this was not the case. Patients randomized to standard therapy could still receive NIV prior to intubation if they had clinical deterioration. In fact, 15% of the patients in the standard treatment group did receive NIV, while only 1% of patients in the standard treatment group were intubated. Therefore, many patients with clinical deterioration in the standard treatment arm were rescued with NIV and did not require intubation. Since it is widely believed that NIV decreases mortality in acute CHF (and in other cases of acute respiratory failure) by avoiding intubation and the related complications of intubation, it is difficult to generalize that NIV does not decrease intubation rates or decrease survival from the 3-CPO trial. While other potential weaknesses have been noted, this has been the major criticism of the 3-CPO trial [13, 14].

Table 1.4.1 Outcomes from the 3-CPO study. (Reproduced with permission [13].)

Noninvasive intermittent positive pressure ventilation (NIPPV) vs. continuous positive airway pressure (CPAP) vs standard oxygen therapy in acute cardiogenic pulmonary edema[a]

Outcomes	NIPPV or CPAP	Standard therapy	RRR (95% CI)	NNT (CI)
Mortality at 7 d	9.5%	9.8%	3% (−41 to 35)	Not significant
Mortality at 30 d	15%	16%	7% (−25 to 32)	Not significant
	NIPPV	CPAP		
Mortality or intubation at 7 d	11.1%	11.7%	5% (−42 to 38)	Not significant
Mortality at 7 d	9.4%	9.6%	3% (−52 to 40)	Not significant
Mortality at 30 d	15.1%	15.4%	2% (−39 to 32)	Not significant

[a]RRR = relative risk reduction, NNT = number needed to treat, CI = confidence interval.

Because other prospective, randomized studies have shown a decrease in the rate of intubation with NIV in acute CHF [9], because the 3-CPO trial did not exclude the use of NIV from the standard treatment arm, and because meta analyses have suggested a great decrease in intubation using NIV [11, 12], it is believed the existing evidence suggests a decrease in the rate of intubation when NIV is used to treat acute CHF. However, the same claim cannot be made regarding the incidence of mortality when NIV is used in acute CHF. No prospective, randomized trial has shown a reduction in mortality. While meta-analysis data are suggestive, they are not confirmatory. As the investigators in the 3-CPO trial felt it would be unethical (reasonably so) to withhold NIV from patients in the standard treatment arm who were decompensating, this question may never be addressed in a large randomized trial.

1.4.5   NIV-PS or NIV-CPAP in acute CHF

Early research raised concern about the possible use of NIV-PS in patients with acute CHF. These small studies showed significant increases in myocardial infarction rates [15] and a trend toward increased mortality [16] in patients with acute CHF treated with NIV-PS compared with NIV-CPAP. However, a follow up study did not find an increased rate of myocardial infarction with NIV-PS compared with NIV-CPAP in patients with acute CHF [17]. While recent meta analyses found no significant difference in the incidence of myocardial infarction between patients treated with NIV-PS and those treated with NIV-CPAP [11, 18], an insignificant trend toward increased myocardial infarction rate in those treated with NIV-PS was found [18]. The authors warned that, at this time, "a small risk for inducing myocardial ischemia with NIV-PS cannot completely be excluded." [18] However, as noted in the physiology section above, these results do not correlate with physiologic rationale (NIV-PS should decrease work of breathing and reduce myocardial ischemia).

The 3-CPO trial enrolled over 300 patients to both NIV-CPAP and NIV-PS. As these patients were prospectively followed over time, this allowed for the most comprehensive comparison of the two modalities. As shown in Table 1.4.1, there was no significant difference in mortality or intubation rates between NIV-CPAP and NIV-PS. Therefore, it is believed that both NIV-CPAP and NIV-PS can be used to treat acute CHF. While NIV-CPAP is cheaper and easier to administer, there are patients who may benefit from NIV-PS over NIV-CPAP.

1.4.6   NIV-PS in acute hypercapnic CHF

Two small studies have analyzed the role of NIV-PS in patients with acute CHF and hypercapnia. As hypercapnic patients in acute CHF have more respiratory muscle fatigue and increased work of breathing compared with eucapneic patients, they would theoretically have more to gain from NIV-PS. In a randomized control trial of NIV-PS plus medical therapy versus medical therapy alone, Nava *et al.* [19] did find a reduced intubation rate in patients with acute CHF and elevated $PaCO_2$ (>45 mm Hg). Recently, Bellone and colleagues [17] studied patients with acute CHF and hypercapnia. They found no difference in rates of mortality or need for invasive ventilation between those treated with NIV-PS and those treated with NIV-CPAP [17]. However, this study included only 36 patients, making a definitive judgment difficult.

1.4.7 Where and how long to treat with NIPPV in acute CHF

In clinical practice, NIPPV is often maintained in a "trial" period for up to 24 hours. However, studies have suggested that reversal of acute cardiogenic edema with NIPPV occurs within the first two hours of treatment. A recent study [20] enrolled consecutive patients with severe CHF and hypoxemic/hypercapnic respiratory failure who had failed conventional medical treatment. Patients were given a 90 minute trial of NIPPV, and 74% of patients had significant respiratory improvement and avoided both intubation and ICU admission. This evidence suggests that acute CHF usually responds quickly to NIPPV and other measures of afterload reduction. It also suggests that longer trials of NIPPV may be less likely to succeed and could place the patient at higher risk. It is agreed that, if NIPPV is used in acute CHF, a short trial with frequent clinical assessment is warranted.

One recent study looked at the benefit of pre-hospital NIV in patients with acute hypoxemic CHF [21]. In this randomized, controlled, prospective study, an emergency physician traveled with the emergency medical services (EMS) team. Patients in acute CHF were randomized to either NIV or conventional treatment. The group treated with NIV ($n = 10$) had higher saturation levels on admission to the hospital and a trend toward lower troponin levels. However, there was no significant difference in mortality or length of hospitalization. As the ability to diagnose acute CHF and start NIV treatment can be complicated, and it is not practical for a physician to travel with an emergency medical services squad, it is anticipated that conventional treatment by emergency medical services, followed by early treatment with NIV in the emergency room, will continue to be the standard of care.

Noninvasive ventilation is frequently used to treat acute respiratory failure in the emergency room and in intensive care units. At some facilities, use of NIPPV has been extended to "step-down" or to designated "respiratory" or "pulmonary" floors. The decision of where to treat someone must be individualized to the hospital and the patient. However, it is noted that NIPPV for acute respiratory failure must be used very carefully outside of the emergency department or the intensive care unit. As these patients are usually not sedated and subject to problems with the orofacial mask, they often require as much or more attention than patients who are endotracheally intubated. It has been shown that monitoring patients with acute respiratory failure of NIPPV in the intensive care setting has been associated with decreased need for intubation and decreased chance of developing pneumonia [22].

Clinical practice guidelines have been shown to improve patient care [23] and decrease unnecessary variation in practice patterns [24], leading to improvements in clinical outcomes [25]. This has led many hospitals to formulate guidelines for the use of noninvasive ventilation in the treatment of acute CHF. In one study looking at patients with acute respiratory failure (with acute CHF being the leading diagnosis), the implementation of guidelines led to improved patient monitoring but did not show an improvement in intubation rates [23]. However, there was a trend toward decreased intubation with use of the practice guidelines in the subset of patients with CHF. Recent research has indicated that the implementation of guidelines to help physicians use NIPPV in acute CHF has not sacrificed the physician's sense of autonomy [26]. As standardization and the reduction of medical errors becomes increasingly important, practice guidelines in the management of NIPPV are likely to grow.

1.4.8 Summary

Physiology supports the use of both NIV-CPAP and NIV-PS in treating acute CHF. However, at this time, the outcomes with NIV-PS have not been superior to NIV-CPAP treatment, but both types of NIV appear safe to use in acute CHF. NIV-CPAP treatment is easier to use and is less expensive that NIV-PS treatment. Therefore, at this time, the routine use of NIV-CPAP in patients with acute CHF and pulmonary edema is recommended, but the use of NIV-PS in those with hypercapnia is recommended. It must also be stressed that NIPPV should be applied in a setting with proper staffing (usually the emergency department or an intensive care unit), and that frequent clinical assessments are needed to determine if endotracheal intubation is warranted.

1.4.9 Case presentation revisited

The patient has acute hypercapnic respiratory failure due to CHF. Management should include NIPPV and other forms of afterload reduction. Because this patient has hypercapnic failure, starting with NIV-PS (it would not be incorrect to use NIV-CPAP) would be advised. The patient should be monitored closely in either an emergency room or an intensive care unit. Clinical examination and arterial blood gases should be assessed frequently. If the patient has not had any improvement in the first two hours, intubation would be appropriate.

References

1. Jessup, M. (2003) Medical progress: heart failure. *N. Engl. J. Med.*, **348**, 2007–2018.
2. Lin, M. (1995) Reappraisal of continuous positive airway pressure therapy in acute cardiogenic pulmonary edema. *Chest*, **107** (5), 1379–1386.

3. Burns, K.E. (2003) Bilevel noninvasive positive pressure ventilation for acute respiratory failure: survey of Ontario practice. *Crit. Care Med.*, **33** (7), 1477–1483.

4. Malik, A. *et al.* (2000) Pulmonary circulation and regulation of fluid balance, in *Murray and Nadel's Textbook of Respiratory Medicine*, 3rd edn (eds J.F. Murray, J.A. Nadel, R.J. Mason and H.A. Bouchery), WB Saunders Company, Philadelphia, pp. 119–154.

5. Opie, L. (2005) Mechanisms of cardiac contraction and relaxation, in *Braunwald's Heart Disease: A Textbook of Cardiovascular Medicine*, 7th edn (eds D.P. Zipes, P. Libby, R. Bonow and E. Braunwald), Elsevier Saunders, Philadelphia, pp. 547–489.

6. DiBenedetto, R.J. (1997) Noninvasive ventilation: a welcome resurgence and a plea for caution. *Chest*, **111** (6), 1482–1483.

7. Baratz, D.M. *et al.* (1992) Effect of nasal continuous positive airway pressure on cardiac output and oxygen delivery in patients with congestive heart failure. *Chest*, **102** (5), 1397–1401.

8. Chadda, K. (2002) Cardiac and respiratory effects of continuous positive airway pressure and noninvasive ventilation in acute cardiac pulmonary edema. *Crit. Care Med.*, **30** (11), 2457–2461.

9. Bersten, A.D. (1991) Treatment of severe cardiogenic pulmonary edema with continuous positive airway pressure delivered by face mask. *N. Engl. J. Med.*, **325** (26), 1825–1830.

10. Gray, A. *et al.* (2008) Noninvasive ventilation in acute cardiogenic pulmonary edema. *N. Engl. J. Med.*, **359**, 142–151.

11. Masip, J. (2005) Noninvasive ventilation in acute cardiogenic pulmonary edema: systematic review and meta-analysis. *JAMA*, **294** (24), 3124–3130.

12. Winck, J. (2006) Efficacy and safety of non-invasive ventilation in the treatment of acute cardiogenic pulmonary edema: a systematic review and meta-analysis. *Crit. Care*, **10** (2), R69. doi: 10.1186/cc4905.

13. Filippatos, G. *et al.* (2008) Noninvasive ventilation improved dyspnea but did not reduce short-term mortality in acute cardiogenic pulmonary edema. *ACP J. Club*, **149** (6), JC6–JC9.

14. Masip, J. (2008) Editorial. *N. Engl. J. Med.*, **359** (19), 2068–2069.

15. Mehta, S. *et al.* (1997) Randomized, prospective trial of bilevel vs continuous positive pressure ventilation in acute cardiogenic edema. *Crit. Care Med.*, **25** (4), 620–628.

16. Wood, K.A. *et al.* (1998) The use of noninvasive positive pressure ventilation in the emergency department: results of a randomized clinical trial. *Chest*, **113**, 1339–1346.

17. Bellone, A. *et al.* (2004) Myocardial infarction rate in acute pulmonary edema: noninvasive pressure support ventilation versus continuous positive airway pressure. *Crit. Care Med.*, **32**, 1860–1865.

18. Ho, K.M. *et al.* (2006) A comparison of continuous and bi-level positive airway pressure non-invasive ventilation in patients with acute cardiogenic pulmonary oedema: a meta-analysis. *Crit. Care*, **10**, R49.

19. Nava, S. *et al.* (2003) Noninvasive ventilation in cardiogenic pulmonary edema: a multicenter randomized trial. *Am. J. Respir. Crit. Care Med.*, **168** (12), 1432–1437.

20. Giancomini, M. *et al.* (2003) Short-term noninvasive pressure support ventilation prevents ICU admittance in patients with acute cardiogenic pulmonary edema. *Chest*, **123**, 2057–2061.

21. Weitz, G. *et al.* (2007) Prehospital noninvasive pressure support ventilation for acute cardiogenic edema. *Eur. J. Respir. Med.*, **14**, 276–279.

22. Confalonieri, M. *et al.* (1999) Acute respiratory failure in patients with severe community-aquired pneumonia: a prospective randomized evaluation of non-invasive ventilation. *Am. J. Respir. Crit. Care Med.*, **160**, 1585–1591.

23. Sinuff, T. *et al.* (2003) Evaluation of a practice guideline for noninvasive positive pressure ventilation for acute respiratory failure. *Chest*, **123**, 2062–2073.
24. Woolf, S.H. *et al.* (1990) Practice guidelines: a new reality in medicine. Recent developments. *Arch. Intern. Med.*, **150**, 1811–1818.
25. Ellrodt, G. *et al.* (1997) Evidence-based disease management. *JAMA*, **278**, 1687–1692.
26. Sinuff, T. *et al.* (2007) Practice guidelines as multipurpose tools: a qualitative study of noninvasive ventilation. *Crit. Care Med.*, **35** (3), 961–961.

1.5 Noninvasive ventilation in acute respiratory failure

Daniel C. Grinnan[1] and Jonathon D. Truwit[2]

[1] Division of Pulmonary and Critical Care Medicine, Virginia Commonwealth University, Richmond, VA, USA
[2] Division of Pulmonary and Critical Care Medicine, University of Virginia, Charlottesville, VA, USA

1.5.1 Case presentation

You are called to evaluate a 37-year-old with a recent diagnosis of acute myeloid leukemia (AML), now 12 days status post initiation of 7 and 3 induction chemotherapy. She had developed new infiltrates yesterday; she had bronchoscopy yesterday afternoon. The bronchoscopy did not show alveolar hemorrhage and the cell count revealed a neutrophilic alveolitis. Serologic studies are significant for a pancytopenia, including a profound neutropenia. Culture results are pending. She has now developed acute respiratory distress and has an arterial blood gas reading 7.31/48/60 while receiving five liters oxygen by nasal canula. On examination, she is tachypneic with accessory muscle use, and she has bilateral crackles over the bases of her posterior thorax. She is alert and calm but able to talk only in fragments. You are asked to transfer her to the intensive care unit and initiate invasive mechanical ventilation. How would you manage this patient? Is noninvasive ventilation safe? Is it preferred over invasive ventilation in such a patient?

1.5.2 Introduction

This chapter focuses on the use of noninvasive ventilation (NIV) in treating acute respiratory failure from causes other than chronic obstructive pulmonary disease

A Practical Guide to Mechanical Ventilation, First Edition.
Edited by Jonathon D. Truwit and Scott K. Epstein.
© 2011 John Wiley & Sons, Ltd. Published 2011 by John Wiley & Sons, Ltd.

(COPD) and congestive heart failure (CHF), as these topics are covered separately. In status asthmaticus and with post pneumonectomy patients, NIV holds promise because these disorders can often be resolved rapidly, and NIV can stabilize their respiratory status while awaiting improvement. In other patient populations (cystic fibrosis and immunosuppression), NIV seems to confer an advantage because it can reduce the likelihood of ventilator associated pneumonia compared with invasive ventilation. Discussed is the evidence supporting the use of NIV in all of these disorders, as well as in patients with early acute respiratory distress syndrome (ARDS). In addition, the role of NIV in pre-oxygentating patients requiring urgent intubation in the intensive care unit is discussed.

1.5.3   Status asthmaticus

The success of NIV in treating COPD complicated by acute hypoxemic or hyper-capnic respiratory failure has led to speculation that NIV might be successful in the treatment of status asthmaticus. Similarly to COPD, status asthmaticus often leads to accessory muscle use, tachypnea, increased work of breathing, respiratory muscle fatigue, and hypoxemic and hypercapnic respiratory failure. However, it has been noted that these two obstructive lung diseases differ physiologically and by their natural history, so that extrapolation of data from COPD studies to asthma patients could be presumptive and dangerous [1]. It is unusual for patients with severe status asthmaticus to die [2], but common to have prolonged hospitalizations. In patients with status asthmaticus requiring endotracheal intubation, hospital stay is prolonged and there is a high incidence of neuromuscular paralysis induced myopathy [3]. In clinical practice, NIV is commonly used to treat status asthmaticus. Many clinicians have personal experiences of improved gas exchange and decreased work of breathing following initiation of NIV. NIV also permits the administration of nebulized treatments and heliox [1]. Unfortunately, there have been no randomized, controlled studies of NIV in status asthmaticus. In one prospective case series of patients with status asthmaticus, 29 out of 76 patients were initially treated with NIV, and only seven of these (23%) progressed to require intubation [2]. Intubation was associated with increased length of hospitalization compared with the group treated with NIV. Similar success at avoiding intubation was found in a second retrospective case series of 22 patients in status asthmaticus treated with NIV. In this series, only three (14%) required intubation [4]. A third case series indicated that gas exchange was improved and the need for intubation was decreased in patients treated with noninvasive ventilation with pressure support (NIV-PS) compared with conventional treatment [5]. However, this study had small patient numbers (17) and was not controlled, making its interpretation difficult. Therefore, patients must be monitored very closely if NIV is used to treat status asthmaticus, as its use in this patient population has yet to be proven. If using NIV, it is recommended using NIV-PS, since it has a sound clinical basis in COPD, the closest disease entity to status asthmaticus.

1.5.4   Immunosuppressed patients with acute respiratory failure

One of the fastest growing patient populations is the immunosuppressed population. Pulmonary complications are common and frequently lead to acute respiratory failure, traditionally treated with supplemental oxygen and, if needed, invasive mechanical ventilation. In the immunosuppressed population, invasive mechanical ventilation has conferred an increased risk of death, primarily due to infectious complications [6]. In 1998, Antonelli and colleagues showed that the incidence of nosocomial pneumonia is significantly decreased when patients with acute hypoxemic respiratory failure are treated with NIV compared with traditional strategies [7]. Therefore, it was soon proposed that using NIV to treat acute hypoxemic respiratory failure in the immunosuppressed would lead to decreased infectious complications and improved outcomes. In 2001, Hilbert *et al.* [8] performed a prospective, randomized, controlled trial of noninvasive mask ventilation versus conventional treatment with supplemental oxygen. Etiologies of immunosuppression included HIV, chemotherapy, and organ transplantation. All patients had pulmonary infiltrates with acute hypoxemic respiratory failure. They found that the NIV treated group had significantly improved oxygenation with decreased complication rates (mostly ventilator acquired pneumonia and sepsis), requirement for intubation, length of stay in the intensive care unit, and mortality rate. While this study was intended to include many etiologies of immunosuppression, the majority of patients had hematologic cancers and neutropenia.

Acute hypoxemic respiratory failure is common in patients following solid organ transplantation, and the survival of patients requiring invasive mechanical ventilation is poor [9]. A prospective, randomized trial assessed the efficacy of NIV in this specific population [10]. It found that, compared with a conventionally treated group, NIV led to a significant decrease in the incidence of mechanical intubation and number of infectious complications and an increased survival.

Acute hypoxemic respiratory failure due to pneumocystis jiroveci pneumonia (PCP) requiring invasive mechanical ventilation has led to poor outcomes due to the high incidence of pneumothoraces and infectious complications. A prospective case-control study investigated the use of NIPPV in this population [11]. They found that the NIV group, compared with conventional treatment, had significantly decreased rates of intubation, pneumothoraces, and intensive care unit mortality. While the study was not randomized and the patient population was small, the results are intriguing and suggest that NIV may play a helpful role in acute hypoxemic respiratory failure from PCP.

Since mask discomfort is the leading cause of discontinuation and treatment failure in acute hypoxemic respiratory failure, more comfortable alternatives to the mask could improve NIV treatment. Rocco *et al.* [12] recently studied helmet NIV (Figure 1.5.1) as an alternative to mask NIPPV in immunocompromised patients with acute hypoxemic respiratory failure. They report significantly improved NIV

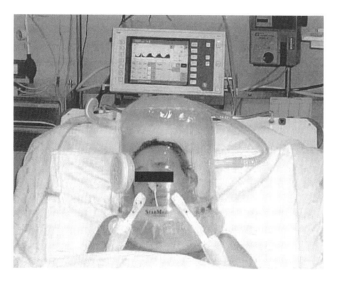

Figure 1.5.1   The helmet device for use with NIPPV as an alternative to mask ventilation. (Reproduced with permission [12].)

tolerance and fewer discontinuations in the group treated with helmet NIV. They also found significantly fewer mechanical complications (mostly due to decreased rate of skin necrosis) in the group treated with helmet NIV. In addition, they found improved oxygenation when treated by helmet. Because the study was small and designed as a case control, further research is needed. However, the use of the helmet is intriguing and should be considered in the immunosuppressed population if available.

In summary, there are significant data to suggest that noninvasive ventilation offers superior results compared with traditional treatment of acute respiratory failure in immunocompromised patients. This includes patients with neutropenia following chemotherapy, patients on immunosuppressive medications following solid organ transplantation, and patients with AIDS and PCP. While the studies that led to this conclusion all used the oronasal mask for NIV, this patient population may benefit further from use of the helmet device, although further research is needed to confirm this statement.

1.5.5   NIV during bronchoscopy

One potential limitation to treating immunosuppressed patients with noninvasive ventilation is the need for bronchoscopy. Bronchoscopy is commonly used to help tailor antibiotics and antifungals in this patient population. It is also valuable to assess for diffuse alveolar hemorrhage, a common cause of respiratory failure following chemotherapy and a relative contra-indication to oronasal mask use.

Traditionally, severely hypoxemic patients are intubated prior to bronchoscopy. This allows a controlled environment during the procedure and is felt to reduce complications of the procedure.

One study assessed the ability to use NIV in this patient population [13]. Patients were placed on NIV-PS during bronchoscopy if they had severe hypoxemic respiratory failure with known immunosuppression, a pH greater than 7.35, and improved oxygen saturation using NIV in a 15 minute trial prior to bronchoscopy. The authors did not have to intubate any of these patients. While limited in patient volume, this study suggests that NIV can be used to avoid intubation in hypoxemic immunosuppressed patients. It should be noted that NIV would not be appropriate in patients with a recent history of hemoptysis or suspected diffuse alveolar hemorrhage (DAH). Similarly, if DAH is found during bronchoscopy, endotracheal intubation would be appropriate.

1.5.6   Respiratory failure after lung resection

Pneumonectomy is traditionally associated with 30-day mortality rates of 11.5%, while lobectomy has 4% 30-day mortality [14]. Complications of post-operative reintubation (bronchopleural fistula, persistent air leak, and pulmonary infection) are a major reason for the high mortality rate [15]. Two studies have confirmed a role for NIV in patients with acute respiratory failure following lung resection. Firstly, it was shown that NIV leads to improved arterial oxygenation compared with conventional supplemental oxygen, and that this improvement is sustained following the discontinuation of NIV [16]. Subsequently, Auriant *et al.* [17] found a decreased rate of invasive ventilation and improved survival with NIV compared with conventional treatment using supplemental oxygen. Therefore, NIV should be considered in patients with respiratory failure following lung resection.

1.5.7   Cystic fibrosis patients with acute respiratory failure

Patients with cystic fibrosis (CF) and acute respiratory failure have poor outcomes when treated with invasive mechanical ventilation, and it is felt that intubation should be a last resort [18]. Significant complications that result from invasive ventilation in CF patients include bacteremia and sepsis, ventilator acquired pneumonia, and pneumothorax [19]. Because NIV has been proven to decrease these complications of invasive ventilation in other patient populations, it is promising for cystic fibrosis. However, the pathophysiology is very different compared with other lung diseases, so it is not safe to extrapolate data to the CF population. In the United States, the lung transplant allocation system has recently changed the waiting list from a time-based system to a disease severity-based system. This may have important implications for the use of NIV in CF patients. Traditionally, CF patients with acute respiratory failure who were bridged to transplantation with invasive or noninvasive ventilation required long periods of mechanical ventilation prior to transplantation. Under the new system, this time period may be reduced, as these patients would have very high lung allocation scores.

Intuitively, it would be assumed that NIV would decrease intubation rates, ventilator pneumonia rates, and barotraumas rates compared with conventional mechanical ventilation. However, few studies have looked at the use of NIV in acute hypoxemic respiratory failure in patients with cystic fibrosis. The best of these studies showed that NIV significantly improved hypoxemia compared to conventional oxygen therapy. In this study, under the old allocation system, 23 of 65 patients with cystic fibrosis and respiratory failure were able to be bridged to lung transplantation [19].

Therefore, NIV may be reasonable in patients who have acute hypoxemic respiratory failure from cystic fibrosis and have already been listed for lung transplantation. It is unclear how the new lung allocation system will affect the use of NIV in this population in the United States.

1.5.8   NIV in early ARDS

Acute respiratory distress syndrome (ARDS) describes the impairment from diffuse pulmonary inflammation and breakdown of the barrier and gas exchange functions of the lung resulting from a myriad of causes. It is clinically defined as radiographic presence of bilateral alveolar infiltrates with profound hypoxemia (P:F < 200) in the absence of left sided heart dysfunction. Acute lung injury (ALI) is a less severe form of the syndrome and is characterized by a P:F between 200 and 300. Advances in invasive mechanical ventilation have led to significant improvement in patient survival from ARDS [20]. Today, the acceptable mortality from ARDS is considered to be 40% or less [20]. Because ALI/ARDS represents the most severe form of hypoxemic respiratory failure, NIV has only recently been studied in this patient population.

Initial publications investigating the feasibility of NIV in ARDS were small case series of nine patients [21] and seven patients [22]. These series found that endotracheal intubation was avoided in 6/9 and 1/7 patients, respectively. Recently, a large cohort study has provided further insight into the feasibility of using NIV in ARDS. Antonelli and colleagues [23] followed 479 patients with ARDS requiring transfer to ICU. The majority (332 patients) required intubation on or before transfer. Of the remaining 147 patients, intubation was avoided using NIV in 79 patients (54%). Factors associated with an increased probability of requiring intubation at baseline included old age, high positive end-expiratory pressure (PEEP) requirement on NIV, or high pressure support requirement on NIV. At the initiation of NIV, a high (>34) Simplified Acute Physiologic Score (SAPS) II indicated a high probability of requiring intubation. After one hour of NIV, having a $PaO_2:FiO_2 < 175$ indicated a high probability of requiring intubation. (Figure 1.5.2) Not surprisingly, in those who avoided intubation, the incidence of pneumonia (2% vs. 20%) was improved

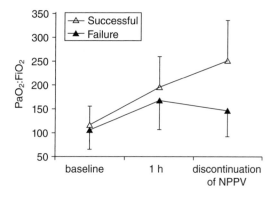

Figure 1.5.2   After one hour of NIV, there was a significant difference (*) in oxygenation between NIV responders and NIV nonresponders. This difference was enhanced at the discontinuation of NIV. (Reproduced with permission [23].)

and ICU mortality was improved. Patients maintained on NIPPV required treatment for an average of 48 h, and most patients received NIPPV via the helmet interface in this study. This study indicated that ARDS remains a disorder which primarily requires invasive mechanical ventilation (the group that was treated successfully with NIV represented 17% of the initial cohort). Using the SAPS II on initial assessment is reasonable, as this will help to avoid treating patients with concurrent sepsis or multi-organ failure with NIV. If NIV is attempted, it is necessary to reassess the patient after one hour. If their $PaO_2:FiO_2$ has not improved, then mechanical ventilation is appropriate. It should also be noted that the majority of treatment failures in this group occurred between 12 and 48 h of NIV [24], indicating that these patients require close observation in an intensive care unit if treated with NIV.

Specific guidelines for starting NIV in patients with ARDS do not exist. However, one physiologic study [25] suggests that NIV-PS is likely superior to NIV-CPAP. In this study, NIV-CPAP was able to increase oxygenation independently, but it was not able to decrease the work of breathing (as determined by neuromuscular drive and inspiratory muscle effort). In addition, dyspnea scores were much improved with NIV-PS compared with NIV-CPAP. Also, NIV-PS has been used in the previously mentioned studies [21–23] using NIPPV in patients with ARDS. Therefore, if NIV is started in a patient with ARDS, using NIV-PS is recommended.

1.5.9   NIV to provide pre-oxygenation before endotracheal intubation

Respiratory failure is very common in the intensive care unit and frequently requires endotracheal intubation. Intubations in the intensive care unit are associated with increased risk [26], including the common occurrence of hypoxemia [27]. Moreover, hypoxemia during intubation has been associated with increased mortality [28, 29]. This led Baillard and colleagues [30] to propose incorporating NIV into the technique of pre-oxygenation, hoping that the safe duration of apnea during intubation would be prolonged and complications would be reduced. In this study, patients randomized to the NIV group received three minutes of pre-oxygenation with NIV-PS at settings of 100% FiO_2, PEEP of 5 cm H_2O, and pressure support to maintain tidal volume of 700–1000 ml. They found that, compared with three minutes of traditional pre-oxygenation, the NIV group had higher oxygen saturation levels at the end of pre-oxygenation. In addition, the number of significant desaturations (less than 80%) was significantly reduced in the NIV group (7%) compared with the conventional pre-oxygenation group (46%). Therefore, in patients in the intensive care unit requiring intubation for hypoxemic respiratory failure, pre-oxygenation using NIV is a valid clinical practice when carried out by an experienced team of clinicians.

1.5.10   Interface selection in acute respiratory failure

As mentioned in the introductory chapter, patients with acute respiratory failure are usually mouth breathers. Patients treated with a nasal mask will usually have a large air leak and less effective ventilation. A recent study showed that 75% of patients in acute respiratory failure who were treated with a nasal mask required transition to an oronasal mask [31]. Therefore, continuous use of the oronasal mask is the standard of care in a patient with acute respiratory failure.

It must be emphasized that close monitoring of patients in acute respiratory failure on NIV is needed. Trials of NIV in acute respiratory failure repeatedly show that patient discomfort is the most common reason for discontinuation of NIV and progression to intubation [31, 32]. Once a patient has shown improvement in physiologic parameters and feels subjective improvement in dyspnea, attempts should be made to use NIV intermittently (instead of continuously). This decreases the chance for skin ulceration and permits intake of food and drink, which will increase patient tolerance. Alternatively, as the patient improves, a nasal mask can be attempted. This will also allow for eating/drinking, talking, and improved tolerance.

1.5.11   Summary

This chapter shows the large impact that NIV has had on the treatment of acute respiratory failure. While the best evidence remains in those patients who have CHF or COPD and acute respiratory failure, a variety of other conditions now have compelling evidence as above. This has led to the recommendation of NIV in patients with acute respiratory failure in clinical practice guidelines (Table 1.5.1) [33, 34]. Clinically, it is not uncommon to treat patients with status asthmaticus,

Table 1.5.1 Recommendations for use of NIV in varying forms of acute respiratory failure.

Underlying disease	Recommendation	Grade of recommendation	Considerations
Immunosuppressed	Use NIV-PS. Decreases incidence of ventilator associated PNA	Strong	Consider the role of bronchoscopy in the patient's care before deciding whether to pursue NIV
Status asthmaticus	Use in patient with accessory use or acidosis without altered mentation	Moderate (little clinical evidence but common clinical practice)	Heliox and nebulizer treatments can be administered via mask
Early ARDS	Continue trial of NIV only if PaO_2:FiO_2 improves after first hour of use	Moderate	Close observation is demanded, as failure rate of NIV is high.
Post pneumonectomy	NIV-PS decreases the rate of intubation	Moderate	
Pre-oxygenation before endotracheal intubation	Decreases hypoxemic events compared with conventional pre-oxygenation	Moderate	Assess for relative contra-indications (facial hair, etc.) before trying. Always have bag-valve mask ready as back up.
Cystic fibrosis	Use NIV-PS. Decreases incidence of VAP	Weak	May help to "bridge" patients to lung transplant, especially under the new lung allocation system

immunosuppression, cystic fibrosis, early ARDS, or following pneumonectomy with NIV. While the clinical evidence is not overwhelming, there is rationale for using NIV in each of these situations as described above. In addition, new evidence supports the use for using NIV as a method of pre-oxygenation before intubation. While this is not yet the standard in most intensive care units, this evidence may soon change the practice of intubation.

1.5.12 Case presentation revisited

The case describes an immunosuppressed patient with bilateral pulmonary infiltrates and acute respiratory failure. As mentioned above, studies have shown that using NIV in this population improves mortality, decreases the length of stay in the intensive care unit, and decreases the incidence of pneumonia and sepsis. Therefore, if this patient can tolerate NIV, it would be recommended. As with any patient who has acute respiratory failure and is using NIV, close observation in an intensive care unit is recommended. Using NIV-PS is recommended, as this is the mode used by Hilbert and colleagues, and NIV-PS should decrease the work of breathing over NIV-CPAP. After starting out at low settings (10 cm H_2O pressure support and 5 cm H_2O PEEP) with an oronasal mask, the settings can be adjusted based on tidal volume (adjust the pressure support for increased volumes), oxygenation (increase PEEP as needed to improve oxygenation, generally not to exceed 12 cm H_2O), and patient comfort and tolerance. The patient should also be closely monitored to determine when continuous NIV can be stopped, when intermittent NIV can be started, and when transition from oronasal mask to nasal mask can be considered.

In this patient, our comfort with using NIV is enhanced by knowing that bronchoscopy has already been performed. It is important to know that diffuse alveolar hemorrhage (DAH) is not the etiology of this respiratory failure, as DAH would be in the differential and would be a relative contra-indication to oronasal mask use. In addition, while bronchoscopy can be performed using NIV in hypoxemic immunosuppressed patients, many centers still prefer endotracheal intubation during bronchoscopy in this population.

References

1. Liesching, T. (2003) Acute applications of noninvasive positive pressure ventilation. *Chest*, **124**, 699–713.
2. Gehlbach, B. *et al.* (2002) Correlates of prolonged hospitalization in inner-city ICU patients receiving noninvasive and invasive positive pressure ventilation in status asthmaticus. *Chest*, **122**, 1709–1714.
3. Leatherman, J.W. *et al.* (1996) Muscle weakness in mechanically ventilated patients with severe asthma. *Am. J. Respir. Crit. Care Med.*, **153**, 1686–1690.
4. Fernandez, M.M. *et al.* (2001) Noninvasive mechanical ventilation in status asthmaticus. *Intensive Care Med.*, **27** (3), 486.
5. Meduri, G.U. *et al.* (1996) Noninvasive positive pressure ventilation in status asthmaticus. *Chest*, **110**, 767–774.
6. Blot, F. *et al.* (1997) Prognostic factors for neutropenic patients in an intensive care unit: respective roles of underlying malignancies and acute organ failure. *Eur. J. Cancer*, **33**, 1031–1037.
7. Antonelli, M. *et al.* (1998) A comparison of noninvasive positive-pressure ventilation and conventional mechanical ventilation in patients with acute respiratory failure. *N. Engl. J. Med.*, **339**, 429–435.
8. Hilbert, G. *et al.* (2001) Noninvasive ventilation in immunosuppressed patients with pulmonary infiltrates, fever, and acute respiratory failure. *N. Engl. J. Med.*, **344**, 481–487.
9. Mermel, L.A. *et al.* (1990) Bacterial pneumonia in solid organ transplantation. *Semin. Respir. Infect.*, **5**, 10–29.

10. Antonelli, M. (2000) Noninvasive ventilation for treatment of acute respiratory failure in patients undergoing solid organ transplantation. *JAMA*, **283**, 235–241.

11. Confalonieri, M. *et al.* (2002) Noninvasive ventilation for treating acute respiratory failure in AIDS patients with pneumocystis carinii pneumonia. *Intensive Care Med.*, **28** (9), 1233–1238.

12. Rocco, M. *et al.* (2004) Noninvasive ventilation by helmet or face mask in immunocompromised patients: a case-control study. *Chest*, **126** (5), 1508–1515.

13. Antonelli, M. *et al.* (1996) Noninvasive positive-pressure ventilation via face mask during bronchoscopy with BAL in high-risk hypoxemic patients. *Chest*, **110**, 724–728.

14. Harpole, D.H. (1999) Prognostic models of thirty-day mortality and morbidity after major pulmonary resection. *J. Thorac. Cardiovasc. Surg.*, **117**, 969–979.

15. Harpole, D. (1996) Prospective analysis of pneumonectomy: risk factors for major morbidity and cardiac dysrhythmias. *Ann. Thorac. Surg.*, **61**, 977–982.

16. Aguilo, R. (1997) Noninvasive ventilatory support after lung resectional surgery. *Chest*, **112**, 117–121.

17. Auriant, I. *et al.* (2001) Noninvasive ventilation reduces mortality in acute respiratory failure following lung resection. *Am. J. Respir. Crit. Care Med.*, **164**, 1231–1235.

18. Texereau, J. *et al.* (2006) Determinants of mortality for adults with cystic fibrosis admitted in the intensive care unit: a multicenter study. *Respir. Res.*, **7**, 14.

19. Madden, B.P. (2002) Noninvasive ventilation in cystic fibrosis patients with acute or chronic respiratory failure. *Eur. Respir. J.*, **19**, 310–313.

20. Brower, R. *et al.* (2000) Ventilation with lower tidal volumes as compared with traditional tidal volumes for acute lung injury and the acute respiratory distress syndrome. *N. Engl. J. Med.*, **342**, 1301–1308.

21. Rocker, G.M. *et al.* (1999) Noninvasive positive pressure ventilation: successful outcome in patients with acute lung injury/ARDS. *Chest*, **115**, 173–177.

22. Ferrer, M. *et al.* (2003) Noninvasive ventilation in severe hypoxemic respiratory failure. *Am. J. Respir. Crit. Care Med.*, **168**, 1438–1444.

23. Antonelli, M. *et al.* (2007) A multiple-center survey on the use in clinical practice of noninvasive ventilation as a first-line intervention for acute respiratory distress syndrome. *Crit. Care Med.*, **35** (1), 18–25.

24. Garpestad, E. *et al.* (2007) Noninvasive ventilation for acute respiratory distress syndrome: breaking down the final frontier? *Crit. Care Med.*, **35** (1), 288–290.

25. L'Her, E. *et al.* (2005) Physiologic effects of noninvasive ventilation during acute lung injury. *Am. J. Respir. Crit. Care Med.*, **172**, 1112–1118.

26. Schwartz, D.E. *et al.* (1995) Death and other complications of emergency airway management in critically ill adults. *Anesthesiology*, **82**, 367–376.

27. Mort, T. *et al.* (2004) Emergency tracheal intubation: complications associated with repeated laryngoscopic attempts. *Anesth. Analg.*, **99**, 607–613.

28. Davis, D. *et al.* (2004) The impact of hypoxia and hyperventilation on outcome after paramedic rapid sequence intubation of severely head injured patients. *J. Trauma*, **57**, 1–8.

29. Davis, D. *et al.* (2003) The effect of paramedic rapid sequence intubation on outcome in patients with severe traumatic brain injury. *J. Trauma*, **54**, 444–453.

30. Baillard, C. *et al.* (2006) Noninvasive ventilation improves preoxygenation before intubation of hypoxic patients. *Am. J. Respir. Crit. Care Med.*, **174**, 171–177.

31. Girault, C. *et al.* (2009) Interface strategy during noninvasive positive pressure ventilation for hypercapnic acute respiratory failure. *Crit. Care Med.*, **37**, 124–131.

32. Carlucci, A. *et al.* (2001) Noninvasive Versus Conventional Mechanical Ventilation An Epidemiologic Survey. *Am. J. Respir. Crit. Care Med.*, **163** (4), 874–880.

33. British Thoracic Society Standards of Care Committee (2002) Non-invasive ventilation in acute respiratory failure. *Thorax*, **57**, 192–211.
34. American Thoracic Society (2001) International Consensus Conferences in Intensive Care Medicine: noninvasive positive pressure ventilation in acute respiratory failure. *Am. J. Respir. Crit. Care Med.*, **163**, 283–291.

1.6 Noninvasive ventilation in chronic respiratory failure associated with COPD

Daniel C. Grinnan[1] and Jonathon D. Truwit[2]

[1] *Division of Pulmonary and Critical Care Medicine, Virginia Commonwealth University, Richmond, VA, USA*
[2] *Division of Pulmonary and Critical Care Medicine, University of Virginia, Charlottesville, VA, USA*

1.6.1 Case presentation

A 58-year-old presents to your office with complaints of extreme dyspnea. Over the past 10 years, he has noticed slow progression of his dyspnea. At present, he is unable to ambulate in large stores or walk around his neighborhood. He cannot climb a flight of stairs without stopping. He has been hospitalized on three occasions in the past year for extreme dyspnea, each time responding to a gradual steroid taper and bronchodilator treatment. Pulmonary function testing reveals an obstructive pattern with FEV1 of 30% predicted, residual volume of 150% predicted, and a low diffusion capacity. An arterial blood gas reveals pH = 7.36, $PaCO_2$ = 61 mm Hg, and PaO_2 = 68 mm Hg. A chest X-ray is consistent with emphysema. He quit smoking two years ago, but he has a 60 pack year history. He is on appropriate inhaled medications. Examination reveals a thin man with body mass index (BMI) of 21, mild accessory muscle use, "barrel chest" appearance, and significantly diminished breath sounds. You are asked to evaluate for "any further treatment of advanced emphysema." What are your recommendations?

A Practical Guide to Mechanical Ventilation, First Edition.
Edited by Jonathon D. Truwit and Scott K. Epstein.
© 2011 John Wiley & Sons, Ltd. Published 2011 by John Wiley & Sons, Ltd.

1.6.2   Introduction

As chronic obstructive pulmonary disease (COPD) progresses, chronic hypercapnic respiratory failure can develop. As the diaphragm flattens and the zone of apposition is decreased, the accessory muscles are forced to participate in respiration. Since the accessory muscles are partially paralyzed during sleep, patients with stable COPD often have nocturnal desaturations, fragmented sleep, and decreased quality of life [1]. As COPD becomes severe, respiratory muscle fatigue can develop and lead to acute exacerbations. As discussed, noninvasive ventilation (NIV) is an effective therapy for the treatment of acute COPD exacerbations. In patients with chronic hypercapnic COPD, continuous supplemental oxygen has been shown to confer a survival advantage [2]. Therefore, it might be assumed that using NIV in patients with severe COPD and stable hypercapnia would be beneficial. Theoretically, NIV should assist with inspiration and decrease the work of breathing, which should lead to improvement in both physiologic parameters (hypercapnia, hypoxemia, number of nocturnal desaturations) and clinical parameters (number of exacerbations, number of hospitalizations, and patient survival). Recent clinical studies provide the strongest support for the use of NIV in chronic hypercapnic COPD, but significant improvement has yet to be proven for several of the above physiologic and clinical parameters.

1.6.3   Physiologic data of NIV in chronic hypercapnic COPD

Many investigators have been eager to show that noctural NIV improves the physiology of patients with severe hypercapnic COPD. Typically, the studies performed have been small, single center, non-randomized trials. The methodology has changed significantly in these trials over the past several years. Until 2005, most studies utilized a relatively low level of inspiratory positive airway pressure (IPAP) with NIV. Subsequently, studies have focused on using high levels of IPAP, usually over 20 cm H_2O. In this chapter, the era of low IPAP is referred to as "pre-intensive NIV," and the recent era of high IPAP as "intensive NIV."

In the pre-intensive NIV era, physiologic assessment yielded very mixed results. Some studies found that NIV in chronic hypercapnic COPD led to improvements in gas exchange [3, 4], lung volumes [3], lung hyperinflation [3], work of breathing [4], polycythemia [5], and COPD cachexia [6]. However, others found no change in sleep fragmentation, nighttime arousals, or gas exchange [7]. In addition, a small meta analysis of four small studies did not find any improvement in gas exchange, pulmonary function, or sleep efficiency with NIV [8].

In 2005, Windisch et al. [9] performed a retrospective analysis of 34 patients with hypercapnic respiratory failure from COPD. They used very high IPAP settings, averaging 28 cm H_2O, which were previously reported to be tolerated in this population [10]. With these settings, they found a decrease in $PaCO_2$ from 53 mm Hg to 46 mm Hg, and an increase in PaO_2 from 51 mm Hg to 57 mm Hg.

In 2007, a meta-analysis of existing trials on the use of NIV in chronic, stable COPD was performed [11]. The authors included studies from the "pre-intensive" and the "post-intensive" era. Six randomized controlled trials and nine non-randomized controlled trials were included (each non-randomized controlled trial had under 20 patients). As the use of NIV was not consistent between trials, it is not surprising that no difference was found in gas exchange as the primary outcome. However, subgroup analysis showed that trials enrolling patients with severe COPD (FEV1 < 30%) and chronic carbon dioxide retention were likely to have improvement in gas exchange. In addition, further analysis found that patients treated with an IPAP > EPAP (expiratory positive airway pressure) by over 15 cm H_2O had a significant reduction of carbon dioxide and residual volume. Therefore, both the degree of hypercapnic respiratory failure and the IPAP to EPAP gradient may be important determinants of whether gas exchange will and pulmonary function will be improved with NIV.

A recent small, randomized, controlled study looked at heart rate variability and natriuretic peptide measurements in patients with severe hypercapnic COPD [12]. In this "intensive NIV" study, patients had an IPAP goal of 20 cm H_2O and an EPAP of 4 cm H_2O. It has long been known that patients with COPD are prone to atrial arrhythmias, especially multifocal atrial tachycardia (MAT). The authors found a significant reduction in heart rate variability (as assessed by Holter monitoring) in the NIV group compared with the conventional therapy group. In addition, the authors found a significant reduction in ANP (and a strong trend in BNP) levels in the NIV group (Figure 1.6.1). While causality cannot be inferred, it raises the hypothesis that decreased work of breathing and afterload reduction created by nocturnal NIV leads to reduced cardiac stress (as reflected by ANP levels), which in turn may lead to a decrease in nocturnal arrhythmias. This small study also found that exertional capacity, as assessed by the six minute walk, is improved in those

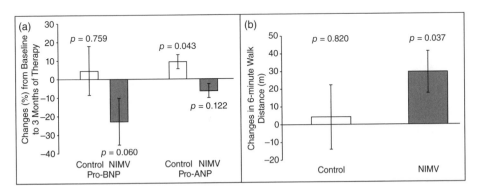

Figure 1.6.1   Changes in (a) daytime plasma natriuretic levels and (b) six minute walk distance in patients with chronic hypercapnic COPD treated with and without NIV over a three-month period [12].

patients with severe COPD on NIV compared with conventional therapy. While interesting and hypothesis generating, there was a significant difference in FEV1 between NIV and conventional group that could influence the results.

1.6.4 Clinical data of NIV in chronic hypercapnic COPD

In the pre-intensive era, there were two large, prospective, randomized controlled trials that have looked at the effect of NIV in COPD. In 2000, Casanova and colleagues [13] followed 52 patients for one year after they were randomized to either NIV plus oxygen or long-term oxygen alone. While they found improvements in the Borg dyspnea scale in patients using NIV, they did not find improvements in gas exchange, hospitalizations, exacerbations, or survival. In 2002, Clini and colleagues [14] performed a multicenter study and followed 90 patients with hypercapnic ventilatory failure from COPD for two years. They found significant improvements in the level of hypercapnia, the resting dyspnea score, and the health care quality of life score in those on NIV compared with those receiving oxygen alone. However, they did not find improvements in survival, hospital admissions, exacerbations, sleep quality, or exercise tolerance. It is important to mention potential limitations of these studies. Firstly, they may not have had enough power to detect differences in survival and hospitalizations. For example, in the Casanova study, 11% of the patients in the NIV arm used NIV for less than three hours a day, significantly reducing the ability to detect a difference in survival with NIV (although lack of adherence with NIV is an important reality). Secondly, the NIV settings were reflective of the pre-intensive era. In the Casanova study, the IPAP to EPAP gradient was 8 cm H_2O on average, while the gradient was 12 cm H_2O on average in the Clini study.

A recent prospective observational study [15] compared patients with chronic hypercapnic respiratory failure from COPD who used NIV (91) versus those who did not use NIV (41). In this study, all patients were offered NIV. Some were able to tolerate NIV and use it long term (the experimental group), while others either declined NIV or were unable to tolerate (the control group). In this intensive NIV study, the average IPAP was 21 mm Hg, while the average EPAP was 5 mm Hg. In this study, the authors found a very significant improvement in survival in the NIV group compared with group receiving standard medical treatment (Figure 1.6.2), even after stratification for risk factors. Patients in this study had extensive obstructive lung disease, with an average FEV1 of 29% predicted and an average $PaCO_2$ of 60 mm Hg. While this study provides some room for optimism regarding the clinical role of NIV in chronic hypercapnic COPD, there are several limitations. Firstly, it is difficult for many to tolerate the high IPAP that was required to achieve the perceived survival benefit. Secondly, those that were adherent with NIV (the experimental group) may have also been more adherent with other therapies, such as continuous oxygen use. Therefore, while this study is hypothesis generating, there still is not strong evidence that NIV in chronic hypercapnic COPD prevents

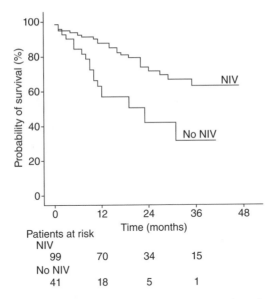

Figure 1.6.2 Kaplan–Meier survival curves from the prospective observational study by Budweiser *et al.* [15], showing an improved survival in the NIV cohort.

hospitalizations or prolongs survival. Clearly the next step in studying the effects of intensive NIV is to perform a large, prospective, randomized study.

Despite the conflicting clinical evidence provided above, NIV has become widespread in the treatment of patients with chronic hypercapnic respiratory failure from COPD. COPD remains the most common use of long-term NIV besides obstructive sleep apnea, in large part as a result of the high prevalence of COPD [16]. At present, in the United States, NIV is approved by Medicare for patients with severe COPD if they have daytime hypercapnia to a level of 52 mm Hg or greater, and they have hypoxemia at night to a saturation of less than 88% for five consecutive minutes while wearing supplemental oxygen. In an effort to better understand the outcomes of patients using long-term NIV in COPD, Budweiser *et al.* [17] recently looked at predictors of mortality in 188 patients. The authors followed spirometry, nutritional status, lung volumes, complete blood counts, serum CRP, gender, exacerbations, age, and blood gas analysis in this cohort of patients. The analysis revealed that only nutritional status (BMI < 25 kg/m^2), hyperinflation (RV/TLC > 73%), and base excess (>9 mmol/l) were predictive of increased mortality. As NIV likely impacts both daytime hyperinflation and base excess, the authors concluded that the use of NIV, together with nutritional consultation and pulmonary rehabilitation, is likely to have clinically meaningful results in chronic, stable COPD. One interesting finding from this study is the predictive value of base excess, but not carbon dioxide, in this cohort. The authors concluded that base excess gives a more representative value of ventilation over time, whereas carbon dioxide is a "snapshot" of ventilation. Therefore, base excess may give a more reliable indication of nocturnal ventilation compared with daytime carbon dioxide measurements.

1.6.5 Daytime NIV in chronic hypercapnic COPD

While looking mostly at physiologic end points rather than clinical outcomes, several small studies have assessed intermittent daytime NIV in patients with hypercapnic COPD. One study found that, after using NIV for three hours a day for three weeks, there was significant improvement in hypercapnia, FEV1, dyspnea, and six minute walk with a reduction in the residual volume [18]. Another study found improvements in the shuttle walk, oxygenation, and the patient assessments of health when NIV was used for at least eight hours a day [19]. However, it should be noted that the routine daytime use of NIV requires significant patient effort and could limit their activities. Before adopting daytime NIV into clinical practice, studies confirming the above findings for a longer duration of time (years) and studies assessing the quality of life with daytime NIV are needed. In addition, it would be useful to know if daytime NIV has any impact on important clinical variables like the number of exacerbations, hospitalizations, and patient survival.

1.6.6 Summary

Definitive studies are lacking to prove a benefit in physiologic and clinical parameters from the use of NIV in chronic hypercapnic COPD. However, recent studies suggest that an IPAP to EPAP gradient of greater than 15 cm H_2O may assist this cohort of patients. In addition, these studies suggest that patients with more severe hypercapnic respiratory failure (FEV1 < 30% predicted and $PaCO_2$ > 55 mm Hg) may receive the most benefit from NIV. Quality of life appears to improve with the use of NIV, and recent studies suggest that markers of cardiac strain (ANP and BNP) and chronic markers of ventilation (base excess) may be improved with NIV. The recent use of intensive NIV in small trials has yielded positive results, and it will be important to continue evaluation of this strategy in large, prospective, randomized trials.

At present, in the United States, nocturnal NIV is approved by Medicare for patients with severe COPD if they have daytime hypercapnia to a level of 52 mm Hg or greater, and they have hypoxemia at night to a saturation of less than 88% for five consecutive minutes while wearing supplemental oxygen. it is agreed that patients with nocturnal abnormalities of gas exchange on supplemental oxygen would be most likely to benefit. If a patient with chronic hypercapnia from COPD is started on NIV, they should be seen in the office within two months to reassess their quality of life and gas exchange since starting NIV. If these parameters are not improved, then NIV should be stopped.

The use of daytime NIV in chronic hypercapnic COPD has yet to be determined. While small studies suggest an improvement in physiologic parameters, it will be important to determine whether or not this time consuming and potentially difficult intervention results in improved quality of life.

1.6.7 Case presentation discussion

Given his significant hypercapnia and severe obstruction, NIV should be discussed as a treatment option. The patient would be likely to have improved quality of life and decreased daytime dyspnea. If he is able to tolerate high IPAP settings of 20 cm H_2O or greater (which many patients cannot), then using NIV may decrease the chance of arrhythmias, improve associated heart failure, improve gas exchange, and may even prolong his life. As with other chronic uses of NIV, a nasal interface would be recommended. In this patient, given his low BMI, consideration should also be given to a nutritional consult, as an increase in his BMI may be beneficial. Lastly, as this patient has developed severe obstruction at a relatively young age, consideration should be given to transplant evaluation, as well as testing for alpha-1 antitrypsin deficiency.

References

1. McNicholas, W.T. (1997) Impact of sleep on respiratory failure. *Eur. Respir. J.*, **10**, 920–933.
2. Nocturnal Oxygen Therapy Trial Group (1980) Continuous or nocturnal oxygen therapy in hypoxemic chronic obstructive lung disease: a clinical trial. *Ann. Intern. Med.*, **93** (3), 391–398.
3. Diaz, O. *et al.* (2002) Effects of noninvasive ventilation on lung hyperinflation in stable hypercapnic COPD. *Eur. Respir. J.*, **20**, 1490–1498.
4. Vitacca, M. *et al.* (2000) The appropriate setting of noninvasive pressure support ventilation in stable COPD patients. *Chest*, **118**, 1286–1293.
5. Sivasothy, P. *et al.* (1998) Mask intermittent positive pressure ventilation in chronic hypercapnic respiratory failure due to chronic obstructive pulmonary disease. *Eur. Respir. J.*, **11**, 34–40.
6. Budweiser, S. *et al.* (2006) Weight gain in cachectic COPD patients receiving noninvasive positive-pressure ventilation. *Respir. Care*, **51** (2), 126–132.
7. Krachman, S.L. *et al.* (1997) Effects of noninvasive positive pressure ventilation on gas exchange and sleep in COPD patients. *Chest*, **112**, 623–628.
8. Wijkstra, P.J. *et al.* (2003) A meta-analysis of nocturnal noninvasive positive pressure ventilation in patients with stable COPD. *Chest*, **124**, 337–343.
9. Windisch, W. *et al.* (2005) Outcome of patients with stable COPD receiving controlled noninvasive positive pressure ventilation aimed at a maximal reduction of $PaCO_2$. *Chest*, **128**, 657–662.
10. Windisch, W. *et al.* (2002) Normocapnia during NIPPV in chronic hypercapnic COPD reduces subsequent spontaneous $PaCO_2$. *Respir. Med.*, **96**, 572–579.

11. Kolodziej, M.A. *et al.* (2007) Systematic review of noninvasive positive pressure ventilation in severe stable COPD. *Eur. Respir. J.*, **30** (2), 293–306.
12. Sin, D.D. *et al.* (2007) Effects of nocturnal noninvasive mechanical ventilation on heart rate variability of patients with advanced COPD. *Chest*, **131**, 156–163.
13. Casanova, C. *et al.* (2000) Long-term controlled trial of nocturnal nasal positive pressure ventilation in patients with severe COPD. *Chest*, **118**, 1582–1590.
14. Clini, E. *et al.* (2002) The Italian multicentre study on noninvasive ventilation in COPD patients. *Eur. Respir. J.*, **20**, 529–538.
15. Budweiser, S. *et al.* (2007) Impact of noninvasive home ventilation on long-term survival in chronic hypercapneic COPD: a prospective observational study. *Int. J. Clin. Pract.*, **61** (9), 1516–1522.
16. Jansenns, J.-P. *et al.* (2003) Changing patterns in long-term noninvasive ventilation: a 7 year prospective study in the Geneva Lake area. *Chest*, **123**, 67–79.
17. Budweiser, S. *et al.* (2007) Predictors of survival in COPD patients with chronic hypercapnic respiratory failure receiving noninvasive home ventilation. *Chest*, **131**, 1650–1658.
18. Diaz, O. *et al.* (2005) Physiological and clinical effects of diurnal noninvasive ventilation in hypercapnic COPD. *Eur. Respir. J.*, **26**, 1016–1023.
19. Garrod, R. *et al.* (2000) Randomized controlled trial of domiciliary noninvasive positive pressure ventilation and physical training in severe chronic obstructive pulmonary disease. *Am. J. Respir. Crit. Care Med.*, **162**, 1335–1341.

1.7 Noninvasive ventilation in chronic respiratory disease

Daniel C. Grinnan[1] and Jonathon D. Truwit[2]

[1] *Division of Pulmonary and Critical Care Medicine, Virginia Commonwealth University, Richmond, VA, USA*
[2] *Division of Pulmonary and Critical Care Medicine, University of Virginia, Charlottesville, VA, USA*

1.7.1 Case presentation

A 22-year-old male with Duchenne's muscular dystrophy presents to your office for further management of shortness of breath. He states that he has had progressive daytime shortness of breath over the past six months. In addition, he has developed morning headaches and daytime somnolence. During the day he is active and utilizes electronic hand controls. He speaks clearly and does not report any difficulty with secretions. His examination is significant for upper extremity contractures, mild scoliosis, clear lungs and a normal cardiac exam. His oxygen saturation is 95% at rest. He just saw his neurologist, who was concerned about his symptoms and ordered an overnight polysomnography study. How should you manage this patient?

1.7.2 Introduction

The long-term use of noninvasive positive pressure ventilation (NIV) has been applied to different patient populations. While NIV is most well studied in its administration to patients with sleep apnea, this review focuses on patients with

A Practical Guide to Mechanical Ventilation, First Edition.
Edited by Jonathon D. Truwit and Scott K. Epstein.
© 2011 John Wiley & Sons, Ltd. Published 2011 by John Wiley & Sons, Ltd.

neuromuscular disease, chronic obstructive pulmonary disease (COPD), and cystic fibrosis. These diseases have very different courses, manifestations, and treatments. Therefore, the role of NIV differs in these populations, and they are discussed separately. In general, good studies are more difficult to perform in patients with chronic respiratory disease than in patients who have acute respiratory failure. Whereas the later group can be studied over a relatively short time, proper studies in the former group take years to complete. While some questions have been answered regarding the use of NIV in patients with chronic respiratory disease, others remain unanswered.

1.7.3   NIV in patients with neuromuscular disorders and skeletal deformity

The conditions that are discussed in this section include skeletal disorders (severe scoliosis or kyphosis), slowly progressive neuromuscular diseases (post-polio syndrome) and the rapidly progressive neuromuscular syndromes (amyotrophic lateral sclerosis (ALS) and Duchenne's muscular dystrophy during teenage years). It should be noted that most of the data for starting NIV in these patient populations come from relatively small case series. Randomized trials in symptomatic patients with chronic respiratory failure are regarded to be unethical, as it would be cruel to withhold the option of mechanical ventilation to the patients in the control arm [1].

In neuromuscular diseases, progressive weakness of the respiratory muscles leads to severe restrictive lung disease. Similarly, severe skeletal disorders lead to progressively impaired lung compliance and severe chest wall restriction. Over time, respiratory impairment progresses to chronic hypercapnic respiratory failure. Because sleep is associated with partial paralysis of the accessory respiratory muscles, hypoxemia and hypercapnia are usually potentiated at night, initially in REM sleep and later in non-REM sleep as well. Therefore, the initial symptoms of chronic hypercapnic failure often mimic those of the obesity hypoventilation syndrome. Patients with neuromuscular disease and hypercapnic respiratory failure often present with daytime somnolence, morning headaches, impaired concentration, and poor sleep.

However, patients with neuromuscular diseases are also susceptible to acute respiratory failure. Acute respiratory failure commonly occurs when bronchitis further compromises already severe lung restriction. Bronchial infections are frequently complicated by mucous plugging and often lead to increased work of breathing and respiratory muscle fatigue. It is important to identify which patients with neuromuscular diseases will be able to protect themselves from mucous plugging and which patients require tracheotomy for frequent suctioning. The former patients may be reasonable candidates for NIV, while the latter patients should be offered tracheotomy and mechanical ventilation. Studies in various neuromuscular diseases have built evidence that the peak cough flow (PCF) can assist with risk stratification for NIV. In patients with a PCF > 160 l/min, acute respiratory failure is unlikely [2, 3]. However, once the peak cough flow is under 160 l/min, patients often have difficulty with mucous plugging and the option of tracheotomy should be pursued. Because the PCF can be done with a peak flow meter, this is a practical test for bedside and home use.

The availability of NIV has provided an alternative to tracheotomy for the treatment of respiratory failure in many patients with neuromuscular diseases. It is usually the preferred treatment of patients who require mechanical ventilation, since it does not require surgery, does not compromise swallowing function, and allows for greater mobility and travel. Usually, NIV is started at night to prevent symptoms of nocturnal hypercapnia. As the disease progresses, NIV is often needed throughout the day to treat symptoms of inadequate gas exchange. Patients on nocturnal NIV generally wear a nasal mask, as this is usually more comfortable than an oronasal mask. The fitting of the mask takes some time to ensure that the right mask is being used and the straps have been adjusted to the proper tension (to avoid excessive air leak and to avoid pressure sores). When a patient requires daytime NIV, a simple mouthpiece is often effective and permits the most freedom for the patient (Figure 1.7.1). If motor control of facial muscles does not permit the simple mouthpiece, then a mouthpiece with lip seal retention can be used (Figure 1.7.1).

In patients with neuromuscular diseases, NIV-PS is the preferred modality, as this decreases the work of breathing considerably over continuous positive airway pressure (CPAP) alone. Moreover, a significant gradient between the inspiratory

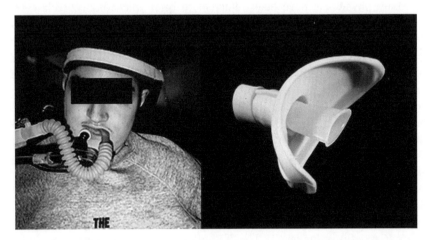

Figure 1.7.1   On the left, a patient uses a simple mouthpiece to deliver NIV for daytime support. On the right, a mouthpiece with lip seal is shown (http://www.uptodate.com/online/content/image.do?imageKey=PULM%2F23854). The lip seal is secured to the patients face with a strap, permitting the patient to use the mouthpiece for daytime NIV use. (Reproduced with permission [34].)

positive airway pressure (IPAP) and the expiratory positive airway pressure (EPAP), called the inspiratory-to-expiratory pressure span, is usually needed to correct symptoms of respiratory failure [4]. When first starting a patient with neuromuscular disease on NIV, it is important to start with comfortable settings. It is standard to begin with an IPAP of 8–12 cm H_2O and an EPAP of 5 cm H_2O [5]. Over time, the IPAP should gradually be increased, increasing the pressure support gradient, until symptoms of hypercapnia have improved or resolved. While it is reasonable to reassess gas exchange parameters after the initiation of NIV, the primary management should be to improve symptoms rather than strictly treating the hypercapnia.

1.7.3.1 Amyotrophic lateral sclerosis (ALS)

Amyotrophic lateral sclerosis is a rapidly progressive neuromuscular disease, with a median survival of 3–5 years from diagnosis [6]. The destruction of motor neurons (and likely cortical neurons) leads to progressive and profound muscular weakness. The resultant weakness usually involves the bulbar and respiratory muscles, in addition to causing limb weakness. Inevitably, as the disease progresses, respiratory muscle weakness leads to hypercapnic respiratory failure. In addition, bulbar muscle weakness can lead to inability to swallow secretions, leading to suffocation. Patients with ALS commonly have respiratory muscle weakness at the time of diagnosis [7]. The vast majority (>80%) of patients with ALS die from respiratory failure due to respiratory muscle fatigue [8].

Prior to noninvasive mechanical ventilation, patients with ALS were given the option of tracheotomy with mechanical ventilation to defer life-prolonging measures. Many physicians have been reluctant to offer tracheotomy, feeling that it prolongs suffering. Traditionally, fewer than 10% of patients with ALS ultimately underwent tracheotomy [9]. In those who receive tracheotomy and mechanical ventilation, it does prolong life by an average of five years [10]. The advent of NIV raised more concerns regarding the ethical use of mechanical ventilation in patients with ALS. There was concern that NIV would prolong suffering, and there was concern that NIV would eventually increase the number of patients with ALS who would receive tracheotomy. These concerns led to a number of case series looking at the quality of life in patients with ALS receiving NIV. The availability of NIV also led to other questions: When in the disease course should NIV be offered? What patient characteristics will prognosticate success with NIV? Can NIV be offered in ALS patients with bulbar symptoms?

Studies that have assessed the quality of life in patients with ALS on NIV are inconclusive but appear promising. One case series studied patients with ALS on NIV for 26 months or longer [7]. They found that quality of life was directly linked to the amount of NIV that patients could tolerate. Higher use of NIV was associated with improved sleep-related problems and improved mental health. There have also been efforts to discern which signs or symptoms will be associated with an improved quality of life. Younger patients and patients with relatively preserved upper arm strength have improved compliance with NIV, likely due to having increased skill at applying and removing the mask [7]. However, since a randomized study in asymptomatic patients with Duchenne's muscular dystrophy (DMD) showed an increase in mortality in a group that was prophylactically treated with NIV, it is difficult to advocate prophylactic use in other neuromuscular disease patients [11]. Moreover, patients with early disease and without significant respiratory complaints consistently had poor compliance with NIV [4].

Guidelines for offering NIV in ALS have traditionally used a $PaCO_2$ of over 45 mm Hg or the presence of nocturnal desaturations as indications [4, 12]. A case series found that the quality if life was improved in patients with hypercapnia and nocturnal desaturation, giving further credibility to these guidelines. However, this study also found that the presence of orthopnea prior to NIV use was the strongest independent predictor of improved quality of life with NIV [7]. Of note, these orthopneic patients did not uniformly have hypercapnia or nocturnal desaturations. In summary, there is increasing consideration being given to the use of NIV in treating symptomatic patients with ALS, as it appears to improve the quality of life in these patients, thus alleviating suffering rather than contributing to suffering.

A recent study by Bourke *et al.* [13] randomized 41 patients with ALS and either orthopnea or daytime hypercapnia to either NIV or conventional therapy. In patients without severe bulbar symptoms, patients treated with NIV had a significant survival benefit (205 days, $p < 0.006$) and improved quality of life. This study suggests that, with the onset of respiratory symptoms (usually orthopnea) or daytime hypercapnia, NIV should be offered to patients with ALS.

Caution must be used with NIV in patients with bulbar weakness. These patients can have significant difficulty controlling oral secretions, leading to suffocation. While NIV may assist with neuromuscular weakness, it does not help with the hypoxemia from upper airway obstruction by oral secretions. Studies have shown that patients with bulbar signs do not live as long on NIV compared with those who do not have bulbar signs [8]. In addition, patients with bulbar symptoms have decreased adherence with NIV and decreased quality of life compared with patients who do not have bulbar weakness [13]. However, some patients with bulbar signs do report an improved quality of life compared with a baseline [13, 14]. While the use of NIV in patients with bulbar signs has not been found to extend life, the subset of patients with both bulbar symptoms and hypercapnia appeared to have a survival advantage in one case series [8]. Therefore, it is necessary to be careful in selecting patients with bulbar signs for NIV. Patients with hypoxemia and shortness of breath caused mainly by secretions would not be good candidates for NIV and should be offered the option of tracheotomy. However, patients with both bulbar signs and significant respiratory muscle weakness (as manifest by hypercapnia) may have improved quality of life with NIV.

1.7.3.2   Duchenne's muscular dystrophy (DMD)

Duchenne's muscular dystrophy is a progressive neuromuscular disorder of X-linked inheritance. Patients are usually wheelchair bound by early adolescence and usually develop respiratory failure by late adolescence. If ventilatory support is not used, the average survival is 9.7 months after the onset of daytime hypercapnia [15]. Prior to NIV and home ventilation, up to 90% of patients with DMD die of respiratory failure by the age of 19 [16].

Case series have shown that NIV likely increases the life span of patients with DMD. One series found one-year and five-year survivals of 85% and 73% [17], while another reported a 36% chance of continuing NIV three years after it was started [18]. When combined with a strict protocol of insufflation–exsufflation use and abdominal thrusts, NIV was found to significantly reduce hospitalizations and time in the hospital compared with conventional tracheotomy and mechanical ventilation [19]. In addition, while no study has been done testing the quality of life before and after starting NIV in DMD, patients with DMD and respiratory failure generally judge their quality of life as satisfactory and similar to age-matched controls [1]. These results have led to the consensus recommendation that NIV should be started in symptomatic patients with DMD and hypercapnia [20].

A randomized study looked at the efficacy of prophylactic NIV in patients with DMD and found that survival was actually worse in the group that received NIV [11]. While this result may be explained by the increased disease severity in the NIV group, it still deters us from recommending prophylactic NIV in DMD. As with patients with ALS, the presence of bulbar signs is considered a relative contraindication to NIV in patients with DMD [1]. However, in hypercapnic patients with bulbar symptoms, NIV may be well tolerated in cases and should be considered before tracheotomy.

Patients with DMD should be followed by serial measurements of spirometry and respiratory muscle strength. A recent study found that following vital capacity over time is a sensitive and specific method of predicting the onset of both nocturnal hypercapnia and the progression to daytime hypercapnia [21]. In this study, a vital capacity of less than than 1820 cc is a sensitive measure of impending nocturnal hypercapnia, while a vital capacity of less than 680 cc is a sensitive measure of impending daytime hypercapnia (despite nocturnal NIV) (Figure 1.7.2). Other studies have found that a vital capacity of less than 30% of predicted is often associated with hypercapnia [1]. Also, maximal inspiratory pressures of less than 30% of predicted are associated with hypercapnia [1]. By following vital capacity, static muscle pressures, and arterial blood gas measurements, clinicians can help determine the right time to recommend NIV use in DMD patients.

1.7.3.3 Kyphoscoliosis

Kyphosis and scoliosis are abnormal curvatures of the spine. Kyphosis is determined by the degree of the spine's anteroposterior angulation, while scoliosis is determined from the extent of the spine's lateral angulation. They are often present in combination and can cause significant disfigurement of the chest wall, impaired

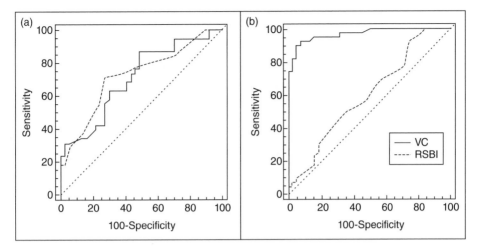

Figure 1.7.2   A:. Receiver operator curve assessing the sensitivity and specificity of a vital capacity of 1820 cc (solid line) compared with the rapid shallow breathing index (dotted line) in predicting nocturnal hypercapnia. B: Receiver operator curve assessing the sensitivity and specificity of a vital capacity of 680 cc (solid line) compared with the rapid shallow breathing index (dotted line) in predicting daytime hypercapnia. (Reproduced with permission [21].)

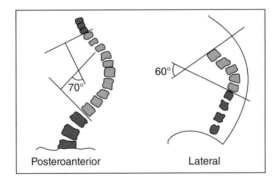

Figure 1.7.3   Measurement of the Cobb angle. A schematic of a posteroanterior radiograph (left) shows measurement of a Cobb angle for scoliosis, while a lateral radiograph (right) shows measurement of a Cobb angle for kyphosis. The angle can be determined either directly from perpendicular lines drawn from the vertebrae (right), or indirectly by drawing sequential perpendicular lines and measuring the inferior angle (left). (Reproduced with permission [22].)

lung compliance, restrictive lung disease, and respiratory failure. The extent of scoliosis or kyphosis can be assessed by measuring the Cobb angle from a posteroanterior or lateral radiograph (Figure 1.7.3). The magnitude of the angle has been used to predict the likelihood of developing respiratory failure, with an angle of >100° increasing the chance of developing respiratory failure [22].

In addition to patients with a large Cobb angle, patients with vital capacity of less than one liter, onset of scoliosis before the age of eight, and a high thoracic curve are at high risk for developing respiratory failure at a future time, usually after the age of 30 [1]. These patients should be watched over time and educated regarding the symptoms of chronic hypercapnic failure.

In patients with chronic respiratory failure from kyphoscoliosis, NIV has been successful. The transition to NIV has been shown to improve gas exchange, respiratory muscle performance, hypoventilation-induced symptoms, and quality of life [23]. It has also been shown to improve lung volumes and improve the quality of sleep [24]. Once NIV is started, treatment is usually well tolerated and survival rates of 90% at one year and 80% at five years have been reported [17, 18].

1.7.3.4   Poliomyelitis (polio)

The second polio syndrome, or post-polio syndrome, is a disease of progressive muscular weakness and joint paint that occurs decades after the initial manifestations of polio. Hypoventilation is the most serious complication of post-polio syndrome and usually manifests during sleep. The use of NIV in this syndrome is not well defined, as this is a relatively rare problem. It has been suggested that the early start of mechanical ventilation or NIV may be beneficial in preventing respiratory muscle fatigue and thus the progression of the post-polio syndrome [25]. One case series looked at a population of patients with post-polio syndrome and compared the efficacy of NIV with mechanical ventilation through tracheotomy [26]. They found that, in the post-polio population, tracheotomy and mechanical ventilation was associated with better alertness, improved sleep, and less pain than those who used NIV. The size and nature of this study make it difficult to extrapolate the data to post-polio patients in respiratory failure.

1.7.3.5   NIV in chronic cystic fibrosis

Cystic Fibrosis (CF) results from a mutation in the CFTR chloride channel. This mutation results in the formation of thick, viscous secretions and severe impairment of mucociliary transport. Over time, this leads to recurrent infections with Staphylococcus, pseudomonas, and other highly resistant bacteria. Bronchiectasis and obstructive physiology invariably develop and eventually lead to chronic respiratory failure. While advances in the assistance of clearing secretions and the treatment of chronic infections have led to improved survival in recent years, most patients develop respiratory failure by the age of 30. Patients develop a rapid shallow breathing pattern in an attempt to reduce the inspiratory muscle load, leading to hypercapnia [27]. Lung transplantation is a viable alternative in patients with poor lung function and respiratory failure, but it can require a wait between the onset of respiratory failure and the time of transplant. NIV is an attractive alternative to invasive ventilation in patients with end-stage pulmonary manifestations of Cystic Fibrosis, since they are prone to pulmonary infections and ventilator acquired pneumonia.

Unfortunately, there is a lack of clinical studies assessing the role of NIV in patients with severe Cystic Fibrosis. To date, there has been no prospective, controlled study performed in this population. The studies that have been done are mostly small case series. Several of these looked at physiologic end points, and the results appear to be favorable. Acutely, authors have reported improvements in oxygen saturation, hypercapnia, and tidal volumes with decreases in the respiratory rate and the work of breathing [28–30].

Small case series suggest that improvements in hypercapnia are maintained over time, and that NIV is generally well tolerated in this population [31, 32]. One other case series used NIV to support patients receiving chest physical therapy (CPT). CPT is an integral part of the management of Cystic Fibrosis, but it creates increased respiratory effort for the patient, and this can lead to respiratory fatigue and gas exchange impairment. One small study found that CPT caused significant hypoxemia, and that the use of NIV-PS was able to significantly reduce this hypoxemia [33].

While these studies are suggestive, they do not confirm a role for NIV in patients with stable Cystic Fibrosis. Many questions remain unanswered at this time. Does NIV improve physiologic parameters and respiratory mechanics compared with oxygen treatment alone? Does the use of NIV in patients with severe Cystic Fibrosis lead to decreased hospitalizations, improved survival, or improved quality of life compared with conventional treatment? When is it appropriate to start NIV treatment – should we wait until patients develop respiratory failure requiring mechanical ventilation (as a bridge to transplant), or could an earlier marker (hypercapnia) indicate the need for starting NIV and prolong the time to transplantation? Unfortunately, these questions remain unanswered at this time.

1.7.4 Conclusion

The use of NIV in patients with DMD and ALS is becoming more defined, as there are several studies and guidelines supporting its use. However, patient selection remains challenging and individual considerations are frequent. In patients with kyphoscoliosis and post-polio syndrome, sufficient evidence exists to recommend its use to improve hypercapnia and to improve the quality of life. Despite the high prevalence of patients with COPD and hypercapnia, the data regarding the use of NIV are sparse. To date, no study has shown that NIV improves survival, decreases hospitalizations, or decreases acute exacerbations compared with long-term oxygen therapy. However, Medicare guidelines do support the use in patients with chronic hypercapnia and persistent nocturnal hypoxemia despite supplemental oxygen. In patients with hypercapnia and Cystic Fibrosis, the use of NIV is theoretically

Table 1.7.1 Guidelines for the use of NIV in chronic respiratory disease [35].

Underlying disease	Recommendation	Grade of recommendation	Considerations
Amyotrophic Lateral Sclerosis	Use in presence of nocturnal desaturations or hypercapnia	Strong	Chin strap? Bulbar symptoms?
Duchenne's muscular dystrophy	Use in the presence of nocturnal desaturations, hypercapnia, or VC <30% predicted	Strong	
Kyphoscoliosis	Use if the presence of hypercapnia	Moderate	
Post-polio syndrome	Use in the presence of hypercapnia	Moderate	
COPD	Use in the presence of hypercapnia and refractory hypoxemia despite long term oxygen therapy	Moderate	Use NIV-PS over CPAP
Cystic Fibrosis	Use as a "bridge" to lung transplantation in patients with hypercapneic respiratory failure	Weak	
Amyotrophic lateral sclerosis	Use in the presence of bulbar muscle weakness or orthopnea with normocapnia	Weak	Adequate cough? Desaturations despite NIV?
COPD	Use in the presence of hypercapnia without a trial of supplemental oxygen	Not recommended	
Cystic Fibrosis	Use in the presence of hypercapnia	Not recommended	Data are lacking

promising (Table 1.7.1). However, the lack of data makes it difficult to understand the role of NIV in Cystic Fibrosis.

1.7.5 Case presentation revisited

At the beginning of the chapter, a patient with DMD and symptoms of nocturnal hypercapnia was described. An arterial blood gas, spirometry, and measures of respiratory muscle strength are indicated. The arterial blood gas revealed daytime hypercapnia ($PaCO_2 = 54$ mm Hg). His forced vital capacity was only 22% of predicted for a patient his height (measured by arm span) and age. His maximum inspiratory mouth pressure (PIMax) was only 12% of predicted. Based on data presented above, each of these measurements indicates that NIV should be beneficial. The overnight polysomnography study was canceled, since it is not needed to start NIV and would be difficult for the patient to tolerate. He was started on NIV-PS, using a BiPAP machine, with an IPAP of 14 cm H_2O and an EPAP of 5 cm H_2O, the pressure support gradient is 9 cm H_2O. After one week, he reported improvement in his symptoms. After one month, a repeat arterial blood gas showed resolution of his daytime hypercapnia. He eventually had recurrence of daytime hypercapnia and required the addition of a simple mouthpiece for daytime NIV. To this time he has not developed bulbar symptoms. Clinic discussions have addressed end of life care issues, and he has elected to defer intubation and tracheotomy should he develop respiratory failure unresponsive to NIV.

References

1. Shneerson, J.M. and Simonds, A.K. (2002) Noninvasive ventilation for chest wall and neuromuscular disorders. *Eur. Respir. J.*, **20**, 480–487.
2. Bach, J.R. (2002) Amyotrophic lateral sclerosis: prolongation of life by noninvasive respiratory aids. *Chest*, **122**, 92–98.
3. Bach, J.R. (1995) Amyotrophic lateral sclerosis: predictors for prolongation of life by noninvasive respiratory aids. *Arch. Phys. Med. Rehabil.*, **76**, 828–832.
4. Bach, J.R., Brougher, P., Hess, D.R. *et al.* (1997) Consensus statement: Noninvasive positive pressure ventilation. *Respir. Care*, **42**, 364.
5. Hill, N.S. and Kramer, N.R. (2007) Practical aspects of noninvasive nocturnal ventilation in neuromuscular and chest wall disease. UpToDate.
6. Elman, L.B. (2010) Clinical features of amyotrophic lateral sclerosis. UpToDate.
7. Bourke, S.C. *et al.* (2003) Noninvasive ventilation in ALS: indications and effect on quality of life. *Neurology*, **61**, 171–177.
8. Farrero, E. *et al.* (2005) Survival in ALS with home mechanical ventilation: the impact of systematic respiratory assessment and bulbar involvement. *Chest*, **127**, 2132–2138.
9. Moss, A.H. *et al.* (1993) Home ventilation for amyotrophic lateral sclerosis patients: outcomes, costs, and patient, family, and physician attitudes. *Neurology*, **43**, 438–443.
10. Bach, J.R. *et al.* (1993) Amyotrophic lateral sclerosis: communication status and survival with ventilatory support. *Am. J. Phys. Med. Rehabil.*, **72**, 343–349.
11. Raphael, J.C., Chevret, S., Chastang, C. and Bouvet, F. (French Multicentre Cooperative Group on Home Mechanical Ventilation Assistance in Duchenne de Boulogne Muscular Dystrophy) (1994) Randomised trial of preventive nasal ventilation in Duchenne muscular dystrophy. *Lancet*, **343**, 1600.
12. Meyer, T.J. *et al.* (1994) Noninvasive positive pressure ventilation to treat respiratory failure. *Ann. Intern. Med.*, **120** (9), 760–770.
13. Bourke, S.C. *et al.* (2006) Effects of non-invasive ventilation on survival and quality of life in patients with amyotrophic lateral sclerosis: a randomized controlled trial. *Lancet Neurol.*, **5**, 140–147.
14. Bourke, S.C. *et al.* (2001) Respiratory function versus sleep disordered breathing as predictors of quality of life in ALS. *Neurology*, **57**, 2040–2044.
15. Vianello, A. *et al.* (1994) Long-term nasal intermittent positive pressure ventilation in advanced Duschenne's muscular dystrophy. *Chest*, **105**, 445–448.
16. Rideau, Y. (1983) Prolongation of life in Duchenne muscular dystrophy. *Acta Neurol.*, **5**, 118–124.
17. Simonds, A.K. *et al.* (1995) Outcome of domiciliary nasal intermittent positive pressure ventilation in restrictive and obstructive disorders. *Thorax*, **50**, 604–609.
18. Leger, P. *et al.* (1999) Nasal intermittent positive pressure ventilation: long term follow up in patients with severe chronic respiratory insufficiency. *Chest*, **105**, 100–105.

19. Bach, J.R. (1997) Prevention of pulmonary morbidity for patients with Duschenne muscular dystrophy. *Chest*, **112**, 1024–1028.
20. Consensus Conference (1999) Clinical indications for noninvasive positive pressure ventilation in chronic respiratory failure due to restrictive lung disease, COPD, and nocturnal hypoventilation- a consensus conference report. *Chest*, **116**, 521–534.
21. Toussaint, M. *et al.* (2007) Lung function accurately predicts hypercapnia in patients with Duchenne muscular dystrophy. *Chest*, **131**, 368–375.
22. Tzelepis, G.E. and McCool, D.F. (2005) The lungs and chest wall disease, in Murray and Nadel's Textbook of Medicine, 4th edn (eds. R.J. Mason, V.C. Broaddus, J.F. Murray and J.A. Nadel), Elsevier Saunders, Philadelphia, Chapter 83.
23. Gonzalez, C., Ferris, G., Diaz, J. *et al.* (2003) Kyphoscoliotic ventilatory insufficiency: effects of long-term intermittent positive-pressure ventilation. *Chest*, **124**, 857.
24. Ellis, E.R., Grunstein, R.R., Chan, S. *et al.* (1988) Noninvasive ventilatory support during sleep improves respiratory failure in kyphoscoliosis. *Chest*, **94**, 811.
25. Agre, J.C. (1994) Local muscle and total body fatigue, in Post Polio Syndrome (eds L.S. Halstead and C. Grimby), Hanley and Belfus Inc., Philadelphia, pp. 35–67.
26. Markstrom, A. (2002) Quality of life evaluation of patients with neuromuscular and skeletal diseases treated with noninvasive and invasive home mechanical ventilation. *Chest*, **122**, 1695–1700.
27. Hart, N. *et al.* (2002) Changes in pulmonary mechanics with increasing disease severity in children and young adults with cystic fibrosis. *Am. J. Respir. Crit. Care Med.*, **166**, 61–66.
28. Granton, J.T. and Kesten, S. (1998) The acute effects of nasal positive pressure ventilation in patients with advanced cystic fibrosis. *Chest*, **113**, 1013–1018.
29. Milross, M.A. *et al.* (2001) Low-flow oxygen and bilevel pressure support: effects on ventilation during sleep in cystic fibrosis. *Am. J. Respir. Crit. Care Med.*, **163**, 129–134.
30. Regnis, J.A. *et al.* (1994) Benefits of nocturnal CPAP in patients with cystic fibrosis. *Chest*, **106**, 1717–1724.
31. Piper, A.J. *et al.* (1992) Nocturnal nasal IPPV stabilizes patients with cystic fibrosis and hypercapnic respiratory failure. *Chest*, **102**, 846–850.
32. Hill, A.T. *et al.* (1998) Long-term nasal intermittent positive pressure ventilation in patients with cystic fibrosis and hypercapnic respiratory failure. *Respir. Med.*, **92**, 523–526.
33. Fauroux, B. *et al.* (1999) Chest physiotherapy in cystic fibrosis: improved tolerance with nasal pressure support ventilation. *Pediatrics*, **103**, 32.
34. Bach, J.R. (1994) Update and perspectives on noninvasive respiratory muscle aids. Part 1: The inspiratory aids. *Chest*, **105**, 1230–1240.
35. British Thoracic Society Standards of Care Committee (2002) Non-invasive ventilation in acute respiratory failure. *Thorax*, **57**, 192–211.

1.8 Weaning from invasive ventilation to noninvasive ventilation

Daniel C. Grinnan[1] and Jonathon D. Truwit[2]

[1] Division of Pulmonary and Critical Care Medicine, Virginia Commonwealth University, Richmond, VA, USA
[1] Division of Pulmonary and Critical Care Medicine, University of Virginia, Charlottesville, VA, USA

1.8.1 Case presentation

A 72-year-old with history of tobacco use and suspected chronic obstructive pulmonary disease (COPD) developed hypoxemic and hypercapnic respiratory failure requiring intubation and mechanical ventilation. His chest X-ray was suggestive of pneumonia, and a sputum sample grew *streptococcus pneumoniae*. After four days of treatment, he is able to pass a spontaneous breathing trial, his mental status is appropriate, and his secretions are minimal. He is extubated to nasal canula, and his initial arterial blood gas following extubation shows a pH = 7.42, CO_2 = 46 mm Hg, and PaO_2 = 75 mm Hg. Two hours later, he appears tachypneic and is using accessory muscles of respiration. He is not coughing and his chest X-ray shows no significant change. Repeat arterial blood gas shows a pH = 7.26, $PaCO_2$ = 66 mm Hg, and PaO_2 = 63 mm Hg. Is noninvasive ventilation (NIV) appropriate or should he be reintubated? If he receives NIV, how should he be followed?

1.8.2 Introduction

The discontinuation of invasive mechanical ventilation has been a challenge for physicians since mechanical ventilation was instituted into clinical practice. Both prolonged intubation and early extubation can cause significant adverse events [1].

A Practical Guide to Mechanical Ventilation, First Edition.
Edited by Jonathon D. Truwit and Scott K. Epstein.
© 2011 John Wiley & Sons, Ltd. Published 2011 by John Wiley & Sons, Ltd.

Many different mechanical factors have been studied to help clinicians accurately predict the success of extubation, but none have proven more effective than the spontaneous breathing trial [2]. Therefore, guidelines suggest using spontaneous breathing trials (T-piece, CPAP, or trach collar trials) prior to discontinuing invasive mechanical ventilation [3]. However, even when guided by spontaneous breathing trial, multiple studies have reported reintubation rates of 15–20% [4–6]. This is concerning, as reintubation clearly leads to worse clinical outcomes. Even after controlling for the severity of illness, reintubation has been associated with an increased mortality [7]. This is likely secondary to the increased risk of nosocomial pneumonia conferred by reintubation [8]. Since NIV decreases nosocomial pneumonia compared with invasive ventilation [9], it seemed likely that NIV would lead to better outcomes by sparing reintubation and preventing nosocomial pneumonias. However, clinical results have shown varied results, some of which have warned clinicians to have great care before proceeding with NIV after recent extubation [10]. In this chapter, the evidence for using NIV following extubation is discussed.

The post-extubation population can be separated into three distinct subpopulations. In the first group, patients are invasively ventilated, on minimal ventilator settings, and have failed a spontaneous breathing trial. The second group includes patients who were recently extubated, only to develop recurrent acute respiratory failure. The last group consists of patients who have just been extubated after passing a spontaneous breathing trial but are at high risk for reintubation. As will be discussed, each of these patient populations should be considered differently when considering the use of NIV.

1.8.3   Using NIV to expedite weaning from invasive ventilation

The spontaneous breathing trial is often used to predict the safety of extubation. Often, patients with prolonged intubation will be on minimal ventilator settings for days, but remain unable to pass a spontaneous breathing trial (SBT). Unfortunately, continued intubation confers the risk of nosocomial pneumonia. NIV offers the theoretical advantage of continuing to provide ventilator support while decreasing the risk of nosocomial pneumonia. In addition, eliminating the endotracheal tube may enhance patient comfort and permit less sedation. In fact, in patients who failed a spontaneous breathing trial (T-piece trial), invasive and noninvasive ventilation were equivalent in their ability to improving gas exchange and reduce inspiratory effort, although noninvasive ventilation resulted in better patient comfort [11]. To date, there have been three randomized studies looking at the benefit of NIV in patients with chronic respiratory failure who have failed a spontaneous breathing trial [12].

The first of these studies looked only at patients with acute COPD exacerbations requiring invasive mechanical ventilation [13]. After 48 hours of intubation, patients who were on minimal ventilator settings and who failed a spontaneous breathing trial were randomized to either continued intubation or extubation and transition to NIV. The NIV group had significant reductions in the number of days requiring mechanical ventilation (either invasive or noninvasive) and in the length of intensive care unit stay. In addition, they also found improved success of weaning in the NIV group and significantly improved 60-day survival in the NIV group.

Girault and colleagues [14] looked at 33 patients with various underlying pulmonary conditions (mostly COPD) leading to chronic ventilatory failure. These patients were on minimal ventilatory support but had failed a spontaneous breathing trial (T-piece trial). Patients were randomized to either continued invasive ventilation or extubation with transfer to NIV. The most important finding was that transfer to NIV had an equivalent rate of successful weaning (76.5%) compared with the invasive ventilation group (75%). Not surprisingly, the group transitioned to NIV had decreased time of invasive ventilation. However, the NIV group had an increase in the average number of days spent weaning (11.54 days) compared with the invasive ventilation group (3.46 days).

The last study enrolled 43 patients with prolonged intubation (>3 days) who had failed a spontaneous breathing trial on three consecutive days [15]. These patients had a variety of underlying conditions, although over half were COPD exacerbations. As in the previous studies, patients were randomized to either extubation with transition to NIV or continued invasive ventilation with daily spontaneous breathing trials. The investigators found several positive outcomes in the NIV group. Patients randomized to NIV had reduced intensive care unit and hospital stays, improved intensive care unit and hospital survival, decreased need for tracheostomy, and decreased incidence of pneumonia and sepsis.

In summary, these results provide evidence that patients with COPD may benefit from early extubation to NIV. However, caution must be used to screen patients with excessive secretions and those unable to cooperate with NIV (not always easy to determine before extubation). It should be noted that up to two-thirds of eligible patients were excluded from Ferrer's study, indicating that careful screening is warranted, and that widespread extrapolation of these data may be dangerous. Also, these studies did not include enough patients with other pulmonary conditions (restrictive lung disease, immunosuppression, etc.) to determine if these populations may benefit. While patients with severe congestive heart failure likely represent another patient population that often fails a spontaneous breathing trial despite minimal ventilator settings, no study to date has investigated early extubation to NIV in this group.

1.8.4 NIV in acute respiratory failure following extubation

The second population includes patients who were recently extubated, but then develop respiratory distress. In these patients, NIV was not part of the initial weaning plan. However, once respiratory distress develops, NIV is started with the hope of preventing reintubation, as reintubation leads to worse clinical outcomes. To date, there have been three studies which have addressed the question of NIV in the setting of acute respiratory failure following extubation.

Hilbert and colleagues [16] performed a historical case-control on 30 patients with COPD who developed hypercapnic respiratory failure after extubation. They found that patients receiving NIV had a significantly lower rate of reintubation (20% versus 67% in the historical control), as well as significantly shorter length of intensive care unit stay. However, the design of this study (using a historical control group) introduces several biases that make extrapolation of the data difficult.

Keenan and colleagues [17] investigated 81 patients in a single center who had been intubated for over two days and developed respiratory failure within two days of extubation. Respiratory distress was defined as either the use of accessory muscles of respiration, respiratory rate over 30 per minute, or an increase in the respiratory rate of over 50% from baseline. Patients were then randomized to receive either NIV or continued supplemental oxygen, and they assessed the rate of reintubation. They did not find a decrease in the rate of reintubation, the length of intensive care unit stay, or the length of total hospital stay. In this study less than 10% of the patients receiving NIV had a diagnosis of COPD, a group that traditionally responds the best to NIV.

Esteban and colleagues [10] performed a multicenter study involving 221 patients from 37 centers that provided further insight and controversy to the use of NIV in this group of patients. The study included a small number of patients with COPD (12%) or congestive heart failure (7%). Similar to the Keenan study, patients who were intubated for over two days and extubated for less than two days were eligible. After the development of respiratory distress, patients were randomized to NIV or conventional treatment with supplemental oxygen. Results parallel that of Keenan *et al.*, there was no difference in the rate of reintubation between those assigned to NIV and those receiving conventional treatment. Surprisingly, this study found a significantly increased mortality rate in the group assigned to NIV. The increased mortality rate was due to a higher rate of death among those reintubated in the NIV group compared with those reintubated in the conventional group. The time from development of respiratory distress to reintubation differed markedly between the NIV group (median of 12 h) and the conventional group (median of 2 h 30 min). Therefore, in this study, delays in reintubation correlate with increased mortality [18].

The results of Esteban's study have raised serious concerns about the use of NIV in patients with acute respiratory failure following extubation. If a practitioner uses NIV in this setting, it is advocated that he/she include only those populations that are known to benefit from NIV in acute respiratory failure (COPD, congestive heart failure, immunocompromised patients with pulmonary infiltrates, and following lung resection). In addition, it is recommended that patients be monitored in an

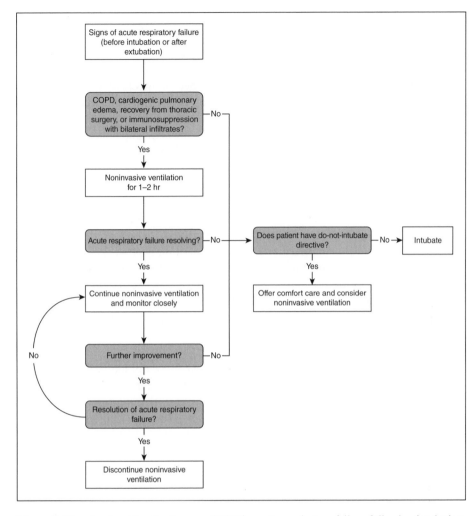

Figure 1.8.1   An algorithm for the use of NIV in acute respiratory failure following intubation. (Reproduced with permission [18].)

intensive care unit so that intubation is not delayed if improvement is not seen after the first 1–2 h of NIV (Figure 1.8.1).

1.8.5   Prophylactic use of NIV following extubation

The relatively high rate of reintubation (10–15%) after successfully completing a spontaneous breathing trial and being extubated has caught the attention of practitioners. Certain populations (chronic heart failure, previous failure of a weaning trial, hypercapnia following extubation) are considered even higher risk of reintubation [7, 19]. Given the known association of reintubation with poor out-comes and the potential danger of using NIV in patients who have developed acute respiratory failure following extubation, attention has been given to the prophylactic use of NIV in patients at high risk for reintubation following extubation. There have been two prospective, randomized studies performed on this patient population.

The first study assessed 93 patients with varying underlying causes of respiratory failure who were extubated [20]. While 56 patients underwent a successful spon-taneous breathing trial prior to extubation, 37 patients had "unplanned extubation," including self-extubation. Patients were randomized to receive either conventional treatment with supplemental oxygen or NIV. While the difference was not signifi-cant, 28% of the patients randomized to NIV required reintubation, while only 15% of the patients randomized to conventional treatment required reintubation.

The second study included only patients who were extubated after passing a weaning trial [21]. Ninety seven patients were enrolled, and all were intubated for over two days and were deemed high risk. If a patient met one of six criteria (Table 1.8.1), he/she was determined to be high risk for reintubation. Patients were rand-omized to NIV or conventional oxygen therapy following extubation. In this study, the NIV group had a significantly lower (8%) rate of reintubation compared with the conventional group (24%). In patients who benefited from NIV, the intensive care unit mortality was significantly reduced ($p < 0.001$).

In a similar study, Ferrer $et\ al.$ [22] examined the application of NIV in patients at risk for recurrent acute respiratory failure (rARF) in a randomized control trial of NIV versus conventional management. At risk patients were identified by: age > 65 years, cardiac failure as etiology of initial respiratory failure or APACHE II score > 12 on day of extubation. Those randomized to NIV had a reduced inci-dence of rARF ($p = 0.029$) but this did not translate into a reduction in reintubation. However, the application of NIV to patients with hypercapnia during the spontane-ous breathing trial prior to extubation resulted in improved survival ($p = 0.006$).

The difference in the results of these studies is likely due to the difference in inclusion criteria. Jiang's study included patients who had self-extubated and had not passed a spontaneous breathing trial, making it impossible to extrapolate the

Table 1.8.1 Inclusion criteria for the study performed by Nava $et\ al.$ [21] highlighting the high-risk scenarios for reintubation.

A. Mechanical ventilation >48 h
B. Successful weaning trial
C. Plus one or more of the following high-risk scenarios for reintubation features:
　1. More than one consecutive failure of weaning trial
　2. Chronic heart failure
　3. $PaCO_2$ >45 mm Hg after extubation
　4. More than one comorbidity (excluding chronic heart failure)
　5. Weak cough defined as Airway Care Score values >8 and <12
　6. Upper airways stridor at extubation not requiring immediate reintubation

results to patients who are high risk and have passed a spontaneous breathing trial. We currently recommend using NIV in these high-risk patients following planned extubation to prevent acute respiratory failure, especially those with COPD and hypercapnia during an spontaneous breathing trial. However, as the patient population in the Nava study was heterogenous (Table 1.8.1), further research on each of these populations (Table 1.8.1) should be done.

1.8.6   Practical considerations

As in any situation where NIV is used, a practitioner must choose an interface, a ventilator, and ventilator settings. As this instance involves the use of NIV in an acute setting, the practitioner should also have an end point to its use. Because most patients with acute respiratory failure are mouth breathers, the oronasal mask has become the interface of choice in treating patients after extubation. While both intensive care ventilators and portable noninvasive ventilators can be used to deliver NIV, portable ventilators have improved leak compensation, thus giving improved patient triggering and decreased dysynchrony [23]. Unless patients have hypoxemia at the time of NIV initiation, portable ventilators may offer an advantage. However, intensive care ventilators allow more accurate titration of FiO_2, making it the preferred ventilator in the setting of acute hypoxemic respiratory failure [24].

The initial ventilator settings will depend on the clinical scenario (the three patient populations discussed earlier in this section). Firstly, there is the patient with COPD who is transitioned from minimal ventilator settings to NIV after failing spontaneous breathing trials. NIV-PS is the mode of choice in this situation. The clinician should make sure that the intubated patient is stable on a pressure support mode prior to the transition. When delivering NIV-PS with a BiPAP machine, the expiratory positive airway pressure (EPAP) should correspond to the positive end-expiratory pressure (PEEP). The pressure gradient between inspiratory positive airway pressure (IPAP) and EPAP should correspond to the pressure support level applied prior to extubation. Similarly, the FiO_2 can be matched with the FiO_2 from invasive ventilation. Initially, the patient should have NIV-PS overnight and for multiple 2–4 h periods during the day (Girault) [14]. Short breaks from NIV during the day (initially 2 h or less using supplemental oxygen) can gradually be lengthened as the patient's status allows.

If NIV is used to prophylactically treat patients at high risk for reintubation or rARF, NIV-PS is again the mode of choice. In this case, the initial settings should be fairly low (when using a BiPAP machine; IPAP of 10 cm H_2O, EPAP of 5 cm H_2O) and titrated as needed for the goal oxygen saturation. If a patient is well after two days, NIV can be discontinued [21]. If they continue to have some distress, NIV should be continued at the discretion of the clinician. If patients remain stable after the initial application of an oronasal mask, some patients may be transitioned to a nasal mask for comfort.

When using NIV on patients who have developed acute respiratory failure after extubation, the settings should be titrated to improve either patient work of breathing, hypoxemia or hypercapnia (or both). While NIV-CPAP could be considered in patients with acute congestive heart failure after extubation, NIV-PS should be used for other causes. In this instance, NIV should be continued until the underlying cause has been addressed and the patient has recovered. Careful monitoring with frequent assessments is essential, as these patients may fail NIV and prompt intubation may be needed.

1.8.7   Summary

The validity of using NIV following extubation depends of the circumstances around the extubation. There is data to support the use of NIV to decrease the duration of endotracheal intubation in patients with COPD on minimal ventilator settings. However, evidence does not yet support the use of NIV to accelerate ventilator weaning in other patient populations. Following planned extubation, patients at high risk for reintubation or rARF may benefit from the prophylactic use of NIV to avoid reintubation. However, in patients who develop acute respiratory failure following extubation, the use of NIV has more risk, and may lead to worse outcomes. If applied in this setting, patients must be closely observed and intubated if not improving with NIV. There is no evidence to support the use of NIV in patients with unplanned extubation. If the clinician chooses to intervene with NIV in this setting, patients should be closely monitored so that the time to reintubation (if needed) is minimized.

1.8.8   Case presentation revisited

This case describes a patient who has developed acute respiratory failure following planned extubation. Of note, he had $PaCO_2 > 45\,mm\,Hg$ after extubation, placing him in a high-risk group that would benefit from the prophylactic use of NIV to avoid acute respiratory failure immediately following extubation. In this case, this was not done and he now has acute respiratory failure. Given his underlying diagnosis of COPD, a trial of NIV is reasonable. However, he must be watched closely in an intensive care unit. If he has not shown improvement in the first 1–2 h, the clinician should not delay reintubation, as this could increase his risk of death [10].

References

1. Gil, B. *et al.* (2003) Deleterious effects of reintubation of mechanically ventilated patients. *Clin. Pulm. Med.*, **10**, 226–230.
2. Grinnan, D. and Truwit, J.D. (2005) Clinical review: respiratory mechanics in spontaneous and assisted ventilation. *Crit. Care*, **9**, 472–484.
3. MacIntyre, N.R. *et al.* (2001) Evidence-based guidelines for weaning and discontinuing ventilatory support: a collective task force facilitated by the American College of Chest

Physicians, the AmericanAssocation for Respiratory Care, and theAmerican College of Critical Care Medicine. *Chest*, **120**, 375S–395S.

4. Esteban, A. *et al.* (1997) Extubation outcome after spontaneous breathing trials with T-tube or pressure support ventilation. *Am. J. Respir. Crit. Care Med.*, **156**, 459–465.

5. Esteban, A. *et al.* (1999) Effect of spontaneous breathing trial duration on outcome of attempts to discontinue mechanical ventilation. *Am. J. Respir. Crit. Care Med.*, **159**, 512–518.

6. Ely, E.W. *et al.* (1996) Effect on the duration of mechanical ventilation of identifying patients capable of breathing spontaneously. *N. Engl. J. Med.*, **335**, 1864–1869.

7. Epstein, S.K. and Ciubotaru, R.L. (1998) Independent effects of etiology of failure and time to reintubation on outcome for patients failing extubation. *Am. J. Respir. Crit. Care Med.*, **158**, 489–493.

8. Torres, A. *et al.* (1995) Reintubation increases the risk of nosocomial pneumonia in patients needing mechanical ventilation. *Am. J. Respir. Crit. Care Med.*, **152**, 137–141.

9. Celis, R. *et al.* (1998) Nosocomial pneumonia: a multivariate analysis of risk and prognosis. *Chest*, **93**, 318–324.

10. Esteban, A. *et al.* (2004) Noninvasive positive pressure ventilation for respiratory failure after extubation. *N. Engl. J. Med.*, **350**, 2452–2460.

11. Vitacca, M. *et al.* (2001) Physiologic response to pressure support ventilation delivered before and after extubation in patients not capable of totally spontaneous autonomous breathing. *Am. J. Respir. Crit. Care Med.*, **163**, 283–291.

12. Navalesi, P. (2003) Weaning and noninvasive ventilation: the odd couple. *Am. J. Respir. Crit. Care Med.*, **168**, 5–6.

13. Nava, S. *et al.* (1998) Noninvasive mechanical ventilation in the weaning of patients with respiration failure due to chronic obstructive pulmonary disease: a randomized, controlled trial. *Ann. Intern. Med.*, **128**, 721–728.

14. Girault, C. *et al.* (1999) Noninvasive ventilation as a systematic extubation and weaning technique in acute-on-chronic respiratory failure: a prospective, randomized study. *AJRCCM*, **160**, 86–92.

15. Ferrer, M. (2003) Noninvasive ventilation during persistent weaning failure: a randomized, controlled trial. *Am. J. Respir. Crit. Care Med.*, **168**, 70–76.

16. Hilbert, G. *et al.* (1998) Noninvasive pressure support ventilation in COPD patients with postextubation hypercapnic respiratory insufficiency. *Eur. Respir. J.*, **11**, 1349–1353.

17. Keenan, S.P. *et al.* (2002) Noninvasive positive-pressure ventilation for postextubation respiratory distress. *JAMA*, **287**, 3238–3244.

18. Truwit, J.D. and Bernard, G.R. (2004) Noninvasive ventilation – don't push too hard. *N. Engl. J. Med.*, **350**, 2512–2515.

19. Epstein, S.K. *et al.* (1997) Effect of failed extubation on the outcome of mechanical ventilation. *Chest*, **112**, 186–192.

20. Jiang, J.S. *et al.* (1999) Effect of early application of biphasic positive airway pressure on the outcome of extubation in ventilator weaning. *Respirology*, **4** (2), 161.

21. Nava, S. *et al.* (2005) Noninvasive ventilation to prevent respiratory failure after extubation in high-risk patients. *Crit. Care Med.*, **33** (11), 2465.

22. Ferrer, M. *et al.* (2006) Early noninvasive ventilation averts extubation failure in patients at risk: a randomized trial. *Am. J. Respir. Crit. Care Med.*, **173** (2), 164–170.

23. Miyoshi, E. *et al.* (2005) Effects of gas leak on triggering function, humidification, and inspiratory oxygen fraction during noninvasive positive airway pressure ventilation. *Chest*, **128**, 3691–3698.

24. Hess, D. (2006) Noninvasive ventilation in neuromuscular disease: equipment and application. *Respir. Care*, **51** (8), 896–912.

Part II
Invasive mechanical ventilation

2.1 Respiratory failure

Kyle B. Enfield and Jonathon D. Truwit

Division of Pulmonary and Critical Care Medicine, University of Virginia, Charlottesville, VA, USA

2.1.1 Case presentation

A 32-year-old male C4-quadriplegic is transferred from a referring hospital for worsening hypoxia of unclear etiology. At baseline he uses BiPAP nocturnally and has for the past four years. Vital signs on arrival show blood pressure 85/30, heart rate 140 beats/min, respiratory rate 32 breaths/min, temperature 39 °C, oxygen saturation by pulse oximetry of 80%. On arrival his arterial blood sample reveals pH 7.26, PaO_2 80, $PaCO_2$ 50 with a chest X-ray showing bilateral infiltrates. He is promptly intubated in the emergency department. What is the cause of his respiratory failure? How does the mechanism of failure help with treatment? What are the outcomes for chronic respiratory failure? This chapter focuses on the mechanisms of respiratory failure and their implications for treatment.

2.1.2 Introduction

Respiratory failure leads to an estimated 1–3 million patients require mechanical ventilatory support outside of the operating room annually [1], with the best estimate of patients living at home with invasive mechanical ventilation being between

A Practical Guide to Mechanical Ventilation, First Edition.
Edited by Jonathon D. Truwit and Scott K. Epstein.
© 2011 John Wiley & Sons, Ltd. Published 2011 by John Wiley & Sons, Ltd.

10 000 and 20 000 [2] Additionally, respiratory failure is associated with significant mortality and morbidity. In 1998, respiratory failure and diseases leading up to respiratory failure accounted for 14.4% of all deaths [3, 4], with approximately 25 000 from acute respiratory distress syndrome (ARDS) [5]. The Study to Understand the Prognoses and Preferences of Seriously Ill Hospitalized Patients (SUPPORT) [6] found that many patients with acute respiratory failure due to pneumonia or ARDS had normal physiologic function and enjoyed a good quality of life before hospitalization. Despite this they had significant in-hospital mortality, 42%, and another 11% died within one year after discharge [7]. Of the ventilated patients who survived hospitalization and lived to six months, 29% rated their quality of life as only fair or poor [8]. Indeed, survivors of ARDS at one year continue to have functional disability and reduced quality of life compared to normal population [9]. Those patients with chronic respiratory failure admitted with an acute exacerbation (defined by the SUPPORT investigators as a $PaCO_2$ of 50 mm Hg or more on admission) had an associated in-hospital mortality of 11% and a one-year mortality rate of 43% [10]. This chapter focuses on a mechanistic approach to respiratory failure, focusing on acute causes.

2.1.3 Patterns of respiratory failure

Distinguishing the basis for respiratory failure is critical for providing appropriate and timely treatment. While hypoxic and hypercarbic respiratory failure account for many cases of respiratory failure, peri-operative respiratory failure and hypoperfusion states should be kept in the differential diagnosis during the initial evaluation [11].

In 1959, Frumen, Epstein, and Cohen showed that oxygenation was independent of gas exchange. In their experiments, healthy volunteers undergoing routine surgical procedures were provided with 100% FiO_2 without ventilation. After 20 minutes of apenic oxygenation, PaO_2 levels remained above normal despite increased $PaCO_2$ with associated respiratory acidosis [12]. This underscores the importance in distinguishing between failures in gas exchange and respiratory failures secondary to intrapulmonary shunt ($\dot{Q}S/\dot{Q}T$).

Clinically, Hypoxic Respiratory Failure (HORF) is recognized as disorders that fill alveoli partially or fully (cardiac and non-cardiac pulmonary edema, pneumonia, alveolar hemorrhage, etc.) or secondary to V/Q mismatch (e.g., pulmonary embolism) [11]. Assessing the degree of shunt is difficult in the critically ill patient. Traditionally the A–a gradient has been used as a surrogate, and while useful in assessing the patient breathing room air, the correlation with Qs/Qt in critically ill patients is less clear (r = 0.58–0.68) [13, 14]. To overcome some of this limitation, the PaO_2/FiO_2 ratio was introduced. This ratio has a normal range of 300 to 500, with values <250 reflecting clinically significant impairment of pulmonary gas exchange [15]. The correlation of PaO_2/FiO_2 with Qs/Qt also has variability across studies (r −0.51 to −0.90) [13, 14, 16, 17] with findings that a $PaO_2/FiO_2 < 200$ correlated with a Qs/Qt > 20% in patients with ARDS [13].

Pulse oximetry is an acceptable means to detect hypoxemia in critically ill patients showing a bias of <2% and a precision of <3% when SaO_2 is ≥90% in healthy volunteers [18, 19]. This has been replicated in critically ill patients [20, 21]; however, in low perfusion states with decreased cardiac output, the bias and precision increases to >4% [22–24] and the accuracy deteriorates even in healthy volunteers when the SaO_2 is less than 80% [18].

Hypercarbic Respiratory Failure (HCRF), occurs when central nervous system depression (e.g., head injuries, opiods), work to dead-space ratio increases, or neuromuscular uncoupling (e.g., myasthenia gravis, Guillain–Barré syndrome, amyotrophic lateral sclerosis, botulism, or muscle relaxing drugs) reduces minute ventilation leading to a rise in the alveolar and arterial partial pressure of carbon dioxide.

In patients with diseases of airflow obstruction [25–27] or restriction [28], alveolar ventilation (V_A) is reduced despite a normal or increased minute ventilation (V_E) because the ratio of dead-space to tidal volume is increased. As the patient compensates for an increase in minute ventilation, there is a concomitant rise in dead-space ventilation and $PACO_2$. In the case of central nervous system depression and neuromsucular uncoupling, the rise in $PACO_2$ develops from the addition of resting production of carbon dioxide to the alveolar ventilation, leading to an increase in the partial pressure of carbon dioxide both arterially and in the alveoli. In all cases, this increase in the $PACO_2$ leads to decrease in PAO_2, easily corrected with small increases in the FiO_2. This contrasts with HORF, in which the hypoxia is refractory even with a FiO_2 of 1.0.

As with all major muscle groups, respiratory muscles can fatigue. When the load is less than one-third maximal strength this fatigue time approaches infinity. An average inspiratory pressure per breath of 10 cm H_2O represents 10% of a normal individual's negative inspiratory force (NIF), which when measured at residual volume is around 100 cm H_2O. However, should the patient have a NIF of 30 cm H_2O with an average inspiratory pressure of 15 cm H_2O, then spontaneous respiration is likely not sustainable. It is not uncommon for patients to have a high mechanical load and an NIF < 30 cm H_2O [29]. The time to fatigue and respiratory failure is further shortened by attendant hypoxia [30].

The relationship between $PaCO_2$ and PaO_2 in respiratory failure is shown in Figure 2.1.1. In this figure, the normal respiratory exchange ratio of 0.8 is represented by the solid line. With hyperventilation, PaO_2 and $PaCO_2$ move towards the letter H and with hypoventilation, such as seen in drug overdose, they move towards letter D on the solid line. This shows that individuals with normal A–a gradients have sufficient oxygen stores to offset increases in $PaCO_2$. Patients with a large A–a gradients, such as those with ARDS or pneumonia, move along line A, hyperventilating to maintain oxygenation. Patients with interstitial lung disease or non-hypercapnic emphysema are unable to reduce $PaCO_2$ further in the face of worsening hypoxemia, as illustrated line B. Patients with lung disease and inadequate alveolar ventilation move along the line C, a rising $PaCO_2$ despite the increased drive associated with hypoxemia [31].

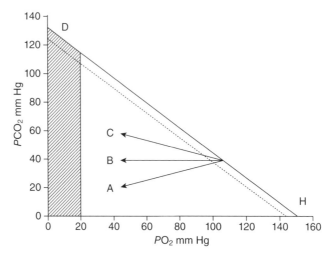

Figure 2.1.1   Relationship between PCO_2 and PO_2 in health and disease. (Reproduced with permission [31].)

The post operative period is typically marked by a alterations in abdominal mechanics leading to a decrease in FRC ($\downarrow$FRC) [32–34] and an increase in closing volume($\uparrow$CV) [32, 35, 36]. The reduced functional residual capacity (FRC) is often below the increased closing volume which results in progressive collapse of dependent lung units. This presents as respiratory failure that can have features of both HORF and HCRF. However, because of its unique mechanism it is labeled as peri-operative respiratory failure (POpRF).

By preventing the common clinical circumstances leading to a decrease in FRC or abnormal airway closure at increased lung volume POpRF can be avoided. This leads to the maxim, attributed to the late Dr T. Petty, that "the lung works best in the upright position." Additionally, patients with HORF and/or HCRF share many of these mechanisms, suggesting the minimizing atelectasis should be part of the management of all patients with respiratory failure. Therapies that achieve this include turning intubated patients, chest physiotherapy, and judicious use of continuous positive airway pressure (CPAP) or positive end-expiratory pressure (PEEP) [35]. Ensuring adequate pain control as well as minimizing abdominal pressure either from internal causes (e.g., ascites) or external causes (e.g., abdominal binders) also helps prevent atelectasis [33, 37]. In the case of lobar collapse, early bronchoscopy and chest physiotherapy have similar results, however, in patients where re-expansion does not occur after vigorous pulmonary hygiene, bronchoscopy to clear obstruction is indicated [38]. Preoperative smoking cessation, at least six weeks prior to elective operations reduces bronchorrhea and atelectasis [39], and avoiding overhydration in peri-operative patients especially vulnerable to atelectasis reduces this problem.

Patients presenting in shock can also require ventilator support for causes not related to HORF, HCRF or POpRF. The hypoperfusion states caused by shock from cardiac, hypovolemic, and septic states can lead to pulmonary problems requiring mechanical ventilator support. The rational for this support in these conditions is to minimize the steal of cardiac output by the increased work of the respiratory muscles until the cause of shock can be reversed [11, 40, 41].

2.1.4 Acute vs. Chronic

Acute respiratory failure distinguishes itself from chronic respiratory failure by the degree of physiologic compensation. Yet, like acute respiratory failure (ARF), chronic respiratory failure (CRF) shares similar mechanisms for hypoxemia (V/Q mismatching) and hypercapnia (load/capacity imbalances). In the latter case, that is a resulting ineffective breathing pattern of a lower tidal volume (V_T) and higher respiratory rate preventing excessive inspiratory effort. In many disorders these two mechanisms overlap, as they do in severe COPD [42].

Both hypoxia and hypercapnia are better tolerated in chronic conditions than in acute conditions as a result of compensatory mechanisms. In the former, compensatory mechanisms including erythrocytosis, angiogenesis, and increased perfused capillary density tend to reduce the ill effects of hypoxemia [43]. Where a normal subject is unlikely to remain conscious with a PaO_2 less than 27 mm Hg, patients with CRF have been noted to remain conscious with PaO_2 values approaching 30 mm Hg. This has also been shown in mountaineers, who have remained conscious as low as a PaO_2 of 20 mm Hg [44].

Patients with chronic hypercapnia are forced to breathe against increased forces imposed by their lung, chest wall, or both. This increase in $PaCO_2$ is most common in COPD; however, the mechanism is not fully understood. Early work suggested that ventilator insufficiency rose from (i) changes in the chemical environment of the respiratory center [45] or (ii) through abnormal mechanics that prevented adequate ventilation [46]. Subsequent work has shown that obtainment of normocapnia by voluntarily increasing ventilation has called into question these theories. It has been shown that a shift in the balance of mechanical impediments leading to the possibility of early fatigue leads to alterations in V_T, and that this leads to changes in medical activation systems to optimize the remaining muscle performance to prevent severe fatigue [47].

Acute respiratory failure can develop in patients with chronic respiratory failure from increased resistance or impaired respiratory drive. Most commonly, dynamic hyperinflation develops secondary to shortened expiratory time or airflow impedance. This hyperinflation leads to ventilation on a steeper portion of the pressure/volume curve of the lung, leading to increased inspiratory load and decreased inspiratory muscle advantage [31]. Similarly, patients with neuromuscular etiology to their chronic respiratory failure can have increased loads secondary to infection, and not necessarily of respiratory etiology, in both cases resulting in excessive energy demands from respiratory muscles compared to available energy and respiratory failure.

2.1.5 Summary

Acute and chronic respiratory failure develop when there is failure of gas exchange, pump, or excessive energy consumption in states of hypoperfusion. With an understanding of the etiology the clinician can tailor treatment. Physicians should recognize that with support for respiratory failure by mechanical ventilation respiratory muscle strength can be weakened, so prompt liberation from mechanical ventilation is key to improving long-term outcomes from acute respiratory failure [48].

2.1.6 Case presentation revisited

Our patient had chronic respiratory failure secondary to quadriplegia. He developed acute hypoxic respiratory failure secondary to infection with 2009 H1N1 requiring support with mechanical ventilation due to energy consumption in excess of available energy. After an attempt at extubation to NIV (a return to his home respiratory support) it was determined that his need for ventilator support was in excess of what he had previously needed. He underwent percutaneous tracheostomy and was discharged with home mechanical ventilation after family education. Prior to tracheostomy it was determined that diaphragmatic pacing was not a viable option.

References

1. McIntyre, N. (1998) Mechanical ventilation: the next 50 years. *Repir. Care*, **43**, 490–493.
2. Make, B.J., Hill, N.S., Goldberg, A.I. *et al.* (1998) Mechanical ventilation beyond the intensive care unit. Report of a consensus conference of the American College of Chest Physicians. *Chest*, **113** (5 Suppl.), 289S–344S.
3. Arias, E. and Smith, B. (2003) Deaths: preliminary data for 2001. *Natl. Vital Stat. Rep.*, **51**, 1–44.
4. Wingo, P.A., Cardinez, C.J., Landis, S.H. *et al.* (2003) Long-term trends in cancer mortality in the United States, 1930–1998. *Cancer*, **97** (12 Suppl.), 3133–3275.
5. Moss, M. and Mannino, D.M. (2002) Race and gender differences in acute respiratory distress syndrome deaths in the United States: an analysis of multiple-cause mortality data (1979–1996). *Crit. Care Med.*, **30** (8), 1679–1685.
6. The SUPPORT Principal Investigators (1995) A controlled trial to improve care for seriously ill hospitalized patients. The study to understand prognoses and preferences for outcomes and risks of treatments (SUPPORT). *JAMA*, **274** (20), 1591–1598.
7. Somogyi-Zalud, E., Zhong, Z., Lynn, J. *et al.* (2000) Dying with acute respiratory failure or multiple organ system failure with sepsis. *J. Am. Geriatr. Soc.*, **48** (5 Suppl.), S140–S145.
8. Hamel, M.B., Phillips, R.S., Davis, R.B. *et al.* (2000) Outcomes and cost-effectiveness of ventilator support and aggressive care for patients with acute respiratory failure due to pneumonia or acute respiratory distress syndrome. *Am. J. Med.*, **109** (8), 614–620.

9. Herridge, M.S., Cheung, A.M., Tansey, C.M. *et al.* (2003) One-year outcomes in survivors of the acute respiratory distress syndrome. *N. Engl. J. Med.*, **348** (8), 683–693.

10. Connors, A.F., Dawson, N.V., Thomas, C. *et al.* (1996) Outcomes following acute exacerbation of severe chronic obstructive lung disease. *Am. J. Respir. Crit. Care Med.*, **154** (4 Pt 1), 959–967.

11. Hall, J., Schmidt, G. and Wood, L. (2005) Principles of Critical Care, 3rd edn. McGraw-Hill, New York.

12. Frumin, M.J., Epstein, R.M. and Cohen, G. (1959) Apneic oxygenation in man. *Anesthesiology*, **20**, 789–798.

13. Covelli, H.D., Nessan, V.J. and Tuttle, W.K. (1983) Oxygen derived variables in acute respiratory failure. *Crit. Care Med.*, **11** (8), 646–649.

14. Cane, R.D., Shapiro, B.A., Templin, R. and Walther, K. (1988) Unreliability of oxygen tension-based indices in reflecting intrapulmonary shunting in critically ill patients. *Crit. Care Med.*, **16** (12), 1243–1245.

15. Horovitz, J., Carrico, C. and Shires, G. (1974) Pulmonary response to majoy injury. *Arch. Surg.*, **108**, 349–355.

16. Räsänen, J., Downs, J.B., Malec, D.J. *et al.* (1988) Real-time continuous estimation of gas exchange by dual oximetry. *Intensive Care Med.*, **14** (2), 118–122.

17. Zetterström, H. (1988) Assessment of the efficiency of pulmonary oxygenation. The choice of oxygenation index. *Acta Anaesthesiol. Scand.*, **32** (7), 579–584.

18. Nickerson, B.G., Sarkisian, C. and Tremper, K. (1988) Bias and precision of pulse oximeters and arterial oximeters. *Chest*, **93** (3), 515–517.

19. Morris, R.W., Nairn, M. and Torda, T.A. (1989) A comparison of fifteen pulse oximeters. Part I: a clinical comparison; part II: a test of performance under conditions of poor perfusion. *Anaesth. Intensive Care*, **17** (1), 62–73.

20. Van de Louw, A., Cracco, C., Cerf, C. *et al.* (2001) Accuracy of pulse oximetry in the intensive care unit. *Intensive Care Med.*, **27** (10), 1606–1613.

21. Webb, R.K., Ralston, A.C. and Runciman, W.B. (1991) Potential errors in pulse oximetry. II. Effects of changes in saturation and signal quality. *Anaesthesia*, **46** (3), 207–212.

22. Clayton, D.G., Webb, R.K., Ralston, A.C. *et al.* (1991) A comparison of the performance of 20 pulse oximeters under conditions of poor perfusion. *Anaesthesia*, **46** (1), 3–10.

23. Smatlak, P. and Knebel, A.R. (1998) Clinical evaluation of noninvasive monitoring of oxygen saturation in critically ill patients. *Am. J. Crit. Care*, **7** (5), 370–373.

24. Vicenzi, M.N., Gombotz, H., Krenn, H. *et al.* (2000) Transesophageal versus surface pulse oximetry in intensive care unit patients. *Crit. Care Med.*, **28** (7), 2268–2270.

25. Wagner, P.D., Dantzker, D.R., Dueck, R. *et al.* (1977) Ventilation-perfusion inequality in chronic obstructive pulmonary disease. *J. Clin. Invest.*, **59** (2), 203–216.

26. Torres, A., Reyes, A., Roca, J. *et al.* (1989) Ventilation-perfusion mismatching in chronic obstructive pulmonary disease during ventilator weaning. *Am. Rev. Respir. Dis.*, **140** (5), 1246–1250.

27. Rodriguez-Roisin, R., Ballester, E., Roca, J. *et al.* (1989) Mechanisms of hypoxemia in patients with status asthmaticus requiring mechanical ventilation. *Am. Rev. Respir. Dis.*, **139** (3), 732–739.

28. Agustí, A.G., Roca, J., Gea, J. *et al.* (1991) Mechanisms of gas-exchange impairment in idiopathic pulmonary fibrosis. *Am. Rev. Respir. Dis.*, **143** (2), 219–225.

29. Roussos, C., Fixley, M., Gross, D. and Macklem, P.T. (1979) Fatigue of inspiratory muscles and their synergic behavior. *J. Appl. Physiol.*, **46** (5), 897–904.

30. Jardim, J., Farkas, G., Prefaut, C. *et al.* (1981) The failing inspiratory muscles under normoxic and hypoxic conditions. *Am. Rev. Respir. Dis.*, **124** (3), 274–279.

31. Roussos, C. and Koutsoukou, A. (2003) Respiratory failure. *Eur. Respir. J.*, **22** (47 Suppl.), 3–14.

32. Alexander, J.I., Horton, P.W., Millar, W.T. *et al.* (1972) The effect of upper abdominal surgery on the relationship of airway closing point to end tidal position. *Clin. Sci.*, **43** (2), 137–141.

33. Ali, J., Weisel, R.D., Layug, A.B. *et al.* (1974) Consequences of postoperative alterations in respiratory mechanics. *Am. J. Surg.*, **128** (3), 376–382.

34. Ford, G.T., Whitelaw, W.A., Rosenal, T.W. *et al.* (1983) Diaphragm function after upper abdominal surgery in humans. *Am. Rev. Respir. Dis.*, **127** (4), 431–436.

35. Craig, D.B., Wahba, W.M., Don, H.F. *et al.* (1971) "Closing volume" and its relationship to gas exchange in seated and supine positions. *J. Appl. Physiol.*, **31** (5), 717–721.

36. Hoeppner, V.H., Cooper, D.M., Zamel, N. *et al.* (1974) Relationship between elastic recoil and closing volume in smokers and nonsmokers. *Am. Rev. Respir. Dis.*, **109** (1), 81–86.

37. Ali, J., Yaffe, C.S. and Serrette, C. (1981) The effect of transcutaneous electric nerve stimulation on postoperative pain and pulmonary function. *Surgery*, **89** (4), 507–512.

38. Marini, J.J., Pierson, D.J. and Hudson, L.D. (1979) Acute lobar atelectasis: a prospective comparison of fiberoptic bronchoscopy and respiratory therapy. *Am. Rev. Respir. Dis.*, **119** (6), 971–978.

39. Warner, M.A., Divertie, M.B. and Tinker, J.H. (1984) Preoperative cessation of smoking and pulmonary complications in coronary artery bypass patients. *Anesthesiology*, **60** (4), 380–383.

40. Ward, M.E., Magder, S.A. and Hussain, S.N. (1992) Oxygen delivery-independent effect of blood flow on diaphragm fatigue. *Am. Rev. Respir. Dis.*, **145** (5), 1058–1063.

41. Gottfried, S.B., Rossi, A., Higgs, B.D. *et al.* (1985) Noninvasive determination of respiratory system mechanics during mechanical ventilation for acute respiratory failure. *Am. Rev. Respir. Dis.*, **131** (3), 414–420.

42. Rossi, A., Poggi, R. and Roca, J. (2002) Physiologic factors predisposing to chronic respiratory failure. *Respir. Care Clin. N. Am.*, **8** (3), 379–404.

43. Beers, M. (1998) Oxygen therapy and pulmonary oxygen toxicity, in Fishman's Pulmonary Diseases and Disorders (eds P.A. Fishman, J.A. Elias, J.A. Fishman *et al.*), McGraw-Hill, New York, pp. 1627–1642.

44. Nunn, J.F. (1993) Hypoxia, in Nunn's Applied Respiratory Physiology (4th edn), Butterworth-Heinemann, Edinburgh, pp. 529–536.

45. Scott, R. (1920) Observations on the pathologic physiology of chronic pulmonary emphysema. *Arch. Intern. Med.*, **26**, 544–560.

46. Christie, R. (1934) The elastic properties of emphysematous lung and their clinical significance. *J. Clin. Invest.*, **13**, 295–231.

47. Bégin, P. and Grassino, A. (1991) Inspiratory muscle dysfunction and chronic hypercapnia in chronic obstructive pulmonary disease. *Am. Rev. Respir. Dis.*, **143** (5 Pt 1), 905–912.

48. Vassilakopoulos, T., Zakynthinos, S. and Roussos, C. (2006) Bench-to-bedside review: weaning failure – should we rest the respiratory muscles with controlled mechanical ventilation? *Crit. Care*, **10** (1), 204–204.

2.2 Airway management

2.2a Bag-Valve-Mask (BVM) assisted ventilation

Drew A. MacGregor

Pulmonary, Critical Care, Allergy, and Immunology, Wake Forest University, Winston-Salem, NC, USA

2.2a.1 Introduction

The primary concept of basic resuscitation begins with Airway, Breathing, and Circulation (ABC). Within any healthcare facility, the primary means of providing support for the initial ABC is to open the airway and use a Bag-Valve-Mask (BVM) system to provide airway support and assistance with breathing. Successful bag-mask ventilation depends on three things: a patent airway, an adequate mask seal, and proper ventilation (i.e., proper rate and tidal volumes for the clinical situation). Providing positive pressure ventilation with a BVM device can be a lifesaving maneuver, and while seemingly simple, the technique requires an understanding of the airway anatomy, the equipment, and the indications, as well as a respect for the potential complications. A full review of Basic Life Support and CPR is beyond the scope of this book [1], but the mechanics of using the BVM device will be reviewed.

A Practical Guide to Mechanical Ventilation, First Edition.
Edited by Jonathon D. Truwit and Scott K. Epstein.
© 2011 John Wiley & Sons, Ltd. Published 2011 by John Wiley & Sons, Ltd.

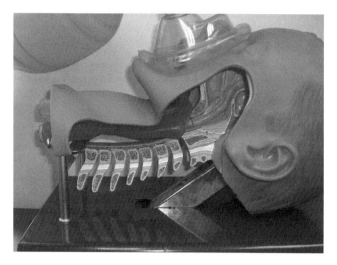

Figure 2.2a.1   Occlusion of the airway caused by excessive downward pressure from the BVM device. Simple downward compression of the mask onto the patient's face may push the mandible and base of tongue posteriorly, which can occlude the airway and make assisted ventilation more difficult.

Providing an adequate airway is the first step in BVM-assisted ventilation, as soft tissue airway obstruction in the unconscious patient is a very common occurrence. Prolapse of the tongue into the posterior pharynx and loss of muscular tone in the soft palate [2, 3] create a functional airway obstruction that prevents gas movement into the trachea. Perhaps the greatest mistake made by providers is to simply press the mask against the face, apply pressure, and begin squeezing the bag. This positioning of the mask and patient applies posterior pressure to the mandible, which further displaces the base of the tongue and larynx backwards worsening the airway obstruction, making adequate ventilation very difficult to achieve (Figure 2.2a.1). This posterior motion of the mandible will not be overcome with the use of a nasal or oral airway. Instead, the optimal positioning to achieve a patent airway is the so-called "sniffing position" that includes forward extension of the lower neck, protrusion of the chin forward and extension of the head posteriorly. Providers of ventilatory support can achieve this position by two common methods – head tilt–chin lift or jaw thrust.

2.2a.2   Head tilt–chin lift

In the provider manual for Basic Life Support for Healthcare Providers [1] the American Heart Association suggests the provider approach the patient from the side and use one hand to press against the forehead and tilt the head back while using two fingers of the other hand under the bony part of the jaw at the mentum

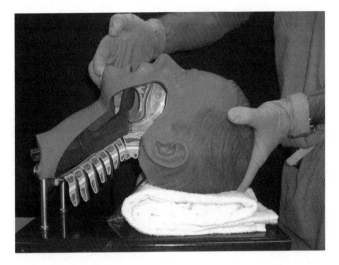

Figure 2.2a.2 Head tilt–chin lift maneuver to open airway. Tilting the head back with one hand while lifting the chin forward with the other hand allows the tongue and soft tissues to be pulled forward, increasing the opportunity for air movement through the pharynx into the trachea.

to lift the chin forward. By pulling the mandible forward, the tongue is also pulled forward and the larynx is brought more into a straight line, and has been shown to significantly improve airway patency [4] (Figure 2.2a.2). In this position the provider can observe the chest for respiratory effort and to listen at the mouth and nose for air movement. In addition, with the rescuer at the side of the patient, the head tilt–chin lift also provides adequate positioning for mouth-to-mouth or mouth-to-mask resuscitation. It is important to recognize that flexion of the lower cervical spine with extension of the head should only be used in patients who do not have cervical spine injuries.

2.2a.3 Jaw thrust

A more efficient way to achieve the sniffing position for use of a BVM is for the provider to be positioned above the patient's head and put the two or three fingertips posterior to the base of the mandible and lift the jaw forward. This maneuver also tends to tilt the head backwards and allows the index fingers and thumbs to form a circle around the mask to apply pressure, allowing for a more complete seal. By using both hands to position the head and jaw, a second person is required to compress the bag for ventilation. If there is no other person to perform this function, a rescuer can use one hand to support the jaw thrust and apply the seal while using the other hand to compress the bag (Figure 2.2a.3). From a practical perspective, this positioning can be described as bringing the face and jaw forward to create a seal with the mask rather than pushing the mask down against the face to create

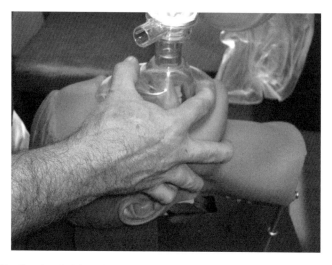

Figure 2.2a.3   One-handed jaw thrust maneuver with BVM-assisted ventilation. The middle, ring and little fingers are positioned along the angle of the jaw, providing anterior movement while the thumb and index finger apply the seal with the mask.

the seal. In addition, two hands combining to pull the jaw forward and seal the mask allows for the provider to use less neck extension for patients with suspected cervical spine injuries, and this maneuver can be used in patients who are still immobilized in a cervical collar.

Another method of two-handed mask technique uses the thenar eminences and bases of the palms to hold the mask in place. With the base of the hands and thumbs on each side of the mask, the four remaining fingers are able to reach the mandible to provide chin lift and jaw thrust maneuvers (Figure 2.2a.4). This technique requires less stress on weaker fingers, minimizing provider fatigue, and enables four fingers to perform the chin lift and jaw thrust. As with any of the airway positioning maneuvers, the provider's palms, fingers, nor the mask cushion should rest on the patient's eyes during bag-mask ventilation, as this can cause damage to the eyes.

2.2a.4   Face mask

The mask used in BVM-assisted ventilation should be sized to make contact with the patient's face in four areas – the bony bridge of the nose, both malar eminences of the cheeks, and the mandibular-alveolar ridge. Too large a mask can allow large air leaks to occur at the sides or air to be blown into the eyelids. Too small a mask can make an adequate seal impossible over the mouth. Most masks have an inflatable cushion that adds flexibility that allows the mask to mold to the facial contours. Over-inflation of the cushion may lessen the adaptability of the mask to mold to

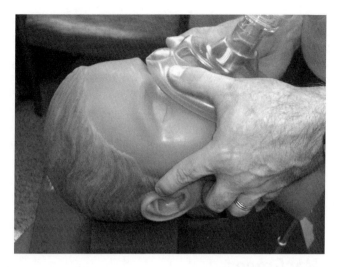

Figure 2.2a.4 Two-handed jaw thrust maneuver for BVM ventilation, with the provider positioned at the patient's side. The thenar eminences and thumbs allow for tight seal against the face, while the fingers can elevate the jaw to maintain airway patency.

the face, while under-inflation may put excessive pressure on the contact points of the face.

2.2a.5 Ventilation

The resuscitation bag that is part of the BVM system, commonly referred to as an "Ambu-bag", should be appropriately sized to provide adequate tidal volumes for the patient. Most adult-sized bags inflate to a volume between 1.0 and 2.0l, but the volume administered by the provider can vary greatly, even with providers who are proficient in resuscitation procedures [5]. Over-ventilation should be avoided, as the subsequent respiratory alkalosis can further complicate the resuscitative efforts, and the American Heart Association Basic Life Support guidelines recommend only six to ten breaths per minute [1]. Adjustments to the depth of ventilation (tidal volume) and the frequency should be made according to the patient's comorbidities and physiologic variables.

References

1. BLS for Healthcare Providers Student Manual. (2006) American Heart Association, Dallas.
2. Shorten, G.D., Opie, N.J., Graziotti, P. *et al.* (1994) Assessment of upper airway anatomy in awake, sedated and anaesthetised patients using magnetic resonance imaging. *Anaesth. Intensive Care*, **22**, 165–169.

3. Mathru, M., Esch, O., Lang, J. *et al.* (1996) Magnetic resonance imaging of the upper airway. Effects of propofol anesthesia and nasal continuous positive airway pressure in humans. *Anesthesiology*, **84**, 273–279.
4. Guildner, C.W. (1976) Resuscitation – opening the airway. A comparative study of techniques for opening an airway obstructed by the tongue. *JACEP*, **5**, 588–590.
5. Lee, H.M., Cho, K.H., Choi, Y.H. *et al.* (2008) Can you deliver accurate tidal volume by manual resuscitator? *Emerg. Med. J.*, **25**, 632–634.

2.2b Endotracheal intubation

Drew A. MacGregor

Pulmonary, Critical Care, Allergy, and Immunology, Wake Forest University, Winston-Salem, NC, USA

2.2b.1 Case presentation

A 50-year-old male with achondroplasia is in respiratory distress from pneumonia. He has had rigors, night sweats and is coughing up green sputum. On examination his blood pressure is 80/60 mm Hg, respiratory rate 36 breaths/min, heart rate 130 beats/min, temperature 39 °C and oxygen saturation 85% on room air. He has E to A changes in the right base. Chest X-ray reveals an infiltrate within right lower and middle lobes. He is felt to be fatiguing and upon discussing options he agrees with intubation. After rapid sequence induction and successful bag-valve-mask ventilation several attempts at intubation are unsuccessful.

Trying to describe all the details of endotracheal intubation is like asking someone to describe the evaluation of a chest radiograph – the techniques can be explained in relatively simple terms, but to fully understand how to do it, it is necessary to develop some experience through trial and error. Along that same logic, there are millions of teaching X-rays out there to look at and learn from, and within any training program there are many different mannequins available for the opportunity to practice the art of intubation. If this segment of the book conveys any message about intubation, it should be to find as many different mannequins (from the bronchoscopy simulators to advanced cardiac life support (ACLS) mannequins to airway cutaways to anesthesiology simulators) as possible, and practice with every

Table 2.2b.1 Anatomical considerations that may indicate difficult intubation.

Short neck, especially if muscular or "thick"
Thyromental distance less than 3 cm (short chin) and/or inability to protrude mandible forward
Presence of "overbite" – maxillary incisors anterior to mandibular
Large upper incisors or poor oral opening (inter-incisor distance)
High arched or narrow hard palate
Poor neck excursion (inability to touch chin to chest or extend neck)
Inability to see uvula on open-mouth examination
Facial fractures, poor dental hygiene, and prior airway injuries

blade, handle, and circumstance that can be created. Also, contact the Pathology Department and ask if they have an anatomy laboratory that will allow intubation skills to be practiced on newly deceased patients (an increasingly common simulation scenario). Finally, remember that the average anesthesiologist intubates between one and 20 tracheas a day, so get to know your colleagues in that department and ask them if they can help teach you, give you pointers, let you intubate patients in the operating rooms, or assist you when you do the procedure outside of the operating rooms.

There are anatomical considerations that have been associated with difficult intubations. These are listed in Table 2.2b.1. Patients with one of more of these variations in anatomy should be considered at risk for failed tracheal intubation, and should alert the provider to prepare more than one plan. The American Society of Anesthesiology has an entire algorithm for difficult airways; this can be accessed on the Web at http://www.asahq.org/publicationsandservices.

A great piece of advice is that evaluation of these risks and consideration for surgical airway as a back-up plan of action should be done early in the planning stage, not when there are two bloody tubes sitting next to the head following failed attempts at intubation, and a patient whose oxygen saturation is falling precipitously.

2.2b.2 Positioning the patient

Proper positioning of the patient for orotracheal intubation requires flexion of the base of the neck combined with extension of the head (the sniffing position, Chapter 2.2a). Limitation in either the flexion or extension needs to be evaluated prior to initiating airway manipulation. Acute trauma commonly requires the patient to be placed into a cervical collar until adequate evaluation for ligamentous injuries of the neck can be performed. Many diseases (e.g., rheumatoid arthritis) cause significant reductions in neck mobility and impose additional risks on the procedure of intubation. In dire crisis situations, an evaluation of patient positioning, airway mechanics, anatomy, and adequate preparation for endotracheal intubation might not be possible. If, however, there is time to plan, proper attention to these variables may save a life, and may prevent future legal actions!

The anatomy of intubation of the trachea involves three different axis lines: the oral axis, which is the plane defined by the hard palate and tongue; the pharyngeal axis that conforms to the posterior pharyngeal wall; and the tracheal axis. In a patient who is lying supine on a horizontal surface without head support, the oral axis is approximately 90° perpendicular to the bed, the pharyngeal axis is on a rising angle from the posterior pharynx to the larynx, and the tracheal axis is on a declining angle moving caudad from the larynx (Figure 2.2b.1). Attempting to intubate the trachea from this position would require >90° angulation from the oral cavity through the vocal cords into the trachea, a very difficult proposition. Instead, placement of pillows, pads, or other positioning aids underneath the occiput of the head brings the head and neck forward. This brings the tracheal and pharyngeal axes into a nearly straight line, which remains at a fairly sharp angle to the oral axis (Figure 2.2b.2). However, when a jaw-thrust head-tilt maneuver is then performed, the oral axis nearly aligns to the pharyngeal and tracheal axes (Figure 2.2b.3). This allows for a much easier line of sight to the larynx and easier passage of an endotracheal tube into the airway.

A very common mistake made by providers with less experience is to put pillows or pads underneath the shoulder blades, or even pull the patient beyond the head of the bed so that the head can fall backwards below the plane of the bed. While this allows an improved visualization of the oropharynx, it moves the tracheal axis to an even greater angle to the oral axis. Providers who attempt intubation in this

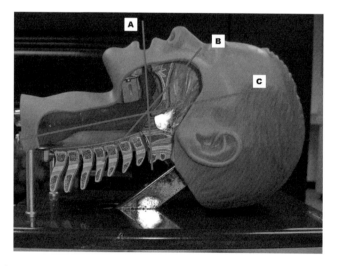

Figure 2.2b.1   Airway axes in a patient resting supine without head support. The cervical spine remains nearly horizontal. The oral axis (A) creates a sharp angle with the pharyngeal axis (B) and even sharper angle with the tracheal axis (C).

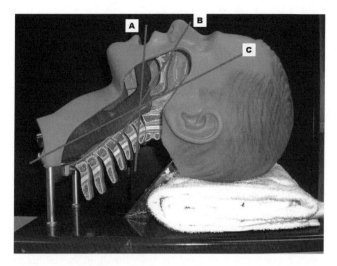

Figure 2.2b.2 Airway axes with patient supine and head support under occiput, the so-called "sniffing position". The cervical spine flexes forward at the shoulders, and the head extends backwards. Note the improved alignment of the oral (A), pharyngeal (B) and tracheal (C) axes, allowing for easier air entry into the trachea.

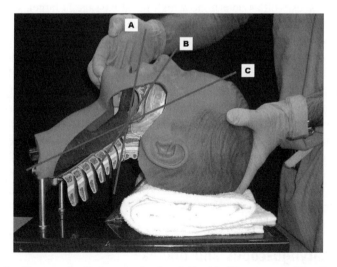

Figure 2.2b.3 Airway axis alignment using head tilt–chin lift maneuver. The alignment of the oral (A), pharyngeal (B) and tracheal (C) axes is greatly improved by this simple maneuver, allowing a more patent airway for assisted ventilation. Also note the increased angulation of the cervical spine with this airway manipulation.

position routinely find that the glottic opening is "too far anterior" to allow for intubation. An experienced airway manager can rectify the situation with the simple act of moving the pillows from behind the shoulders to behind the occiput, bringing the head forward and creating a much more desirable view of the vocal cords.

2.2b.3   Nasotracheal intubation

Any provider facing the potential of obtaining an artificial airway for the use of mechanical ventilation should be familiar with intubating the trachea through the nose. In its simplistic form, the skills required to accomplish nasotracheal intubation are the ability to push an endotracheal tube through the nose and the ability to recognize if the tube is in the trachea. This maneuver does not require special positioning of the patient – which may be ideal for patients with neck injury, or patients trapped in the field following trauma. However, difficulty or mistakes during the intubation process may result in uncontrollable nasal bleeding, inability to achieve tracheal intubation, and trauma to the glottic structures, which may make subsequent oral intubation much more difficult.

For nasotracheal intubation, the patient must continue to breathe spontaneously. If time allows, using a vasoconstrictive agent (neosynephrine nasal spray, oxymeta-zoline, others) and a topical anesthetic (lidocaine, cocaine, others) will decrease the bleeding potential and increase patient tolerance of the procedure. While cotton swabs can reach deeper into the nasal passages, application of lidocaine jelly to a gloved little finger that is inserted into the nares can help dilate and anesthetize the nasal structures, as well as determine which nasal passage is larger. Once the nose is anesthetized, a lubricated endotracheal tube is inserted, with the direction of passage being parallel to the hard palate (not superiorly) with gentle pressure and twisting to assist with passage. As the distal end of the tube reaches the glottic region, exhaled gas will cause "fogging" of the tube. The tube should be advanced during inhalation, and successful intubation of the trachea is commonly associated with coughing, ongoing misting of the tube during exhalation, and carbon dioxide that can be verified using a disposable carbon dioxide detector. Esophageal intuba-tion should be recognized by the absence of audible breath sound through the tube, no misting in the tube, and no exhaled carbon dioxide detection. It is not uncom-mon that several passes will be required for ultimate success, but excessive attempts are likely to induce more damage to the glottic structures, and should not be done if other alternatives are available.

2.2b.4   Laryngoscopes and blades

Dozens of creative engineers have attempted to perfect the laryngoscope used to intubate the trachea and, as such, there are many different models – far more than can be described in this book. Virtually all models of intubating laryngoscopes are

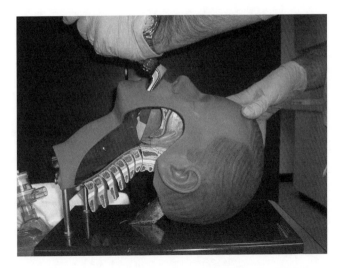

Figure 2.2b.4 Visualization of the vocal cords using a Miller (straight) laryngoscope blade. Moving the handle at 45° away from the provider (in the plane of the handle) raises the base of the tongue and anterior pharynx out of the line of site, allowing for direct visualization of the glottic structures.

designed as variations of two blades: the Miller (straight) laryngoscope blade or the MacIntosh (curved) laryngoscope blade. Each has potential advantages and limitations, but the blade of choice is almost always the one that the individual feels most comfortable with and has the most experience using (remember the practice on different mannequins!)

The Miller blade is straight, and the tip is somewhat pointed, which allows the blade to be used to directly lift the epiglottis anteriorly, giving a straight-on view of the vocal cords. For this view to be obtained, the oral, pharyngeal and tracheal axes need to be virtually in a straight line, giving a good view of the vocal cords (Figure 2.2b.4). Once this view is achieved, placement of the endotracheal tube through the cords is very easy. Another advantage of the straight blade is that the height of the manifold (the portion closest to the handle) is lower than the curved blades. Thus, less separation of the teeth is required to place the laryngoscope into the pharynx. Disadvantages of the straight blade include the fact that the side wall of the blade is curved, so the view down the blade is nearly circular, creating the sense of looking into a tunnel. Large tongues and swelling in the laryngeal area may lessen the view as tissues surround the distal end of the blade, limiting the view of the glottic structures. Another potential problem is the fact that the straight blade exits the oropharynx directly in line with the upper teeth, which leads to the risk of using the teeth as a fulcrum to direct the tip of the laryngoscope.

The MacIntosh (Mac) blade is curved similar to the natural airway. The blade has greater width than the straight blade, the side of the blade is straight, and the

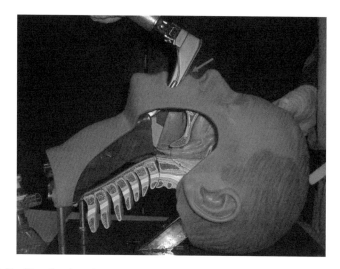

Figure 2.2b.5 Visualization of the vocal cords using a MacIntosh (curved) laryngoscope blade. Care should be taken to avoid a "rocking" motion with the laryngoscope as the blade is in very close proximity to the front incisors (arrow), but rather, the handle should be lifted forward and upward along the plane of the laryngoscope handle.

tip is broader. These features allow for a considerably wider view of the laryngeal structures. The tip is designed to slide into the vallecula anterior to the epiglottis, which is then lifted to expose the vocal cords and glottis (Figure 2.2b.5). The curved design of the Mac blade lessens the proximity of the manifold to the front incisors, but the manifold is also much taller with the curved blades, requiring greater oral opening and separation of the teeth. As with the straight blade, the nature of the curved blade is to use the front incisors as a fulcrum to "rock" the blade to improve airway visualization. Either blade can easily damage the teeth, but an additional risk of this movement of the blade against the teeth is to take the distal end of the blade further out of view from the mouth, thus worsening the intubating view.

For either blade, the size of the blade is dependent upon the anticipated distance from the incisors to the epiglottis – a distance that is *not* usually significantly affected by obesity. For short necks, thyromental distances less than three finger breadths long, and individuals with small chins, a Mac No. 2 (82 mm, measured inside the blade, from the handle to the tip) or Miller #1 (79 mm) are usually adequately long to visualize the glottis. Mac#3 (101 mm) and Miller #2 (132 mm) blades are the most common sizes used for "normal" sized adults. The Mac #4 (135 mm) and the Miller #3 (172 mm) are quite long and reach much deeper into the glottis, raising the potential for traumatic injury to the vocal cords and other structures. A Miller #4 (182 mm) is extremely long, at its use should be reserved for individuals with great experience in airway management (i.e., anesthesiologists).

Choosing which blade to attach to the laryngoscope is similar to choosing between an automatic transmission and a manual gear shift in a car – each has theoretical advantages and disadvantages. Being skilled in the use of both types of blades is ideal, allowing for maximal chances of successful airway visualization in a multitude of different clinical settings, and again, multiple sessions practicing on different mannequins offers the best opportunity to define which blade works best for an individual.

2.2b.5   Preparation of the ETT

The size of the endotracheal tube (ETT) directly correlates with laryngeal injury during mechanical ventilation, so there is a balance between using a tube large enough to ensure unobstructed air movement and potential insertion of a broncho-scope or other airway devices yet small enough to minimize potential laryngeal and vocal cord injury. Most bronchoscopes will pass through a 7.0 mm inner diameter ETT, but there will be insufficient cross-sectional area to allow adequate air move-ment around the scope to provide ventilation to the patient. Thus, most intensive care unit practitioners prefer at least a 7.5 mm ETT. The cuff that seals the ETT against the tracheal wall should be verified as functional prior to insertion, but care should be taken to not contaminate the distal end of the ETT prior to its placement into the airway. Lubrication of the ETT and cuff commonly makes insertion through the vocal cords easier.

The ETT tends to be very flexible and, when holding the proximal end, the distal end is somewhat difficult to direct into the airway. Therefore, a flexible, malleable stylet is commonly used to provide stability to the tube. It is common to apply some curvature to the stylet for insertion, the degree of which depends, in part, on the blade being used for intubation. For straight (Miller) blades, the ETT should remain fairly straight to allow for direct insertion. For curved (Mac) blades, a curve that mimics the angle of the blade may allow for easier coursing into the trachea. It has been suggested that ETTs be soaked briefly in hot water to make them softer and more malleable or ice water to make them stiffer and easier to manipulate. If either of these techniques appears to be required, it is suggested that a better view and better alignment of the axes be accomplished instead!

2.2b.6   Laryngoscopy

It is important to remember the three axes involved in endotracheal intubation. A common mistake once the laryngoscope blade is introduced into the posterior pharynx is to rock the handle of the scope towards the provider. This action changes the pharyngeal axis out of the optimal plane, pushing the maxilla posteriorly while moving the base of the tongue and pharynx anteriorly, out of view. This commonly results in failure due to the airway appearing to be "too anterior", as well as increasing the risk of injuring the front incisors. Instead, the movement of the laryngoscope should be to lift the handle forward at an angle of approximately 45° away from the provider with the goal of aligning the oral axis with the pharyngeal axis by moving the tongue and anterior pharynx forward, providing a view of the vocal cords. The angle of movement is usual the plane defined by the handle of the laryngoscope. The goal is to manipulate the tip of the laryngoscope blade, not the handle, to bring the appropriate glottic structures into view.

2.2b.7 Cricoid pressure and BURP

The concept of cricoid pressure to assist with endotracheal intubation is fairly simple – by using the cartilage-supported trachea to compress the esophagus, the provider will lessen the chance of regurgitation of gastric contents into the glottis, and the posterior movement of the trachea will help bring the tracheal axis into better alignment with the oral and pharyngeal axes, making intubation easier. The difficulties of cricoid pressure include the fact that the esophagus at the level of the cricoid cartilage is commonly off to the side, and not directly behind the trachea, and the amount of pressure required to occlude the esophagus to actually prevent emesis from reaching the glottis is sometimes difficult to achieve without compromising the airway. Also, when someone other than the provider using the laryngoscope is pressing on the cricoid, proper alignment of the trachea with the laryngoscopic view is very difficult. The manipulation of the cricoid that tends to be more useful for intubation is the acronym BURP – meaning **B**ackward, **U**pward, **R**ightward **P**ressure on the cricoid. Movement of the cricoid in this fashion tends to bring the trachea more in line with the intubating view to facilitate intubation. Ideally, the provider attempting intubation can hold the laryngoscope with the left hand and use the right hand to manipulate the cricoid. Once the proper alignment is achieved, a second provider can assume the cricoid pressure and hold the position during placement of the ETT. There is considerable debate as to how much pressure to apply to the cricoid cartilage during these maneuvers, but most of the studied reports recommend the equivalent of between 5 and 10 pounds of pressure.

Suggested Reading

1. Benumof, J.L. (1996) *Airway Management: Principles and Practice*, Mosby, St. Louis.
2. Roberts, J.T. (1983) *Fundamentals of Tracheal Intubation*, Grune & Stratton, New York.
3. Longnecker, D.E., Brown, D.L., Newman, M.F. and Zapol, W.M. (2008) *Anesthesiology*, McGraw Hill Professional, New York.

2.2c Cuff leak and laryngeal edema

Scott van Poppel[1] and Drew A. MacGregor[2]

[1] *Critical Care Division, Wake Forest University, Winston-Salem, NC, USA*
[2] *Pulmonary, Critical Care, Allergy, and Immunology, Wake Forest University, Winston-Salem, NC, USA*

2.2c.1 Introduction

Reintubation after a planned (or unplanned) extubation is an independent factor for increased mortality in the intensive care unit patient. One of the most common, and often most frightening, causes of acute respiratory failure immediately after extubation is stridor secondary to laryngeal edema. The speed of the patient's decline is often impressive and, by definition, the situation is now a "difficult airway" scenario. The incidence of post-extubation laryngeal edema/stridor has been placed between 2 and 16% [1]. Those patients at high risk include self-extubations, those who have had prolonged mechanical ventilation (≥10 days), and patients that were intubated in an emergent or traumatic situation [2]. It should be noted that stridor due to laryngeal edema can occur as late as 48 hours after extubation.

The "cuff leak test" was initially developed in children with croup who had significant laryngeal edema. If the child had an audible air movement around an endotracheal tube (ETT) when the cuff was deflated and the child coughed on positive pressure ventilation, extubation was likely to be successful [3]. This was extrapolated to the adult with the same concept: the amount of edema around the deflated cuff of an ETT should be inversely proportional to the air leak around the cuff. Absence of such a cuff leak suggests that edema may already be present and airway occlusion or stridor may occur after extubation. Use of a cuff leak test in every intubated patient is controversial, but it can certainly be useful as an additional piece of information in planning extubation in patients at high risk.

2.2c.2 Measurement

Cuff leak measurements can be done either qualitatively or quantitatively. Both measures have classically been done on using volume control ventilation at with large tidal volumes set on the ventilator (10–15 cc/kg) when the ETT cuff is deflated. Qualitative measurement is simply listening to the trachea for any upper airway sounds or phonation during exhalation of the patient when the ETT cuff is deflated. This qualitative measure can often be enhanced by disconnecting the patient from the ventilator, deflating the cuff, and occluding the tube while asking them to exhale. A potential pitfall of this method is that there may be edema of the larynx that would prevent air movement outside the ETT with passive exhalation, but under high expiratory pressures (i.e., cough) sound may be heard.

Quantitatively the measurement of the cuff leak is made by comparison of the measured inspiratory tidal volume (V_T) and expiratory tidal volume on the above settings. Measurements should be made on the 5–10 breaths following the cuff deflation, and then averaged. The literature is mixed with different set points for expiratory tidal volume changes to define a cuff leak. The numbers used most recently include between 110 and 140 ml. Also, percentages of between 10 and 15% of lost volume have been used in place of absolute numbers [4]. There are no studies looking at a volumetric cuff leak for patients on tidal volumes that are now considered more appropriate in the intensive care unit (i.e., 5–7 cc/kg).

The advantage of the qualitative measurement over the quantitative measurement is its ease of use. Assuming a stable volume control mode, deflating the cuff and listening can be accomplished by nursing and respiratory staff on a frequent and reproducible basis.

A third method of checking for a cuff leak is to deflate the cuff, occlude the ETT and ask the patient to inhale. Patients who can inhale around the ETT with a deflated cuff likely will have maintained airway patency when the ETT is removed. The inhalation cuff leak test has not been studied in the literature, but in our own anecdotal experience in 200 planned extubations, the three patients who failed this mode of cuff leak test and were extubated anyway required urgent reintubation for airway obstruction.

All methods of testing for a cuff leak have potential risk. Secretions from the oropharynx can pool in the recess formed between the ETT and the inflated cuff, and when the cuff is deflated these secretions can be aspirated into the lower airway. Careful suctioning of the oral cavity and back of the throat may lessen the volume of secretions along the ETT. In addition, asking the patient to inhale immediately prior to deflation of the cuff (allowing the patient to potentially cough up any material that falls into the airway) may lessen the potential for aspiration.

2.2c.3 Effectiveness

As mentioned above, the cuff leak test should be used as another variable to weigh into extubation decision making, especially for patients who are at high risk for difficult reintubation. Its *isolated* use in preventing extubation should be carefully weighed with the patients overall course. In three of the more recent studies, including a varied patient population, the sensitivity of predicting extubation failure using a cuff leak ranged between 75 and 88%. The specificity ranged between 72 and 90% [4].

2.2c.4 Treatment of laryngeal edema

Experience in animal studies, and further studies in children have shown improvement in laryngeal edema with the use of corticosteroids. Two recent studies have discussed the use of variable doses of steroids *prior* to extubation and their effect on post-extubation laryngeal edema. Lee and colleagues describe a prospective randomized controlled trial using scheduled dosing of Dexamethasone (5 mg IV every 6 h for four doses) 24 hours prior to planned extubation in response to having no cuff leak. Not only did they show improvement in the incidence of post-extubation laryngeal edema, but they also showed a direct improvement on cuff leak after the first dose of steroids [5]. Francois and colleagues described a regimented low dose of methylprednisolone (20 mg × 4 doses) prior to extubation for all patients (cuff leak was not used). Their results also showed improvement in the incidence of post-extubation laryngeal edema [6].

Thus, it seems that the majority of studies suggest that the lack of either a qualitative of quantitative cuff leak correlates with laryngeal edema and post-extubation stridor or need for reintubation, and dosing steroids for the 24 hours period prior to extubation may offer protective benefit.

References

1. Chung, Y.H., Chao, T.Y., Chiu, C.T. and Lin, M.C. (2006) The cuff-leak test is a simple tool to verify severe laryngeal edema in patients undergoing long-term mechanical ventilation. *Crit. Care Med.*, **34**, 409–414.
2. Jaber, S., Chanques, G., Matecki, S. *et al.* (2003) Post-extubation stridor in intensive care unit patients. Risk factors evaluation and importance of the cuff-leak test. *Intensive Care Med.*, **29**, 69–74.
3. Adderley, R.J. and Mullins, G.C. (1987) When to extubate the croup patient: the "leak" test. *Can. J. Anaesth.*, **34**, 304–306.
4. De Backer, D. (2005) The cuff-leak test: what are we measuring? *Crit. Care*, **9**, 31–33.
5. Lee, C.H., Peng, M.J. and Wu, C.L. (2007) Dexamethasone to prevent postextubation airway obstruction in adults: a prospective, randomized, double-blind, placebo-controlled study. *Crit. Care*, **11**, R72.
6. François, B., Bellissant, E., Gissot, V. et al.; Association des Réanimateurs du Centre-Ouest (ARCO) (2007) 12-h pretreatment with methylprednisolone versus placebo for prevention of postextubation laryngeal oedema: a randomised double-blind trial. *Lancet*, **369**, 1083–1089.

2.2d The difficult airway

Jonathon D. Truwit

Division of Pulmonary and Critical Care Medicine, University of Virginia, Charlottesville, VA, USA

2.2d.1 Introduction

Encountering a difficult airway amid intubation in a critically ill patient is a terrifying experience. The inexperienced operator commonly follows one of two pathways, both occurring while his or her pulse is racing: (i) persistent attempts to intubate while using direct laryngoscopy or (ii) oxygenation and ventilation with bag-valve-mask (BVM) while mentally processing through an array of adjuncts for a difficult intubation that could be used. An experienced operator approaches the case differently by following an algorithm that calls for assessing the need for intubation, likelihood of a difficult airway, preparing for a difficult intubation and knowing how to access backup support. After a limited number of unsuccessful attempts the experienced operator returns to oxygenating and ventilating with BVM, as he or she did before and between attempts, and calmly returns to the algorithm.

2.2d.2 Assessing the need for intubation

Patients may require intubation for ventilator or oxygenation failure as well as for airway protection. The decision to intubate requires clinical judgment, evaluating the risks and benefits to the patient. While laboratory data can be helpful in making decisions, there are no threshold values that dictate when to intubate. When intubation is for reasons other than protection of airway or upper airway obstruction, a trial of noninvasive mechanical ventilation should be considered.

2.2d.3 Assessing likelihood of difficult intubation

The time permitted for evaluation of a patient's airway is inversely correlated with the urgency of need for intubation. In the critical care arena time is limited when the moment arrives, but often assessments can be done prior to the development of emergent conditions. In the emergency department airway assessments are more difficult to complete, as patients are often unable to follow commands or have their cervical spine restricted. Levitan *et al.* found that only 32% of patients intubated in an urban emergency department were able to follow commands while also not having their cervical spine restricted [1]. Thus more than two-thirds could not be assessed for Mallampati scores and neck mobility.

Factors influencing difficult intubations include long upper incisors, prominent overbite, inability of patient to bring mandibular incisors in front of maxillary incisors, Mallampati class >II, narrow shape of palate, stiff mandibular space, thyromental distance <3 finger breadths (7 cm), short or thick neck, unstable neck, and reduced neck mobility as measured by inability of patient to touch chin to chest or extend the neck [2, 3]. While no variable, nor combination of variables, is reliably predictive of a difficult intubation, their absence is reassuring. As only 30% of emergent intubations can be assessed as such, Murphy and Walls introduced LEMON airway assessment protocol: **l**ook, [**e**] **M**allampati class, **o**bstruction and **n**eck mobility [4].

2.2d.4 Preparing for the difficult intubation

Three parts of preparation are environment, plan of action, and an alternate plan of action for unsuccessful intubation. Environment means do you have the right personnel, assignments and equipment. Environment and plan of action are addressed in the endotracheal intubation and BVM ventilation chapters. However, not all intubations go smoothly and a backup plan is needed. The difficult airway algorithm developed by the American Society of Anesthesiologists (ASA) serves this purpose [5]. Familiarity with it and use in simulations should improve operator choices under the stressful circumstances of failed intubations. The first instruction is "call for help," and this may be the most important. Sometimes a different set of hands results in successful intubation alone. It is worth remembering that while critical care physicians may successfully perform several tracheal intubations during a month, anesthesiologists and certified nurse anesthetists commonly perform tracheal intubations several times per day, and utilization of that experience and training can be the most valuable step in addressing the difficult intubation.

The ASA guideline provides many options as to next steps if the initial attempts at tracheal intubation are unsuccessful and separates conditions into emergent and non-emergent. However, it clearly favors use of a laryngeal mask airway (LMA) as the next step if noninvasive ventilation (NIV) or awakening the patient is not appropriate. A different algorithm, put forth by Reynolds and Heffner, moves toward blind nasal tracheal intubation (BNTI) before other adjuncts such as LMA, Gum Elastic Bougie (GEB) or fiberoptic guidance [2].

Combes *et al.* tested another algorithm that separated situations into "cannot intubate" or "cannot ventilate." [6] Those unable to be intubated after two attempts by a senior anesthesiologist but successfully ventilated with BVM ventilation were considered "cannot intubate" and the operator then utilized a GEB. If failing after two attempts with a GEB then an intubating LMA (ILMA) was used. Of those failing to be intubated and unsuccessfully ventilated with BVM, "cannot ventilate", an ILMA was used and the GEB bypassed. Unsuccessful placement of an ILMA was to be followed by percutaneous transtracheal jet ventilation (PTJV). One hundred of 11,257 intubations were recorded as unexpected difficult airways (0.9%). Of the 100 patients, 89 were successfully oxygenated and ventilated with BVM and six required ILMA. In three patients the algorithm was not followed and two patients were awakened. Of the 89 "cannot intubate" patients successfully ventilated with BVM, eighty were intubated using GEB and nine by ILMA after failing with GEB. It appears this simpler protocol was quite successful.

However, often a GEB is not available in intensive care units and critical care physicians may not be as skilled with GEB. Thus, an even simpler algorithm is proposed; (1) call for help, (2) ventilate and oxygenate with BVM, (3) insert an ILMA or LMA, (4) be prepared to use PTJV and (5) regroup at all steps. Should help arrive early, and with a GEB, the GEB can be used as step 2b. After gaining control of the airway at steps 2b or 3, intubation should be pursued and, if at step 4, cricothyroidectomy or tracheostomy should be considered. Although the standard LMA does not permit conversion to an endotracheal tube (ETT) as easily as an ILMA, it does permit the operator to inert a GEB or tube changer for exchange or a bronchoscope loaded with an ETT (requires a large size LMA, removal of struts prior to placement and removal of ventilator tubing-ETT adapter). This algorithm simplifies the decision nodes and requires less expertise at the bedside. However, LMA and PTJV training is needed and simulation is recommended.

Ferson reports that anesthesiologists trained to use an ILMA can successfully intubate patients, following ILMA placement [7]. Blind intubation success rates were 96.5% and with fiberotpic assistance, 100%. The study was carried out at four institutions with operators facile with ILMAs. Of the 254 patients, 70 patients were in Philadelphia collars for unstable cervical spines and another 50 had distorted airways. Another twelve patients were wearing stereotactic frames.

Rosenstock noted that residents with an average of 60 months of training reported they were unable to recall the ASA difficult airway algorithm and half could not demonstrate how to apply PTJV [8]. Three quarters had however, already established an airway with an LMA during emergent conditions when intubation was unsuccessful. Ezri *et al.* published survey results from 452 respondents attending the 1999 ASA annual meeting [9]. 62% were attending anesthesiologists. 86% were familiar and skilled with LMA, 61% with ILMA, 78% with BNTI and only 24% with GEB. Similar data for critical care physicians are lacking.

2.2d.5   Percutaneous Jet Transtracheal Ventilation

Percutaneous Jet Transtracheal Ventilation, which dates back to the 1950s, is a means of maintaining oxygenation along with ventilation. A 12 gage angiocatheter

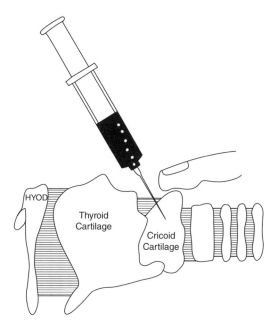

Figure 2.2d.1 Gaining access to the trachea through the cricothyroid membrane for percutaneous transtracheal jet ventilation. After insertion of angiocatheter and needle, the angiocatheter is advanced. Liquid within the syringe makes entry into trachea easily recognizable, as air will bubble into the syringe. (Reproduced with permission [11].)

needle is inserted through the cricothryoid membrane. After entry into the trachea, the angiocatheter is advanced, the needle removed, the angiocatheter secured and tubing from a wall oxygen source (50 psi) is attached. The operator then depresses a valve to open flow from the wall source at a frequency of 12–20 breaths per minute [10]. Expiration occurs passively when oxygen is not jetted in. Boyce and Peters suggests a vessel dilator be used instead of an angiocatheter, as the latter may become kinked and obstruct flow (Figures 2.2d.1 and 2.2d.2) [11]. Kindopp and Nair have devised a setup that relies on items commonly found in the intensive care unit or operating room setting (Figure 2.2d.3) [12]. Once the emergent use of PJTV is accomplished and additional support has arrived, the Seldinger technique can be used to facilitate use of a dilating cricothyrotomy catheter for percutaneous tracheostomy (Chapter 2.2e).

2.2d.6 Conclusion

As most intubations are uncomplicated the clinician might become complacent. However, a difficult airway in a patient with limited reserve, the critically ill patient, is a frightening prospect. To minimize the risk, patients' airways should be assessed

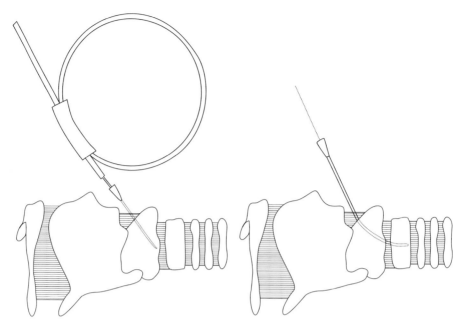

Figure 2.2d.2 The guide wire is inserted through the angiocatheter and after a small incision a vessel dilator from an 9F introducer kit is advanced. (Reproduced with permission [11].)

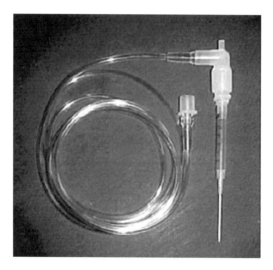

Figure 2.2d.3 Applying percutaneous transtracheal jet ventilation. The oxygen source is usually a wall outlet with 50 psi. Instead a special setup requiring depression of a manual trigger, a 90° elbow adapter with a monitoring port is connected to oxygen tubing. With the monitoring port open, oxygen flows by and does not enter the airway. Occluding the monitoring port with one's thumb allows for inspiration. In the figure an angiocatheter is attached to a syringe, plunger removed, but could as well be a vessel dilator. (Reproduced with permission [12].)

and the operator and bedside team should have a plan of action and alternate plan of action. This chapter was designed to help with the latter.

2.2d.7 Case resolution (from chapter 2.2b, endotracheal intubation)

After successfully oxygenating and ventilating with BVM, an LMA was successfully placed. After maintaining oxygenation and ventilation a GEB was inserted into the trachea though the LMA. The LMA was removed and an endotracheal tube was inserted over the GEB. The ETT was secured and connected to the mechanical ventilator circuit.

References

1. Levitan, R.M., Everett, W.W. and Ochroch, E.A. (2004) Limitations of difficult airway prediction in patients intubated in the emergency department. *Ann. Emerg. Med.*, **44** (4), 307–313.
2. Reynolds, S.F. and Heffner, J. (2005) Airway management of the critically ill patient: rapid-sequence intubation. *Chest*, **127** (4), 1397–1412.
3. Walz, J.M., Zayaruzny, M. and Heard, S.O. (2007) Airway management in critical illness. *Chest*, **131** (2), 608–620.
4. Walls, R.M. and Murphy, M.F. (2008) *Manual of Emergency Airway Management*, 3rd edn. Wolters Kluwer Lippincott Williams & Wilkins, Philadelphia, p. xv.
5. Practice guidelines for management of the difficult airway: an updated report by the American Society of Anesthesiologists Task Force on Management of the Difficult Airway. *Anesthesiology*, 2003, **98** (5), 1269–1277.
6. Combes, X. Le Roux, B., Suen, P. et al. (2004) Unanticipated difficult airway in anesthetized patients: prospective validation of a management algorithm. *Anesthesiology*, **100** (5), 1146–1150.
7. Ferson, D.Z., Rosenblatt, W. H., Johansen, M. J. et al. (2001) Use of the intubating LMA-Fastrach in 254 patients with difficult-to-manage airways. *Anesthesiology*, **95** (5), 1175–1181.
8. Rosenstock, C., Østergaard, D., Kristensen, M. S. et al. (2004) Residents lack knowledge and practical skills in handling the difficult airway. *Acta Anaesthesiol. Scand.*, **48** (8), 1014–1018.
9. Ezri, T., Szmuk, P., Warters, R. D. et al. (2003) Difficult airway management practice patterns among anesthesiologists practicing in the United States: have we made any progress? *J. Clin. Anesth.*, **15** (6), 418–422.
10. Patel, R.G. (1999) Percutaneous transtracheal jet ventilation: a safe, quick, and temporary way to provide oxygenation and ventilation when conventional methods are unsuccessful. *Chest*, **116** (6), 1689–1694.
11. Boyce, J.R. and Peters, G. (1989) Vessel dilator cricothyrotomy for transtracheal jet ventilation. *Can. J. Anaesth.*, **36** (3 Pt 1), 350–353.
12. Kindopp, A.S. and Nair, V.K. (2001) A new setup for emergency transtracheal jet ventilation. *Can. J. Anaesth.*, **48** (7), 716–717.

2.2e Cricothyroidotomy

Mark R. Bowling

Division of Pulmonary, Critical Care, and Sleep Medicine, University of Mississippi, Jackson, MS, USA

2.2e.1 Introduction

Cricothyroidotomy is a safe and fast technique to secure an airway in a situation where traditional oral or nasal tracheal intubations have failed. It is the final pathway in The Difficult Airway Society 2004 guidelines for the cannot intubate/ cannot ventilate emergencies [1]. Reports have suggested that this procedure can be safely performed in two minutes and compared to tracheostomy has a considerably lower risk of complications in an emergent situation [2]. Cricothyroidotomy can be a life saving technique and the physician who will be caring for patients in respiratory distress should be proficient in this procedure. This section reviews the indications, contra-indications, placement, and complications of performing cricothyroidotomy.

2.2e.2 Indications

1. Any patient requiring airway management who cannot be intubated by the oral or nasal route [3].
2. Trauma patients whose cervical spine has a possible injury and where manipulation of the neck is contra-indicated [4].
3. Severe maxillofacial trauma [5].
4. Edema of the glottis and inability to visualize the vocal cords [5].
5. Severe oropharyngeal or tracheobronchial hemorrhage [5].
6. Fracture of the base of the skull [5].
7. Foreign body obstruction [5].
8. Creating an emergency airway where equipment is lacking and where oral and nasotracheal intubation cannot be performed rapidly and safely [5].
9. Technical failure to intubate [5].
10. Clinched teeth [5].
11. Masseter spasm following succinylcholine [5].

2.2e.3   Contra-indications

1. A less invasive method is possible to secure a patient airway [3].
2. Patients under five years of age.
3. Fracture of the larynx and existing pathology of the larynx [6].
4. Transection of the trachea with retraction of distal end of the trachea into the mediastinum [3].
5. Anatomical barriers, like a vast hematoma or massive subcutaneous emphysema in the region, which makes palpation of the anatomical landmarks impossible [3].
6. Acute laryngeal pathology [6].

2.2e.4   Anatomy

Before discussing the techniques of the cricothyroidotomy procedure, it is necessary to understand the basic and pertinent anatomy of the neck. Important landmarks and anatomical danger zones are demonstrated in Figure 2.2e.1.

2.2e.5   Placement

There are two general approaches for performing a cricothyroidotomy: needle or surgical (Tables 2.2e.1 and 2.2e.2). In general, the difference between the two approaches includes the insertion of a 12–14 gage cannula vs. a cuffed endotracheal or tracheostomy tube.

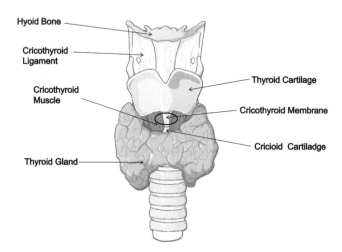

Figure 2.2e.1   Anatomy of the neck: important landmarks and anatomical danger zones.

Table 2.2e.1 Surgical cricothyroidotomy [3].

1. Place the patient in a supine position with the neck in a neutral position. Palpate the thyroid notch, cricothyroid membrane, the sternal notch, and hyoid bone for orientation. Assemble the necessary equipment.
2. Surgically prepare and anesthetize the area if the patient is conscious.
3. Stabilize the thyroid with the nondominant hand, keeping the skin taunt over the thyroid notch. This is important in order not to lose the anatomical landmarks during the procedure.
4. Make a vertical skin incision (2 cm) over the cricothyroid membrane. Locate the membrane and then carefully incise horizontally (1.5 cm) through the lower half of the membrane in order to avoid the cricothyroid arteries. Make sure only the tip of scalpel blade enters the airway, to avoid injury to the posterior cricoid cartilage. The tracheal hook can be used to stabilize the larynx, especially in a patient with a fat neck or hypermobile larynx.
5. Insert the scalpel handle into the incision and rotate it 90 degrees to open the airway. Extend the incision laterally for approximately 1 cm on each side of the midline.
6. Insert an appropriately sized, cuffed endotracheal tube or tracheostomy tube into the cricothyroid membrane incision, directing the tube distally into the trachea. The tube should always be aimed downwards in order not to injury the vocal cords above.
7. Inflate the cuff and ventilate the patient.
8. Observe bilateral lung inflation and auscultate the chest for adequate ventilation.
9. Perform suction of the trachea.
10. Secure the endotracheal tube to the patient to prevent dislodging.
11. Caution – do not cut or remove the cricoid or thyroid cartilages.

Table 2.2e.2 Needle cricothyroidotomy [3].

1. Place the patient in a supine position with a non-twisted neck.
2. Assemble a 12 or 14 gage over-the-needle catheter attached to a 5 ml syringe.
3. Surgically prepare the neck using antiseptic swabs.
4. Identify the cricothyroid membrane, between the cricoid cartilage and the thyroid cartilage. Stabilize the trachea with the thumb and forefinger of one hand to prevent lateral movement of the trachea during performance of the procedure.
5. Puncture the skin in the midline with a needle attached to the syringe, directly over the cricothyroid membrane. A small incision with a No. 20 scalpel may facilitate passage of the needle through the skin.
6. Direct the needle at a 45° angle inferiorly to avoid injury to the vocal cords, while applying negative pressure to the syringe and carefully insert the needle through the lower half of the cricothyroid membrane.
7. Aspiration of air signifies entry into the tracheal lumen. This is important because it assures that the posterior tracheal wall was not penetrated and it assures that the catheter tip is not embedded in the tracheal mucosa, avoiding tracheal mucosa damage.
8. Remove the syringe and withdraw the needle while advancing the catheter downward into position, being careful not to perforate the posterior wall of the trachea.
9. Attach the oxygen tubing over the catheter needle hub.
10. Intermittent ventilation can be achieved by occluding the open hole. The ventilator rate should be about 20 breaths/min, with the inspiratory phase lasting about 1 s. The expiratory phase should be at least 2 s.

Needle Technique

- **Equipment**
  - 12 or 14 gage cannula
  - 2 ml syringe
  - Oxygen tubing
  - Oxygen source (cylinder or wall suction)
- **Ventilation**

The needle technique can achieve ventilation via either a low pressure or high pressure ventilation system. Low pressure ventilation is achieved by allowing oxygen (flow rate of 15 l/min) to jet into the patient for one second by intermittently occluding an opening in the tubing that is connected to the needle cannula. This will cause the chest to rise and by releasing the occlusion (usually for 4 s) the chest wall will recoil back to a resting position. High pressure ventilation (45–50 psi) can be achieved by using a jet ventilator [7].

Surgical

- **Equipment**
  - 6 mm high volume low pressure cuff tracheostomy tube
  - Scalpel and blade
  - Tracheal spreaders
  - Local anesthetic
- **Ventilation**

The surgical technique can achieve adequate ventilation by utilizing bag masked ventilation or traditional positive pressure ventilation [7].

2.2e.6 Needle vs. Surgical: What is better?

It is unclear if one technique of cricothyroidotomy is superior, but Scarse and Woolard suggested that in the pre-hospital setting the needle technique provides inadequate ventilation unless ventilation is achieved by the high pressure system [8].

2.2e.7 Complications

There have been several complications reported in the literature, including perforated esophagus [4], tracheo-bronchiocephalic vein fistula formation [3], and aspiration [4]. The overall complication rate has been reported to be between 6.1 and 8.6% for elective cricothyroidotomies compared to 40% in the emergency department [5]. This section reviews the most pertinent complications related to cricothyroidotomy and techniques on how to avoid them.

   I. Misplacement of the tube.
      (a) The most common complication is incorrect placement of the tube through
          the thyrohyoid membrane [5].
          • Solution: Vertical incision so that the cricothyroid membrane can be
            easily located [5].
          • Identification of all landmarks: cricoid cartilage, thyroid cartilage, crico-
            thyroid membrane, and hyoid bone [3].
  II. Bleeding.
      (a) Severe bleeding is an uncommon occurrence [9], but the most common
          source of bleeding is from a superficial venous plexus injury [3].
          • Solution: Midline vertical incision directly over the cricothyroid mem-
            brane [3, 10].
      (b) There have been reports of fatal hemorrhage due to cricothyroid artery
          lacerations during cricothyroidotomy. These arteries course through the
          superior half of the cricothyroid membrane and are close to the thyroid
          cartilage [5, 11, 12].
          • Solution: Incision should be made through the inferior half of the mem-
            brane and closer to the cricoid cartilage [3, 5, 11, 12].
 III. Subglottic stenosis.
      (a) Uncommon but does occur [9]. The fear that cricothyroidotomy causes
          devastating subglottic stenosis was championed by the two landmark arti-
          cles by Jackson in 1909 and 1921 [13, 14]. The majority of these patients
          suffered from an infectious disease such as tuberculosis, diphtheria, or
          Ludwig's angina. Jackson described the technique for the standard trache-
          ostomy with insertion of a tracheostomy tube through the second or third
          tracheal ring, which resulted in reduced mortality, thus suggesting that the
          cricothyroidotomy procedure was harmful [15]. It has been suggested that
          the incidence of subglottic stenosis in Jackson's era could have been
          related to the inflammatory process produced by these infections coupled
          with poorly performed procedures rather than to the cricothyroidotomy
          procedure itself [6]. This concept has lead to the belief that prolonged
          cricothyroidotomy should be used in patients free from laryngeal pathol-
          ogy, which includes an already injured larynx due to prolonged endotra-
          cheal intubation [6, 15, 16].
          • Solution: If a patient requires long-term cricothyroidotomy, the patient
            should be free from laryngeal pathology [3, 6, 15, 16].
 IV. Laceration of the vocal cords.
      (a) This can result in dysphonia and occurs if the incision is made too close
          to the thyroid cartilage [17].
          • Solution: Incision should be made along the superior border of the
            cricoid cartilage [12].
  V. Tracheal cartilage fracture.
      (a) This complication is due to the insertion of an oversized endotracheal
          tube [5].

- Solution: The outer diameter of the tube should not exceed 8 mm [5, 18].

VI. Recurrent laryngeal nerve injury leading to vocal cord paralysis [3].

(a) These nerves lie between the trachea and the esophagus at the level of the cricoid cartilage and enter the larynx posteriorly.

- Solution: Maintain a midline incision and be careful not injure the posterior wall of the subglottic airway.

References

1. Henderson, J.J., Popat, M.T., Latto, I.P., Pearce, A.C. and Difficult Airway Society (2004) Difficult Airway Society guidelines for the management of the unanticipated difficult intubation. *Anaesthesia*, **59**, 675–694.

2. Boyd, A.D., Romita, M.C., Conlan, A.A. *et al.* (1979) A clinical evaluation of cricothyroidotomy. *Surg. Gynecol. Obstet.*, **149**, 365–368.

3. Boon, J.M., Abrahams, P.H., Meiring, J.H. and Welch, T. (2004) Cricothyroidotomy: a clinical anatomy review. *Clin. Anat.*, **17**, 478–486.

4. Jorden, R.C. (1988) Percutaneous transtracheal ventilation. *Emerg. Med. Clin. North Am.*, **6**, 745–752.

5. McGill, J., Clinton, J.E. and Ruiz, E. (1982) Cricothyrotomy in the emergency department. *Ann. Emerg. Med.*, (11), 361–364.

6. Brantigan, C.O. and Grow, J.B. Sr. (1982) Subglottic stenosis after cricothyroidotomy. *Surgery*, **91**, 217–221.

7. Greaves, I., Porter, K.M. and Ryan, J.M. (2001) *Trauma Care Manual*, Arnold, London.

8. Scrase, I. and Woollard, M. (2006) Needle vs. surgical cricothyroidotomy: a short to effective ventilation. *Anaesthesia*, **61**, 962–974.

9. Brantigan, C.O. and Grow, J.B. Sr. (1976) Cricothyroidotomy: elective use in respiratory problems requiring tracheostomy. *J. Thorac. Cardiovasc. Surg.*, **71**, 72–82.

10. Little, C.M., Parker, M.G. and Tarnopolsky, R. (1986) The incidence of vasculature at risk during cricothyroidostomy. *Ann. Emerg. Med.*, **15**, 805.

11. Schillaci, R.F., Iacovoni, V.F. and Conte, R.S. (1976) Transtracheal aspiration complicated by fatal endotracheal hemorrhage. *N. Engl. J. Med.*, **295**, 488–490.

12. Walls, R.M. (1988) Cricothyroidotomy. *Emerg. Med. Clin. North Am.*, (6), 725–736.

13. Jackson, C. (1909) Tracheotomy. *Layngoscope*, **18**, 285–290.

14. Jackson, C. (1921) High tracheotomy and other errors. The chief causes of chronic laryngeal stenosis. *Surg. Gynecol. Obstet.*, **32**, 392–398.

15. Rehm, C., Wanek, S.M., Gagnon, E.B. *et al.* (2002) Cricothyroidotomy for elective airway management in critically ill trauma patients with technically difficult challenging neck anatomy. *Crit. Care*, **6**, 531–535.

16. O'Connors, J.V., Reddy, K., Ergin, M.A. and Griepp, R.B. (1985) Cricothyroidotomy for prolonged ventilatory support after cardiac operations. *Am. Surg.*, **56**, 353–354.

17. Gleevson, M.J., Pearson, R.C., Armistead, S. and Yates, A.K. (1984) Voice changes following cricothyroidotomy. *J. Lryngol. Otol.*, **98**, 1015–1019.

18. Kress, T.D. and Balasubramaniam, S. (1982) Cricothyroidotomy. *Ann. Emerg. Med.*, **11**, 197–201.

2.3 Ventilator mechanics

David L. Bowton[1] and R. Duncan Hite[2]

[1] *Critical Care Anesthesia, Wake Forest University, Winston-Salem, NC, USA*
[2] *Pulmonary, Critical Care, Allergy, and Immunology, Wake Forest University, Winston-Salem, NC, USA*

2.3.1 History

The first descriptions of artificial ventilation supporting life include those of Vesalius, who in 1542 described placing a reed into an animal's trachea and blowing into it to maintain life while examining the animal's thoracic contents, and of Robert Hooke, who in 1642 similarly described maintaining a dog by using a pump attached to a tube in the dog's trachea to inflate the lungs with air [1]. However, the widespread application of mechanical ventilation in humans had its origins in the support of patients with respiratory insufficiency due to polio. Drinker reported the use of a tank ventilator to support a girl with polio and respiratory insufficiency in 1929. These tank ventilators, so-called "iron lungs", surrounded the patient, with only the head protruding, applying negative pressure to produce inspiration and positive pressure for exhalation. The provider can attend to the patient's head, which extends through a flange at the end of the iron lung, and his/her body through a limited number of portholes built into the side of the ventilator. Further, the application of negative pressure could produce peripheral venous pooling resulting in decreased cardiac output and hypotension, termed "tank shock" [2].

The application of positive pressure ventilation to large numbers of patients was first described during an epidemic of polio in Copenhagen in 1952 [3]. The airways

A Practical Guide to Mechanical Ventilation, First Edition.
Edited by Jonathon D. Truwit and Scott K. Epstein.
© 2011 John Wiley & Sons, Ltd. Published 2011 by John Wiley & Sons, Ltd.

of these patients were established by tracheostomy, and ventilation achieved by manual bag ventilation. Each day, over the several months of the epidemic, 40–70 patients were ventilated by up to 200 medical students working in shifts. This became the impetus for the development of powered positive pressure mechanical ventilators. The first positive pressure ventilators were electrically powered bellows capable of delivering a fixed tidal volume in a sinusoidal flow pattern and monitoring only airway pressure. These primitive, yet effective, devices have evolved into our modern microprocessor-controlled devices capable of delivering volume or pressure limited ventilation with a variety of flow patterns and instantaneous monitoring of inspiratory and expiratory pressures, volume and flow.

2.3.2 Ventilators

While older mechanical ventilators used pistons or bellows to limit and control the volume and pattern of gas delivery to the patient, modern ventilators most often employ electromagnetic proportional solenoid valves (Figure 2.3.1) controlled by microprocessors to control gas flow to the patient using measurements of flow and pressure to modulate gas delivery. Microprocessor technology provides for many more options and accuracy within those options. Today's ventilator provides a level of complexity that extends far deeper than early positive pressure ventilators. Hence, it is useful to develop a pattern for setting ventilator controls.

The operator should begin with the mode of ventilation: controlled, spontaneous or a combination. With the advent of responsive demand valves, combination modes are the most frequently used, whereby the patient is able to breathe spontaneously in between ventilator mandated breaths determined by the set rate. Examples of combination modes include assist control (AC) and synchronized intermittent mandatory ventilation (SIMV). In each, the patient is assured a minimum number of breaths whose timing and characteristics are determined by the ventilator set-

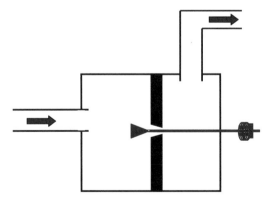

Figure 2.3.1 Electromagnetic proportional solenoid.

tings, while the number of breaths in excess of this is dependent upon patient effort. The character of these "extra" breaths will vary with the mode chosen.

The next choice is usually the manner in which breaths are targeted: pressure or volume. Combination modes are also available, such as (volume targeted) intermittent mandatory ventilation plus (pressure targeted) pressure support (SIMV + PS). Also present are selections to limit the peak airway pressure, control the inspiratory flow pattern (square wave, decelerating ramp, or sinusoidal), control the rate of rise of inspiratory flow rate (when a decelerating flow pattern is selected) or the actual flow rate (when a square wave pattern is selected). Controls also enable the operator to vary the duration of inspiration, either directly through setting the inspiratory time, or indirectly by setting an inspiratory : expiratory (I : E) ratio or the inspiratory flow at which exhalation begins (by opening the exhalation valve). If inspiratory flow is used to determine when exhalation is begun, it is usually set as a percentage of the maximal inspiratory flow (often between 5 and 60%).

To effect this remarkable control of ventilatory parameters, a mechanical ventilator must be able to measure and analyze flow and pressure data in the inspiratory and expiratory limbs of the ventilator circuit repetitively and rapidly, and to provide tight control of the flow of gas to and from the patient. Pressure is measured in the ventilator itself (commonly at the inspiratory and expiratory gas outlets and inlets, respectively) or within the ventilator circuit. Importantly, ventilator or circuit pressure is not equal to alveolar pressure except when zero flow conditions exist, which occurs most commonly at end-inspiration and end-expiration. When flow is present, the difference between alveolar pressure and ventilator-measured pressure is largely dependent on the flow-resistive properties of the airways and ventilator circuit and, to a much smaller extent, on the inertial or viscoelastic properties of the chest wall and lung parenchyma.

Both pressure and volume targeted ventilator modes use software algorithms to control gas flow to the patient. These algorithms assess the current circuit pressure, the volume of gas delivered to the patient and the timing of the gas flow with respect to the breath cycle to determine how much gas flow the solenoid valves meter to the patient. In volume targeted ventilation, most ventilators permit selecting the shape of the inspired flow pattern – usually at least between a square wave pattern and a decelerating wave pattern (Figure 2.3.2). In the square wave pattern (Figure 2.3.2a), the gas flow on initiation of inspiration is immediately increased to the set flow and then, on triggering of exhalation, turned off – thus achieving the square pressure waveform. If a decelerating pattern is selected (Figure 2.3.2b), the flow rate on initial inspiration is higher and then tapers to low flows (or zero flow) during the course of inspiration. This more nearly mimics the natural pattern of flow during spontaneous breathing. The slope of the decelerating waveform is controlled by the software specific to each ventilator. In pressure targeted ventilation (Figure 2.3.3), the flow pattern is nearly always decelerating, with the initial flow rate being very high to rapidly achieve the targeted airway pressure and then rapidly decreasing to maintain the targeted airway pressure as the distal lung units fill. Again, this

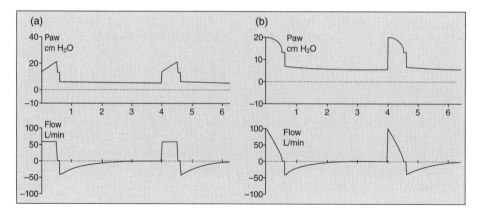

Figure 2.3.2 Volume targeted ventilation: (a) square wave pattern; (b) decelerating wave pattern.

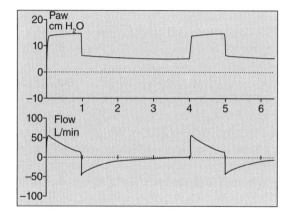

Figure 2.3.3 Pressure targeted ventilation.

requires that the ventilator sample airway pressure repetitively and that the ventilator makes rapid adjustments to flow rates to maintain airway pressure at the targeted level. This responsiveness is a function of many factors including the frequency of pressure sampling, the site of pressure sampling, the response times of the demand valves, and the controlling software.

2.3.3 Humidification

Air and oxygen for mechanical ventilators are obtained from high pressure gas sources that deliver dry gas at room temperature. Gas is most commonly delivered to the patient by an endotracheal tube or tracheotomy tube; the warming and humidifying actions of the nose and nasopharynx are bypassed. Room air (22 °C, relative humidity 50%) has a water vapor content of about 10 mg per liter. In the trachea, the nose and pharynx have typically warmed and humidified the inspired air to 32–34 °C, 100% relative humidity, containing about 36–40 mg of water per liter. Humidification of inspired gases during mechanical ventilation is usually achieved by a heated humidifier (HH) or a heat moisture exchanger (HME). HHs have the ability to deliver gas containing more water due to the ability to heat the gas to higher temperatures than those achievable passively by HMEs. The actual amount of water in inspired gas is dependent upon a number of variables. For HHs, this is primarily related to the temperature of the inspired gas at the "Y" of the ventilator circuit. For HMEs water content is dependent upon: 1) minute ventilation and tidal volume (with higher minute ventilation or tidal volume typically resulting in lower water content due to greater cooling of the HME during inspiration), 2) ambient temperature (again due to greater cooling of gas) and 3) patient temperature (which is the driving force for warming gas by HMEs). Under usual operating conditions, water content of inspired gases commonly ranges from 22 to 28 mg/l using an HME, while it is commonly 30–40 mg/l with a HH.

One problem associated with the use of HHs is the condensation of water vapor in the inspiratory limb as the heated humidified gases are cooled in the circuit on the way to the patient. This condensate can rapidly become colonized with bacteria originating from the patient's oropharyngeal flora, and can thus act as a potential contributor to nosocomial pneumonia when colonized condensate rolls down the endotracheal tube into the patient's lung. Condensate can be reduced, if not eliminated, by using ventilator circuits with embedded heating coils that can warm the circuit to maintain water in gas phase until the humidified gases reach the patient.

Studies examining the relative merits of HHs versus HMEs are generally conflicted. Of three recent meta analyses comparing the risk of ventilator-associated pneumonia (VAP) with HHs versus HMEs, two found reduced rates of VAP with HMEs, while the most recent found no difference in the rate of VAP [4]. These discordant results likely are a consequence of the studies available for inclusion, the duration of mechanical ventilation, the type of HH (with or without a heated circuit), and how VAP was diagnosed. Importantly, there have been no consistently described differences in mortality or duration of mechanical ventilation between these two humidification modes. The lower humidity achievable with HMEs can lead to increased deposition of adherent secretions on the inner surface of the endotracheal tube. While most studies have not demonstrated an increased rate of endotracheal tube occlusion due to these secretions, one recent study suggests that HMEs are associated with more endotracheal tube narrowing and an increased resistance to airflow in patients mechanically ventilated for an average of 10 days [5]. Our practice is to use HMEs in patients likely to require mechanical ventilation for a short time period and HHs with heated circuits in patients likely to require longer term mechanical ventilation.

2.3.4 Inhaled gas mixture

The blending of oxygen and air to achieve the desired F_iO_2 is most commonly done by one of two different methods. In the first method, the gases are delivered to a mixing chamber using a blender that controls the relative pressures of oxygen and air that are delivered, and then the mixed gas is delivered from the mixing chamber to the patient through a single proportional solenoid valve. Air and oxygen are admitted into the mixing chamber until the desired operating pressure is reached, which will be the sum of the partial pressures of the individual gases. This system is used by Hamilton ventilators (Galileo and Veolair). The other method employs two proportional solenoids that meter the flow of air and oxygen into the mixing chamber whose gas is then delivered to the patient (Puritan Bennett 7200, Draeger Evita 2 and 4, Servo 300). The relative flow of air and oxygen controlled by each solenoid determines the F_iO_2. Both methods use oxygen analyzers in the inspiratory limb to ensure that the delivered F_iO_2 is the same as the set F_iO_2.

Heliox is a mixture of helium and oxygen. Helium is an inert gas with a low atomic weight and density. The density of helium is 0.18 g/l, while the density of air and oxygen are 1.3 and 1.4 g/l, respectively. The lower density favors laminar flow, with a lower resistance for a given airway radius, and results in higher flow rates for any given driving pressures under conditions of turbulent flow. Thus, the work (or pressure) required to deliver a defined flow or volume of heliox will be lower than that for air or oxygen. The impact of helium–oxygen mixtures on work of breathing is directly related to the percentage of helium in the mixture. Heliox is commonly available as 80:20, and 70:30 (helium : oxygen) mixtures, with densities of 0.43 and 0.55 g/l, respectively. In non-intubated patients, heliox has been shown to relieve dyspnea and reduce work of breathing in patients with asthma and chronic obstructive pulmonary disease (COPD) [6, 7]. The impact on other outcomes, such as need for intubation, length of stay, or other morbidities, has not been well studied. There are no prospective controlled trials demonstrating improved outcomes using heliox in mechanically ventilated patients. Further, there are significant technical issues with regard to the use of heliox in mechanically ventilated patients. *In vitro* modeling has demonstrated improved lung deposition of aerosols delivered either by nebulization or by metered dose inhaler (MDI) [8]. Reduced $PaCO_2$ and increased pH have been reported in small series of mechanically ventilated asthmatics after initiation of heliox [8]. Similarly, in patients with COPD, heliox has been shown to reduce intrinsic positive end-expiratory pressure (PEEP) and trapped gas volume, and may reduce the work of breathing following extubation. However, the technical issues surrounding heliox use during mechanical ventilation should not be ignored.

Ventilator behavior changes with heliox, and each model or type of ventilator behaves differently according its pneumatics and monitoring paradigms [9]. The primary change is that the delivered tidal volume is different from the set tidal volume, sometimes by more than 20%. In some ventilators (e.g., Hamilton), correction factors can be applied, while other ventilators (e.g., PB 7200) simply will not function properly with heliox. It is important that, prior to consideration of use of heliox in a mechanically ventilated patient, these data are reviewed and carefully considered. Because of safety considerations, a helium tank (100% helium) should never be connected to a mechanical ventilator or other device interfaced with a patient. While heliox may play an adjunctive role in highly selected patients with severe airflow obstruction, it is a temporizing measure only, reducing dyspnea and work of breathing, until the underlying disease process improves or resolves.

2.3.5 Conclusion

Changes in technology have transformed mechanical ventilators, yet the principle in application to the patient remains the same. The application of mechanical ventilation is to be used to support a patient who is unable to maintain respiratory homeostasis and to do so safely. The process requires the clinician to assess the accuracy of delivered tidal volumes, minute volumes, oxygen content, patient–ventilator interactions (pressures, asynchrony), and patient comfort.

References

1. Baker, A.B. (1971) Artificial respiration, the history of an idea. *Med. Hist.*, **15**, 336–351.
2. Chen, K. *et al.* (1998) Mechanical ventilation: past and present. *J. Emerg. Med.*, **16**, 453–460.
3. Young, J.D. and Sykes, M.K. (1990) Artificial ventilation: history, equipment and techniques. *Thorax*, **45**, 753–758.
4. Siempos, I.I. *et al.* (2007) Impact of passive humidification on clinical outcomes of mechanically ventilated patients: a meta-analysis. *Crit. Care Med.*, **35**, 2843–2851.
5. Jaber, S. *et al.* (2004) Long-term effects of different humidification systems on endotracheal tube patency: evaluation by the acoustic reflection method. *Anesthesiology*, **100**, 782–788.
6. Diehl, J.-L. *et al.* (2003) Helium/oxygen mixture reduces the work of breathing at the end of the weaning process in patients with severe chronic obstructive pulmonary disease. *Crit. Care Med.*, **31**, 1415–1420.
7. Ho, A.M. *et al.* (2003) Heliox vs air-oxygen mixtures for the treatment of patients with acute asthma: a systematic overview. *Chest*, **123**, 882–890.
8. Hurford, W.E. and Cheifetz, I.M. (2007) Respiratory controversies in the critical care setting. Should heliox be used for mechanically ventilated patients? *Respir. Care*, **52**, 582–591.
9. Tassaux, D. *et al.* (1999) Calibration of seven ICU ventilators for mechanical ventilation with helium-oxygen mixtures. *Am. J. Respir. Crit. Care Med.*, **160**, 22–32.

2.4 Modes of mechanical ventilation

R. Duncan Hite

Pulmonary, Critical Care, Allergy, and Immunology, Wake Forest University, Winston-Salem, NC, USA

2.4.1 Case presentation

You are called from the intensive care unit (ICU) to assist with the initial management of a 28-year-old man with no significant past medical history other than alcohol abuse who presented less than an hour ago with acute respiratory failure from community acquired pneumonia. On examination, the patient demonstrated marked dyspnea (respiratory rate of 40 bpm), febrile at 103.5 °F and an altered mental status. His initial arterial blood gas on room air was pH = 7.12, $PaCO_2$ = 22 and PaO_2 = 45, which prompted the emergency room to intubate him and admit to the medical intensive care unit (MICU). His chest X-ray reveals dense left lower lobe consolidation and some otherwise patchy bilateral infiltrates, a well-positioned endotracheal tube and a normal cardiac silhouette. His vital signs are: sinus tachycardia at 140 bpm, BP = 100/60 mm Hg on 15 µg/kg/min of norepinephrine. Laboratory studies are remarkable for a white blood cell count of 19.5/mm^3 with 20% bands and elevated blood urea nitrogen (42 mg/dl) and creatinine (3.4 mg/dl). Some questions for you to consider regarding your selection of mechanical ventilation mode are:

- What mode and settings should you select now? Why?
- Will this be the mode you will use throughout the patient's ICU course?

A Practical Guide to Mechanical Ventilation, First Edition.
Edited by Jonathon D. Truwit and Scott K. Epstein.
© 2011 John Wiley & Sons, Ltd. Published 2011 by John Wiley & Sons, Ltd.

- Should you pick a mode that will permit you to start weaning the patient tomorrow morning?
- What modes would you consider if the patient's condition did not respond well to your initial choice?

2.4.2   Introduction

The principal indication for mechanical ventilation is to support patients with respiratory failure, including failure of either ventilation (hypercarbic) or oxygenation (hypoxic) or both. Although hypoxia is common in patients with respiratory failure, the majority of patients who require mechanical ventilation require it for support of ventilation [1]. Although the patient above presented with hypoxia, his principal indication for intubation in the emergency room was his severe acidosis for which he was not able to adequately compensate despite an apparent markedly elevated work of breathing. Although not tested, his hypoxia may have been adequately corrected with supplemental oxygen alone, which is the case for most pure hypoxic respiratory failure.

The inspiratory phase of spontaneous ventilation occurs through the creation of negative intrathoracic pressure (negative pressure ventilation, NPV) via the diaphragm and other muscles of respiration, while exhalation is a passive process driven by the elastic recoil of the lung parenchyma and chest wall. There are mechanical forms of NPV (e.g., iron lung, cuirass, pneumowrap), which have been and can still be utilized to provide ventilatory assistance, but their use has become increasingly uncommon. Over the past two to three decades, the vast majority of devices providing mechanical assistance to ventilation have utilized forms of positive pressure ventilation (PPV), in which inspiration occurs via the creation of a positive airway pressure [2, 3]. In all forms of mechanical ventilation, exhalation remains a passive process similar to that in spontaneous NPV [4].

Multiple modes of PPV are now available and it is the purpose of this chapter to review the mechanics of these modes. Although this chapter discusses some principles of application of the modes to unique disease states, further details regarding the application of these modes to specific patients is provided in subsequent chapters. As outlined in Table 2.4.1, the most commonly utilized modes of PPV are typically separated into two general categories: volume cycled and pressure cycled. More recent modes of ventilation including dual modes (combine aspect of pressure- and volume-cycled modes) and patient-tailored modes (modes that automatically adjust to changes in the patient's clinical condition) are also discussed. It should be noted, that evidence behind the efficacy and safety of these newer modes is far less, so routine use of these modes in broad patient populations is currently discouraged.

Although most PPV modes are distinguished by how they control either volume or pressure, it is critical to understand that in all PPV modes the variables of

Table 2.4.1 Modes of mechanical ventilation.

Volume-cycled modes	Assist Control (AC)
	Intermittent Mandatory Ventilation (IMV)
	Synchronized Intermittent Mandatory Ventilation (SIMV)
Pressure-cycled modes	Pressure Support Ventilation (PSV)
	Pressure Controlled Ventilation (PCV)
	Airway Pressure Release Ventilation (APRV)
Dual modes	Pressure-Regulated Volume Control (PRVC)
Patient-tailored modes	Proportional Assist Ventilation (PAV)
	Adaptive Support Ventilation (ASV)
	Neurally Adjusted Ventilatory Assist (NAVA)

volume, pressure, flow and time are involved and important for effective and safe delivery of ventilation. The rationale for categorizing modes into volume or pressure cycled is simply to identify the variable that the operator is able to control, while the opposing variable will be determined by the physiology or pathophysiology of the patient's lung parenchyma, airways and chest wall [5]. In that regard, the reader should refer to Chapter 2.5 on lung physiology for details regarding lung compliance and the relationship between pressure and volume during mechanical ventilation. It is essential to understand these principles in order to effectively apply each mode of PPV to any given patient or disease state.

Although not technically a mode of ventilation, continuous positive airway pressure (CPAP) or positive end-expiratory pressure (PEEP) are also described later in this chapter. PEEP is typically utilized simultaneously with virtually all modes of ventilation [6]. Although PEEP often has overlapping effects on the response of a diseased lung to a chosen ventilation mode, the management and titration of PEEP should generally be considered separately from ventilation mode. The mechanics and goals for management of oxygen delivery or the fraction of inspired oxygen (FiO_2) during mechanical ventilation are discussed in Chapter 2.5.

Clinicians should also be aware that the application of the principles outlined below for the unique modes of ventilation that are available may differ slightly between the multiple brands of mechanical ventilators that they will experience in their practice. The most common manufacturers of mechanical ventilators include: Drager®, General Electric®, Hamilton®, Maquet® and Puritan Bennett®. Since each of these companies has unique sets of engineers and approaches to device development, their respective ventilators reflect those differences. In addition, not all ventilators from the same manufacturer are built to deliver all modes of mechanical ventilation. Inclusion of all modes is often a choice of the purchaser, since each mode may require additional software which it may not be cost effective to include in all ventilators within a given institution. These variations in devices can be confusing to clinicians once they become familiar with a specific brand. Consequently, it is important for intensivists to become familiar with multiple ventilator brands. The ability to comfortably operate all devices generally results in an enhanced understanding of the physiologic principles behind mechanical ventilation.

2.4.3   Volume-cycled ventilation modes

Volume-cycled modes of mechanical ventilation are characterized by the operator being able to select a preset tidal volume (V_T), while peak inspiratory or dynamic pressure (P_D) will be determined by the dynamic compliance (C_{dyn}) of the patient's respiratory system [7]. In these modes, a decrease in C_{dyn} thru either a decrease in lung or chest wall compliance (e.g., pulmonary edema, patient agitation) or an increase in airway resistance (e.g., bronchospasm), will lead to an increase in P_D, but generally no change in the delivered V_T (Figure 2.4.1). In volume-cycled modes, the operator is able to set an alarm limit for P_D and should this threshold be reached during inspiration flow is discontinued with resultant delivered volume only a fraction of the desired V_T. Of note, as P_D increases, some reduction may be seen in V_T due to the distensibility of the inspiratory tubing from the ventilator, although this effect is minimal, 3 ml/cm H_2O, over the ranges of P_D typically used in clinical practice.

In volume-cycled modes, the operator is also required to determine a respiratory rate (RR), and it is this characteristic that most readily distinguishes the commonly

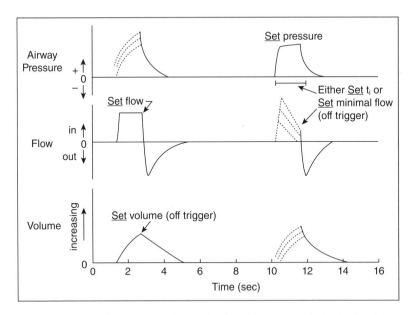

Figure 2.4.1   Representative pressure, flow and volume time curves during both volume-cycled (left) and pressure-cycled (right) modes of ventilation. (Reproduced with permission from N. McIntyre.)

utilized volume-cycled modes including assist control (AC) and synchronized inter-mittent mandatory ventilation (SIMV) [8]. A common limitation of volume-cycled modes is the fixed nature of inspiratory flow, which is set by the operator. Should inspiratory flow be set at a level below the patient's desired level, it can result in air hunger and increased respiratory work of breathing (WOB).

2.4.3.1 Assist control (AC)

When the operator selects a RR, the ventilator translates it to a maximum time interval that the ventilator will wait to deliver the preset V_T in the event no spon-taneous respiratory effort is triggered by the patient during that interval [9]. For instance, in an apneic patient, when a ventilator RR of 12 breaths per minute (bpm) is selected, the ventilator will wait a maximum of five seconds since the onset of the preceding breath before delivering the next breath. In this example, since the patient is apneic, a total of 12 bpm will be delivered and total minute ventilation (V_E) will be 12 times the preset V_T. Since most ICU patients are not apneic, the total RR of the patient is typically not the same as the RR set by the operator. If a patient triggers a spontaneous respiratory effort earlier than the time interval created by the chosen RR in AC mode, the ventilator will deliver the preset V_T at that time, and will then reset the time interval to await the next breath. It is important to note that in AC mode, ALL breaths are delivered at the volume set by the operator regardless of whether the breath is initiated by the patient or the ventilator, which is not the same for all volume-cycled modes (Figure 2.4.2).

For example, in the patient described at the beginning of this chapter, the V_E will be markedly elevated due to his fever and sepsis, and will require a high RR (e.g., V_E might be 15 lpm and with $V_T = 500$ ml, total RR will be 30 bpm). If this patient's central nervous system respiratory drive is intact, he will get a total RR of 30 bpm regardless of whether his AC rate is set anywhere between 2 to 30 bpm. With set RR far less than patient desired RR (2–12 bpm), most if not all of the breaths would be triggered by the patient and not by the ventilator since the time interval would be unlikely to elapse. If a rate above 30 were selected in this example, the ventila-tion being delivered would exceed the patient's V_E, leading to little or no breaths triggered by the patient. Since the time interval between each spontaneous breath triggered by a patient is typically not constant, at most settings (12–28 bpm in this example), the total RR provided during AC mode is frequently a mixture of breaths initiated both by the ventilator and patient. The ideal rate to set is typically deter-mined by several clinical variables but is typically set at a rate below the patient's V_E requirements so that sedation can be titrated to avoid apnea. However, when heavy sedation is required to maximize patient–ventilator synchrony, then setting a rate that matches the patient's V_E is appropriate.

In AC mode, the operator is also allowed to control the percentage time that a patient spends during inspiration (Ti) while the V_T is being delivered. The time a patient spends in expiration (Te) is a passive process that is driven by the elastic

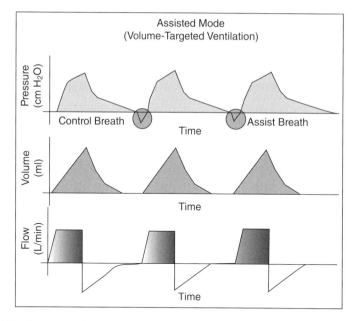

Figure 2.4.2　Pressure, volume and flow curves in Assist Control ventilation with breath #1 delivered without patient triggering (Control) and breaths #2 and #3 WITH patient triggering (Assist). (Reproduced with permission from Dr Byrd.)

recoil of the lung and chest wall, and therefore beyond the control of the operator. The relationship of Ti to Te is typically referred to as the I : E ratio. The mechanism by which an operator controls Ti in AC mode is through control of the inspiratory flow rate (e.g., increasing inspiratory flow rate will decrease Ti). An operator should also be aware that inspiratory airway pressures are likely to change with adjustments to inspiratory flow as a result of airway resistance. Further discussion regarding appropriate selection of I : E ratios for specific respiratory conditions is included in other chapters (e.g., obstructive and restrictive lung disease).

Given its ability to provide a complete V_T with each spontaneous inspiratory effort, AC mode performs as an ideal mode for patients in acute distress, providing adequate ventilation with reduced patient effort. On the other hand, the same characteristics make AC mode not a suitable mode for gradual "weaning" of a patient from mechanical ventilation. Despite its inability to serve as a mode for gradual weaning from mechanical ventilation, patients can be switched directly from AC mode to a spontaneous breathing trial (SBT) and return back to AC mode if the SBT is unsuccessful.

2.4.3.2　Synchronized intermittent mandatory ventilation (SIMV)

Similar to AC mode, SIMV has a minimum number of machine breaths that will be delivered, and these breaths will have an operator determined tidal volume [10].

However, if the patient's respiratory rate exceeds the set rate, tidal volumes are determined by a combination of the patient's spontaneous effort and any additional modes of ventilation that might also be active, such as pressure support ventilation (PSV), which are discussed in more detail later on. Although it is more typical for operators to use SIMV in combination with PSV, it is important to note that SIMV was originally designed prior to the PSV mode being available on most mechanical ventilators, and it is quite feasible to provide mechanical ventilation to a patient on SIMV in the absence of PSV. For clarity, the following discussion regarding SIMV assumes the absence of PSV unless otherwise stated.

As for the initiation of the breaths within the set rate, these can be initiated by either the patient or the ventilator, since SIMV mode attempts to "synchronize" as many of the mandatory breaths with a spontaneous effort as it is able [11]. As demonstrated in Figure 2.4.3, this is accomplished by the operator's set rate establishing a time interval (e.g., rate of 12 corresponds to a time interval of 5 s), similar to AC mode. In contrast to AC, in SIMV mode, a preset fraction of the time interval is reserved to deliver the set V_T with a spontaneous effort. If a breath is taken during that period, then any additional spontaneous efforts initiated during the same time interval are not further supported by SIMV. If the patient is also on PSV mode, then these additional breaths will be supported by PSV (Figure 2.4.4). If a breath is not taken during the initial phase of the time interval, then a mandatory breath is initiated by the ventilator without being triggered by the patient in order to guarantee the preset number of breaths chosen by the operator.

In general, any mandatory breath delivered without triggering by a patient is less tolerated by patients who are sufficiently alert and aware of their respirations. As a result, SIMV is a mode that might be less well tolerated by alert and awake patients, particularly since the regularity of the time interval between spontaneous breaths is not constant over the entire respiratory cycle. Additionally, patients with acute respiratory distress have high ventilator demands and SIMV will only supply guaranteed tidal volumes at the selected rate while A/C provides a guaranteed tidal

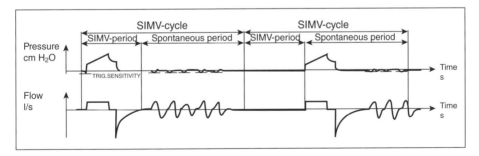

Figure 2.4.3 Pressure and flow time curves for SIMV ventilation with examples in which the patient does and does not trigger a breath during the SIMV period. The pressure and flow changes during the additional patient efforts during the spontaneous period are not supported by the ventilator and represent spontaneous patient effort.

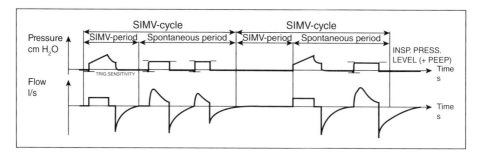

Figure 2.4.4   Pressure and flow time curves for SIMV ventilation when PSV mode is also activated with examples in which the patient does and does not trigger a breath during the SIMV period. The pressure and flow changes during the additional patient efforts during the spontaneous period are supported by the PSV mode.

volume at all breaths, even when the patient's RR exceeds the set ventilator rate. Unfortunately, there are no available equations that permit a clinician to accurately estimate V_E, so it is much easier for the operator to select a rate that is either inadequate or excessive for the patient's V_E, and requires more frequent arterial blood gas (ABG) monitoring during initial stabilization of the patient.

At the time of its development, the advantage of SIMV over AC was its ability to slowly wean a patient from mechanical ventilation by reducing the number of pre-set breaths per minute, which results in a gradual increase in the percentage of total V_E that the patient must generate through spontaneous breaths [12]. As such, SIMV remains a viable mode for this type of weaning. However, other modes, in particular PSV, are available and perform at least as well for this purpose. Furthermore, slow gradual weaning of patients from mechanical ventilation is much less commonly performed with performance of daily SBTs having replaced this approach [13]. Slow gradual weaning approaches are now primarily reserved for patients with prolonged respiratory failure and typically with severe acute and/or chronic lung disease. Of note, one subset of these patients that can be most well suited for SIMV mode are patients with intermittent CNS respiratory drive (e.g., Cheyne–Stokes respiration) who frequently trigger alarms for either apnea or excessive V_E when placed on AC mode.

2.4.4   Pressure-cycled ventilation modes

Pressure-cycled modes of mechanical ventilation are characterized by the operator being able to select a preset inspiratory pressure (ΔP). Upon delivery, the ΔP results in a V_T that will be variable and is determined by C_{dyn}, as described earlier (Figure 2.4.1), since C_{dyn} is the relationship between the change in inspiratory volume and the change in inspiratory pressure ($\Delta V/\Delta P$) [14]. Consequently, when the ΔP selected in a pressure-cycled mode is similar to the pressure (P_D−PEEP) generated by a V_T in a volume-cycled mode, the resulting V_T will typically be approximately the same [15]. For example, in a patient receiving $V_T = 500$ ml in AC mode which leads to a $P_D = 25$ cm H_2O with PEEP $= 5$ cm H_2O, their $\Delta P = 20$ cm H_2O. If the patient were changed to a pressure-cycled mode with $\Delta P = 20$ cm H_2O, then the resulting V_T would be approximately 500 ml. This simple example also illustrates that the level of support being provided with each breath by the ventilator after this change is made has not decreased.

A limitation for all pressure-cycled modes is that pathologic alterations in C_{dyn} typically lead to decreased V_T (rather than P_D too high in volume-cycled modes), and potentially a subsequent increase in RR to maintain V_E. Importantly, gas exchange is more dependent on a volume of gas being delivered to the distal airways than generation of an airway pressure, so changes in C_{dyn} in pressure-cycled modes can lead to more substantial changes in oxygenation and ventilation, and may require more frequent ABG monitoring, at least in the early phases of managing a new patient with acute respiratory failure. In pressure-cycled modes, alarm limits are set to draw attention when V_T and/or V_E get too low.

The ability of the operator to set RR in pressure-cycled modes is variable, and represents an important distinction between the various modes.

2.4.4.1 *Pressure support ventilation (PSV)*

In PSV, the operator determines an increase in pressure (above PEEP) which is triggered by a patient's spontaneous inspiratory effort. The operator cannot set a RR in PSV and the mode requires the patient to have a respiratory drive. Since the amount of pressure that can be delivered can be readily titrated to meet an individual patient's V_E requirements and C_{dyn} tolerance to achieve a desirable V_T and RR, PSV serves as a reliable mode for gradual weaning of mechanical ventilation. Since all breaths must be initiated by the patient, the mode is typically more comfortable for patients, and leads to better patient–ventilator synchrony, than the inconsistent nature of breaths delivered in SIMV mode as described previously. The reduction in ventilator support is typically more gradual than with SIMV and lead to a slower rise in the patient's work of breathing [16]. The comfort of PSV can also be recognized through its inclusion and common utilization as the inspiratory pressure in the design and delivery of biphasic positive airway pressure (BiPAP) devices in noninvasive ventilation (Chapter 1.5).

The primary disadvantage to PSV, as described above for all pressure-cycled modes, is the inability to guarantee a consistent V_E. Since neither V_T nor RR are fixed in PSV mode, changes in the patient's status, including C_{dyn} or V_E requirement (e.g., CO_2 production), can lead to significant changes in the patient's RR and work of breathing. As a result, PSV is less commonly utilized in unstable patients with either worsening respiratory function (decreasing C_{dyn}), evolving infection (increasing V_E) or declining neurologic function (impaired respiratory drive) [17].

Furthermore, since no RR can be set in PSV, its use should also be minimized when patients are being heavily sedated.

When gradual weaning from mechanical ventilation is desirable and respiratory drive is intact, PSV is a reliable and heavily utilized mode. If transitioning from AC to PSV, the selection of initial ΔP is typically estimated by the ΔP (P_D – PEEP) during the AC assisted breaths. Although many health care providers incorrectly conclude that PSV is a mode that provides less support than AC, the similarity of the patient's respiratory status during this transition step provides an excellent illustration that contradicts that commonly oversimplified view of PSV mode. Once the transition has been completed, the level of ΔP can be decreased as the patient's C_{dyn} and V_E improve, which generally result from effective management toward the etiology of the patient's acute respiratory failure.

Some clinicians choose to use PSV in combination with SIMV as a (albeit poor) substitute for AC. In this setting, the patient receives the set number of volume-cycled breaths from the set SIMV rate as described above. Unlike SIMV alone, when the patient generates an additional respiratory effort during the refractory period in which no additional volume-cycled breath will be given, the patient's effort is assisted by the ΔP set in PSV. Although this approach to ventilator support can be very effective for providing support, its disadvantages are the same as those outlined in SIMV and PSV respectively and will depend on what percentage of a patient's V_E is being supported by SIMV or PSV at any given time. An additional disadvantage to this combined approach when being used for slow weaning from mechanical ventilation is that clinicians can become confused as they titrate two separate modes; this can lead to uncertainty about the response of the patient's underlying disease process to ongoing therapies. In general, a weaning approach using either PSV or SIMV alone or predominantly is recommended.

Shortly after its introduction, a common early application of PSV was to use a low level (~5 cm H_2O) to overcome the resistance of the ventilator circuit as a means to assess spontaneous breathing, now referred to as a spontaneous breathing trial [18]. Many current ventilators continue to use this concept and refer to it as *tube compensation*. Tube compensation adjusts the level of PSV based on the size of the endotracheal tube, which must be entered by the operator and the set level of inspiratory flow.

2.4.4.2 Pressure control ventilation (PCV)

In PCV, the operator determines the ΔP (similar to PSV) to be delivered on each breath [19]. However, PCV differs from PSV in the ability of the operator to select a set respiratory rate, such that either a minimum or absolute number of breaths is delivered. Most ventilators provide options for the control of respiratory rate to be similar to either of the two volume-cycled modes (AC and SIMV). In other words,

PCV can be set up to have all breaths deliver the pre-set ΔP (similar to AC) or only for the number of pre-set breaths while all additional breaths are driven by the spontaneous negative inspiratory pressure that the patient is able to generate (similar to SIMV).

The principal advantage of PCV mode over volume-cycled modes is its ability to control airway pressures and, thereby, prevent excessive P_D. However, its disadvantage over AC mode is the inability to guarantee the delivery of a sufficient V_T to maintain gas exchange, which typifies all pressure-cycled modes. More careful monitoring of ventilation with more frequent arterial blood gas analysis is typically required in PCV. The inability or ability to use PCV modes for a slow weaning approach is similar to those discussed for AC and SIMV respectively. Although SBTs can be performed on patients receiving PCV, the type of patients for which it is typically reserved is those sufficiently unstable that SBTs are not being performed. As these patients improve, most clinicians convert to PSV mode before SBTs are attempted.

Although PCV can function similarly to both AC and SIMV in many ways, it is utilized less frequently and in a more limited spectrum of settings by most clinicians. The most common setting in which PCV mode is considered is in patients requiring full ventilator support for acute respiratory failure from acute lung injury (ALI) or acute respiratory distress syndrome (ARDS). In the setting of ALI/ARDS, trials have demonstrated no clear benefit of AC mode versus PCV mode, assuming equivalent pressure and volume goals are achieved [20]. Nonetheless, the use of PCV mode, often in combination with inverse ratio ventilation (IRV, discussed more later) has declined over recent years since the development of the low tidal volume strategy of the ARDS Network.

In addition to selecting pressure, PCV requires the operator to provide a desired I : E ratio by selecting specific times for each (e.g., Ti = 1.0s and Te = 1.0s for I : E ratio of 1:1 and a total RR = 30). As mentioned earlier, I : E ratios are controlled by the operator in AC mode through titration of inspiratory flow rates. In reality, the ventilator also controls I : E ratios in PCV mode through the same mechanism of changes to inspiratory flow, but how the operator interfaces with the individual device to achieve this change often differs. As mentioned, it was once popular to combine PCV with inverse ratio ventilation (IRV), which is defined as an I : E ratio in which Ti > Te (e.g., I : E = 1.5–2:1) [21]. Although some references consider IRV a separate mode of ventilation, this is a misnomer, as it only relates to the I : E ratio and must be combined with another form of ventilation. It is also possible to adjust I : E ratios in volume-cycled modes such as AC but is seldom done. The clinical benefit of IRV is enhanced oxygenation, which typically occurs through air trapping and the creation of intrinsic PEEP (auto-PEEP). However, the benefits of intrinsic PEEP versus machine-generated (extrinsic) PEEP are unproven and inherently more difficult to measure and maintain constant. For most patient with ALI/ARDS, a target I : E of 1:1 with extrinsic PEEP being titrated as needed is appropriate [22].

2.4.4.3 Airway pressure release ventilation (APRV)

In its simplest forms, APRV can be described as the operator selecting two levels of PEEP (P_{high} and P_{low}) and the time duration that the patient spends at each PEEP level (T_{high} and T_{low}) [23]. The time durations set establish the total time spent during a cycle between both pressures and, therefore, dictate the number of cycles per minute (Figure 2.4.5). While at either level of PEEP, the patient is able to make spontaneous respiratory efforts but will generally receive no inspiratory assistance (either pressure cycled or volume cycled). The advantage of APRV is the ability to use high levels of PEEP without risking unacceptably high levels of P_D and risk of barotrauma. Consequently, the use of APRV has been most common in (but not limited to) the setting of severe restrictive lung diseases such as ALI/ARDS, in which problems with severe hypoxemia exist. Ventilation in APRV is achieved through the combined exchange of gas volumes that occur during both the patient's spontaneous efforts as well as the volume of gas released and delivered during transitions between P_{high} and P_{low}. As in other pressure-cycled modes, the volume of gas exchanged will be dependent on C_{dyn}.

Although optimal settings for APRV have not been established, Figure 2.4.5 provides a typical pressure–time waveform in APRV. To optimize alveolar recruitment and prolong alveolar patency for oxygen diffusion across the alveolar–capillary barrier, P_{high} is frequently set at 25–30 cm H_2O and T_{high} is typically maintained for the large majority (80–90%) of the cycle (e.g., 5–5.4 s for a cycle

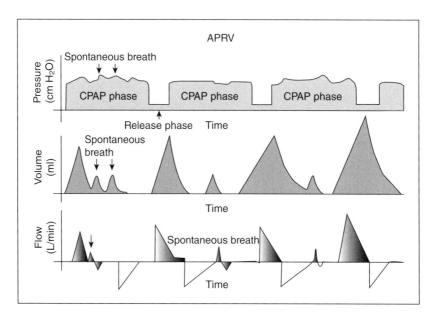

Figure 2.4.5 Pressure, volume and flow waveforms during airway pressure release ventilation (APRV).

rate of 10 per minute). To maximize ventilation and carbon dioxide removal, P_{low} is set low (e.g., 0–5 cm H_2O). The short T_{low} times usually result in incomplete exhalation with resulting air trapping, and consequently APRV can be considered an IRV approach.

Although APRV does not involve the delivery of a preset ΔP during inspiration, it has been included in pressure-cycled modes since the operator's decision involves the titration of pressures without the ability to establish a preset V_T. This characteristic lends APRV to some of the same potential disadvantages of other pressure-cycled modes. Due to its typical utilization of an IRV approach, use of APRV in obstructive lung diseases is generally not recommended, owing to the risk of severe hyperinflation and barotrauma. Patient comfort with APRV is highly variable, with literature supporting the need for both more and less sedation than conventional modes. These discrepancies likely reflect differing delivery approaches among the reporting investigators. APRV has gained increasing popularity over recent years, but its efficacy remains uncertain [24]. Most reports of APRV suggest benefits on oxygenation and hemodynamics in patients with severe hypoxemia from ALI/ARDS, while the impact on duration of mechanical ventilation and length of ICU stay has not been consistently demonstrated, and no trial has demonstrated a benefit on mortality.

Although not available on all ventilators, newer modes of ventilation similar to APRV are available including: biphasic ventilation (different than BiPAP), BiLevel ventilation and intermittent mandatory airway pressure release ventilation (IMPRV) [25]. In IMPRV, the timing of the cyclic changes between P_{high} and P_{low} are synchronized with the patient's spontaneous efforts, which may improve patient comfort. Biphasic ventilation typically utilizes longer T_{low} times and may lead to less hyperinflation and be able to serve a broader range of respiratory failure patients. BiLevel ventilation provides a combination of synchronized cycling (between P_{high} and P_{low}) and PSV support of spontaneous respiratory efforts. No trials currently exist to demonstrate superiority for these modes of ventilation over conventional modes of ventilation (APRV or otherwise), but they might provide additional options for optimizing management in select ICU patients.

2.4.5 Dual control modes

Many newer ventilators now include modes that attempt to combine the advantages of both pressure-cycled and volume-cycled ventilation. In general, these modes attempt to achieve a target or minimum V_T while adjusting the pressure to find the minimum pressure required to achieve V_T. These goals are achieved through continuous analysis of airway flow, pressure and volume during the interaction between the patient and ventilator. Some modes make adjustments as a breath is being delivered (within breath) or at the time the next breath is delivered (breath-to-breath). A key difference between these modes is the shape of the flow curve during inspiration. In normal VC modes, the flow curve is square-waved, meaning inspira-

tory flow is constant, but in these modes inspiratory flow adjusts creating a decelerating ramp flow waveform. The clinician should beware that the names of these
modes are different for many of the available brands.

2.4.5.1 Pressure-regulated volume control (PRVC)

As described above, pressure-regulated volume control (PRVC) is a mode designed
to deliver a targeted or minimum V_T while adjusting inspiratory pressure and flow
to identify the optimal settings by which peak dynamic and static airway pressures
(P_D and P_S) are minimized and does so on a breath-to-breath basis (Figure 2.4.6)
[26]. This mode, by the name of PRVC, is only available on the Maquet Servo-i®
and Servo 300®, but is characteristic of all ventilators with dual modes, such as:
Volume Control Plus (VC+, Puritan Bennett®), *Autoflow* (Drager®) and P-CMV
(Hamilton®). In these modes, the operator not only chooses a target or minimum
V_T similar to VC modes, but must select a maximum delivered pressure which is
typically set as 5 cm H_2O below the pressure alarm limit. The operator also selects
a preset respiratory rate, and PRVC will deliver the set V_T for all breaths triggered
by the ventilator or the patient similar to AC mode. However, the automated feature
of adjusting inspiratory pressure and flow, makes slow gradual weaning more feasible than AC mode.

   The potential advantages of PRVC can be easily appreciated by its ability to
provide a guaranteed V_T and V_E while adjusting pressure and flow to optimize

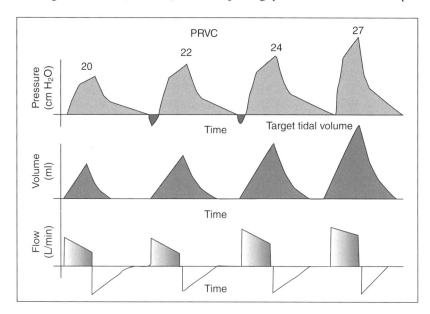

Figure 2.4.6 Pressure, volume and flow waveforms for pressure-regulated volume control
(PRVC) ventilation. On a breath-to-breath basis, inspiratory pressures are adjusted to achieve the
targeted tidal volume.

delivery of the V_T, reduce risk of barotrauma and meet the patient's inspiratory flow demands, which lead to enhanced patient–ventilatory synchrony and comfort. However, the major disadvantage of PRVC is in patients whose inspiratory effort is highly variable. In these situations, V_T will not be truly guaranteed when a strong inspiratory effort is followed by a significantly weaker effort. A second disadvantage is the potential for generating auto-PEEP when a patient actively exhales, and, therefore, will likely limit its application in patients with obstructive lung disease. A recent adaptation in PRVC to address problems with variable respiratory effort is *Automode*, which can alternate between PRVC and VC based on continuous analysis of patient effort [27]. Although PRVC may be a mode with increasing utilization in the future, there are currently no trials to demonstrate its superiority over the more conventional VC or PC modes.

2.4.6 Patient-tailored modes

The recent evolution of mechanical ventilators has been influenced by two key factors: techniques of ventilating and weaning patients have become more standardized with available published guidelines and the continued refinement of microprocessors and in-line devices. These microprocessors continuously analyze pressure, volume and flow and can adjust based on the individual patient's lung mechanics and respiratory demands, even as the patient's condition improves or declines. The operator is required to provide the patient's ideal body weight to permit the calculations of respiratory mechanics.

These modes offer potential advantages that may be able to optimally deliver ventilation on a breath-by-breath basis and serve to optimize many aspects of a patient's experience while on mechanical ventilation, including comfort and length of time ventilator support is required. The relatively recent introduction of these ventilator modes has not permitted enough opportunity for large clinical trials to as yet prove such benefits.

2.4.6.1 *Proportional assist ventilation (PAV)*

In proportional assist ventilation (Puritan-Bennett®), all breaths are patient triggered, pressure controlled and flow cycled, but the ventilator adjusts the pressure and flow based on patient demand and continuous measurements of airway resistance and compliance [28]. The operator must set the percentage of total work of breathing that the ventilator must provide, which then dictates the necessary adjustments in flow and pressure. This mode is typically used only for weaning of a patient, and weaning is accomplished by gradual lowering of the percentage work of breathing.

The advantages of proportional assist ventilation (PAV) include its ability to better synchronize the patient's respiratory effort with the assist being provided by the patient, which enhances patient comfort and even sleep quality. Limitations of PAV include the requirement for all breaths to be patient triggered, which can lead to problems with inadequate or excess ventilation in patients whose respiratory effort is not appropriate for their actual V_E. In addition, impediments to accurate estimates of airway resistance or compliance (e.g., secretions, air leak) can result in incorrect ventilator adjustments.

2.4.6.2 Adaptive support ventilation (ASV)

During adaptive support ventilation (Hamilton®), the ventilator continuously monitors and adjusts the pressure, rate and flow to achieve a minimum or desired minute ventilation [29]. A key variable that the ventilator monitors is the expiratory time constant (RCe), which dictates the targeted tidal volume (increased RCe as in COPD leads to larger V_T). The operator is required to provide a minimum respiratory rate and the range (low and high) of inspiratory pressures. From these settings, the ventilator will then adjust inspiratory pressure and the ratio of mandatory : spontaneous breaths to the minimum levels required to achieve the minute ventilation needs, and therefore serves as a mode that supports more than just weaning patients, unlike PAV. In adaptive support ventilation (ASV), breaths are delivered in a PSV mode when patients are able to spontaneously trigger a breath or in a PCV mode when patients do not.

The principal advantages of ASV are its ability to adapt to varying CNS respiratory drives and its ability to reduce the number of adjustments in ventilator settings required of the operator. As yet, no trials have clearly demonstrated a reduction in ventilator days using ASV mode over more conventional modes. Workflow and preferences of ICU teams toward daytime extubation may limit recognizing the full benefits of modes like ASV.

2.4.6.3 Neurally adjusted ventilatory assist (NAVA)

The neurally adjusted ventilatory assist (NAVA) mode of ventilation has been developed by Maquet® and requires the placement of a unique gastric catheter that measures the electrical signal leading to diaphragmatic stimulation by the vagus nerve (Edi) [30]. The strength of the signal, along with measures of respiratory mechanics, is used to adjust the level of support provided to the patient. The potential advantage of NAVA will be to maximize patient–ventilator synchrony, but disadvantages include the expense of the unique gastric tube and the unclear patient populations in which accurate measurements of Edi can be reliably obtained.

2.4.7 High frequency ventilation (HFV)

Despite the frequent utilization of various modes of high frequency ventilation (HFV) in neonatology and pediatric critical care, the use of HFV in adult critical care remains limited [31]. Given its inherent complexity and unproven benefits in adults, extensive discussion on HFV in this chapter is not prudent. An inexperienced operator should always seek supervision from a clinician with experience in HFV before considering its use in a patient. Further details regarding HFV can also be found in Chapter 2.8, Ancillary Modalities.

The basic principles of HFV combine supraphysiologic respiratory rates (>60 breaths per minute) with tidal volumes that are less than anatomic dead space to maintain airway and alveolar patency while limiting risk of volutrauma [32]. Gas exchange occurs primarily through diffusion of gases across the continuous column of air from proximal to distal airways.

Four types of HFV exist, including: high frequency jet ventilation (HFJV), high frequency oscillatory ventilation (HFOV), high frequency percussive ventilation (HFPV) and high frequency positive pressure ventilation (HFPPV). In HFJV, a jet of gas (35 psi) is delivered via a small cannula that is introduced through the endotracheal tube at a respiratory rate of 100–150 breaths per minute, with inspiratory fraction calculated as a percentage of total time for all breaths. For HFOV, an oscillatory pump is connected to the endotracheal tube and delivers a rate of 180–900 breaths per minute, creating such small V_T changes that airway pressures simply oscillate within a small amplitude around a mean airway pressure that the operator titrates by adjusting inspiratory flow and expiratory back pressure (Figure 2.4.7). HFPV combines HFOV superimposed on conventional PCV mode using a phasitron, which cycles the oscillatory changes at 200–900 breaths per minute and varies the mean airway pressure between the inspiratory and expiratory pressure targets of PCV at a rate of typically 10–15 breaths per minute. Due to the development of these other HFV modes, use of HFPPV is very rare and can be described

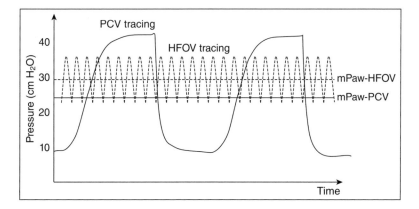

Figure 2.4.7 Pressure waveforms for high frequency oscillatory ventilation (HFOV) compared to waveforms in pressure control ventilation (PCV). (Reproduced with permission from Dr Mehta.)

simply as the delivery of HFV using conventional ventilators and modes set at maximal rates and minimal volumes or pressures.

As mentioned previously, the advantages of HFV in adults are not well proven. Their use is most commonly considered as an option for "salvage therapy" in the management of severe, refractory ALI/ARDS, which is also its most common neonatal intensive care unit (NICU) and pediatric intensive care unit (PICU) use [33]. However, no currently available clinical trials demonstrate a clear advantage of HFV as compared to conventional approaches or other salvage therapy approaches, such as extracorporeal support (e.g., ECMO). Management of large bronchopleural fistulas (BPF) is another less common use for HFV, in particular HFJV, which is Food & Drug Administration approved for this indication. A major disadvantage and risk of all modes of HFV is the development of air trapping (auto-PEEP) and subsequent barotraumas. As a result, use of HFV in patients with obstructive lung diseases should be avoided. Finally, management of airway humid-ification and secretions in HFV is highly problematic and can lead to ineffective ventilation and necrotizing tracheobronchitis. HFPV may have somewhat reduced problems with clearance of airway secretions.

2.4.8   Continuous positive airway pressure (CPAP)

Although frequently mis-stated, CPAP is not a mode of ventilation, and simply refers to the continuous delivery of a fixed level of positive airway pressure during both inspiration and expiration. Consequently, there is no functional or mechanical difference between CPAP and Positive End-Expiratory Pressure (PEEP). The term CPAP primarily refers to the application of noninvasive positive pressure ventila-tion (NIPPV) both for long-term use in patients with upper airway abnormalities, such as obstructive sleep apnea, or short-term use in some patients with acute res-piratory failure in which intubation might be avoided. Bilevel positive airway pressure (BiPAP) refers to the combination of CPAP and PSV. For further details on the application of CPAP and BiPAP, refer to the chapters on Noninvasive Ventilation.

The term PEEP primarily refers to application in acute respiratory failure requir-ing intubation and invasive mechanical ventilation, and serves principally to enhance and maintain alveolar recruitment resulting in improved oxygenation and overall gas exchange [6]. A frequent misconception of PEEP, and why some con-clude it is not equivalent to CPAP, is that PEEP it is not applied during inspiration. However, shortly after increasing PEEP, P_D will typically rise by an equivalent amount. If an increased level of PEEP leads to more alveolar recruitment and improved lung compliance, the change in P_D may be less than the absolute amount of PEEP applied but, nonetheless, PEEP remains present during inspiration. A disadvantage of PEEP is its potential for negative impact on cardiac output due to reduced ventricular filling as a consequence of the higher intrathoracic pressures during diastole.

The optimal levels of PEEP ("Best PEEP") that should be used vary widely for specific clinical conditions (e.g., obstructive versus restrictive lung diseases) and can be highly variable for any specific patient [34]. Titration of PEEP typically must consider its impact on gas exchange, airway pressures and hemodynamics. It is also important to remember that PEEP can be present as a result of both intentional ventilator-generated (extrinsic) PEEP or as a result of incomplete expiration of a given V_T which leads to "air trapping". When PEEP is present as a result of air trapping, it is referred to as intrinsic PEEP or auto-PEEP, and is most commonly seen in patients with obstructive lung diseases, but can also result from inverse ratio ventilation as described earlier in this chapter. There is no evidence to suggest that the impact of intrinsic versus extrinsic PEEP on gas exchange and hemodynamics is different. Accurate quantitation of intrinsic PEEP involves a brief pause at end-expiration, but cannot be performed in all ventilator modes and can often be challenging due to clinical conditions (e.g., high respiratory rates). Intrinsic PEEP can also be quantified from the airway pressure tracing at the zero flow crossing point between expiration to inspiration. These challenges and limitations should motivate clinicians to adjust their treatment approach (ventilator and otherwise) to remove or minimize intrinsic PEEP when possible.

Although many clinicians refer to a low level of PEEP ($\leq 5\,cm\ H_2O$) as being "physiologic", this remains controversial. The routine use of a low level of PEEP began many years ago, as a means to compensate for the resistance of the ventilator circuit, since most ventilators at that time were not otherwise capable. Although most current ventilators have methods to adjust inspiratory airflow and/or pressure to overcome the ventilator circuit, use of a low level of PEEP remains common. Although the need for this level of PEEP is uncertain, no negative impact on patient outcomes has been reported.

2.4.9 Summary

As this chapter has detailed, there are many ways in which a clinician/operator can provide adequate ventilatory support for the majority of patients who require intubation and mechanical ventilation for both hypercapnic and hypoxemic respiratory failure. For each of these modes, the operator must remain aware that all key parameters including volume, pressure and flow are involved in each mode, even when a particular mode does not permit the operator to control it. Most operators will be best served by utilizing a few very common and well understood modes (e.g., AC and PSV), which will meet the needs of the majority of patients with all varieties of acute respiratory failure, including both the initial phase of decompensation requiring high level support as well as during the recovery phase and weaning. Additional benefits of these modes also include the familiarity of the ICU support staff (e.g., respiratory therapy and nursing) assisting the physician in the management of the patient. Often the lack of desirable results at any clinical time point is more related to the patient's underlying condition (e.g., increasing pulmonary edema) or other aspects of their management (e.g., sedation) that require adjustment than changing to alternative modes of ventilation. Once the operator becomes fully familiar with the strengths and limitations of these "workhorse" modes of ventilation, the appropriate settings to consider the numerous alternative modes of ventilation that are available become easier to recognize. It is reasonable to anticipate that, as experience grows with the newer computer-driven patient tailored modes of ventilation, these modes may substantially enhance the ability to optimize patient comfort and reduce the duration and morbidities associated with mechanical ventilation.

2.4.10   Case presentation revisited

Shortly after arrival to the MICU, the patient had a repeat chest X-ray, which revealed progressive bilateral infiltrates consistent with the acute respiratory distress syndrome. He was placed on volume-cycled assist control mode with a tidal volume of 6 mg/kg of predicted body weight, respiratory rate = 20 bpm, FiO_2 of 0.80, PEEP = 12 cm H_2O and inspiratory flow rate to achieve an I : E ratio of approximately 1 : 1. On those settings, the patient demonstrated a total respiratory rate of 30–32 bpm, SaO_2 = 94–97% and peak inspiratory pressures of 25–30 cm H_2O. An ABG obtained on those settings revealed pH = 7.24, $PaCO_2$ = 20 mm Hg and PaO_2 = 76 mm Hg. Assist control mode was chosen in this setting due to its ability to: 1) provide a guaranteed V_T of a size that is known to reduce ventilator induced lung injury and 2) permit the patient to take as many machine supported breaths as needed to achieve the desired minute ventilation. Neither PSV or SIMV can consistently provide this combination in a patient with this degree of ARDS. Although weaning and liberation from mechanical ventilation can be achieved directly from AC mode once a patient has passed an SBT, it is likely this patient would be transitioned to a weaning mode, most likely PSV, once his oxygenation requirements and demand for V_E had reduced sufficiently. Choosing a weaning mode from the onset would not be appropriate, as it would be unlikely to reduce length of time on the ventilator and significantly increase the risk of inadequate ventilation and oxygenation during the early ICU course. Should the patient not improve or deteriorate on AC mode, common options that could be considered as alternate strategies would be either PCV or APRV.

References

1. Hinson, J.R. and Marini, J.J. (1992) Principles of mechanical ventilator use in respiratory failure. *Annu. Rev. Med.*, **43**, 341–361.
2. Tobin, M.J. (1994) Mechanical ventilation. *N. Engl. J. Med.*, **330**, 1056–1061.
3. Slutsky, A.S. (1993) Mechanical ventilation. American College of Chest Physician's Consensus Conference. *Chest*, **104**, 1833–1859.

4. Lourens, M.S., van den Berg, B., Aerts, J.G. *et al.* (2000) Expiratory time constants in mechanically ventilated patients with and without COPD. *Intensive Care Med.*, **26**, 1612–1618.
5. MacIntyre, N.R. (1986) Respiratory function during pressure support ventilation. *Chest*, **89**, 677–683.
6. Rossi, A. and Ranieri, M.V. (1994) Positive end-expiratory pressure, in *Principles and Practice of Mechanical Ventilation* (ed. M.J. Tobin), McGraw-Hill, New York, pp. 259–303.
7. Marini, J.J., Smith, T.C. and Lamb, V. (1988) External work output and force generation during synchronized intermittent mechanical ventilation: Effect of machine assistance on breathing effort. *Am. Rev. Respir. Dis.*, **138**, 1169–1179.
8. Groeger, J.S., Levinson, M.R. and Carlon, G.C. (1989) Assist control versus synchronized intermittent mandatory ventilation during acute respiratory failure. *Crit. Care Med.*, **17**, 607–612.
9. Mador, M.J. (1994) Assist-control ventilation, in *Principles and Practice of Mechanical Ventilation* (ed. M.J. Tobin), McGraw-Hill, New York, pp. 207–219.
10. Sassoon, C.S.H., Del Rosario, N., Fei, R. *et al.* (1994) Influence of pressure- and flow-triggered synchronous intermittent mandatory ventilation on inspiratory muscle work. *Crit. Care Med.*, **22**, 1933–1941.
11. Gurevitch, M.J. and Gelmont, D. (1989) Importance of trigger sensitivity to ventilator response delay in advanced chronic obstructive pulmonary disease with respiratory failure. *Crit. Care Med.*, **17**, 354–359.
12. Weisman, I.M., Rinaldo, J.E., Rogers, R.M. *et al.* (1983) Intermittent mandatory ventilation. *Am. Rev. Respir. Dis.*, **127**, 641–647.
13. Esteban, A., Ferguson, N.D., Meade, M.O. *et al.* (2008) Evolution of mechanical ventilation in response to clinical research. *Am. J. Respir. Crit. Care Med.*, **177**, 170–177.
14. MacIntyre, N.R. (1994) Pressure-limited versus volume-cycled breath delivery strategies. *Crit. Care Med.*, **22**, 4–5.
15. Marini, J.J., Crooke, P.S. and Truwit, J.D. (1989) Determinants of pressure-preset ventilation: a mathematical model of pressure control. *J. Appl. Physiol.*, **67**, 1081–1092.
16. Banner, M.J., Kirby, R.R., Blanch, P.B. *et al.* (1993) Decreasing imposed work of the breathing apparatus to zero using pressure-support ventilation. *Crit. Care Med.*, **21**, 1333–1338.
17. Tokioka, H., Saito, S. and Kosaka, F. (1989) Comparison of pressure support ventilation and assist control ventilation in patients with acute respiratory failure. *Intensive Care Med.*, **15**, 364–367.
18. Fiastro, J.F., Habib, M.P. and Quan, S.F. (1988) Pressure support compensation for inspiratory work due to endotracheal tubes and demand continuous positive airway pressure. *Chest*, **93**, 499–505.
19. Rappaport, S.H., Shpiner, R., Yoshihara, G. *et al.* (1994) Randomized, prospective trial of pressure-limited versus volume-controlled ventilation in severe respiratory failure. *Crit. Care Med.*, **22**, 22–32.
20. Esteban, A., Alia, I., Gordo, F. *et al.* (2000) Prospective randomized trial comparing pressure-controlled ventilation and volume-controlled ventilation in ARDS. *Chest*, **117**, 1690–1696.
21. Lain, D.C., DiBenedetto, R., Morris, S.L. *et al.* (1989) Pressure control inverse ratio ventilation as a method to reduce peak inspiratory pressure and provide adequate ventilation and oxygenation. *Chest*, **95**, 1081–1088.
22. Shanholtz, C. and Brower, R. (1994) Should inverse ratio ventilation be used in adult respiratory distress syndrome? *Am. J. Respir. Crit. Care Med.*, **149**, 1354–1358.

23. Varpula, T., Valta, P., Niemi, R. *et al.* (2004) Airway pressure release ventilation as a primary ventilatory mode in acute respiratory distress syndrome. *Acta Anaesthesiol. Scand.*, **48**, 722–731.

24. Seymour, C.W., Frazer, M., Reilly, P.M. and Fuchs, B.D. (2007) Airway pressure release and biphasic intermittent positive airway pressure ventilation: are they ready for prime time? *J. Trauma*, **62**, 1298–1308.

25. Dries, D.J. and Marini, J.J. (2009) Airway pressure release ventilation. *J. Burn Care Res.*, **30**, 929–936.

26. Guldager, H., Nielsen, S.L., Carl, P. and Soerensen, M.B. (1997) A comparison of volume control and pressure-regulated volume control ventilation in acute respiratory failure. *Crit. Care*, **1**, 75–77.

27. Holt, S.J., Sanders, R.C., Thurman, T.L. and Heulitt, M.J. (2001) An evaluation of Automode, a computer-controlled ventilator mode, with the Siemens Servo 300A ventilator, using a porcine model. *Respir. Care*, **46**, 26–36.

28. Xirouchaki, N., Kondili, E., Vaporidi, K. *et al.* (2008) Proportional assist ventilation with load-adjustable gain factors in critically ill patients: comparison with pressure support. *Intensive Care Med.*, **34**, 2026–2034.

29. Arnal, J.M., Wysocki, M., Nafati, C. *et al.* (2008) Automatic selection of breathing pattern using adaptive support ventilation. *Intensive Care Med.*, **34**, 75–81.

30. Lellouche, F. and Brochard, L. (2009) Advanced closed loops during mechanical ventilation (PAV, NAVA, ASV, SmartCare). *Best Pract. Res. Clin. Anaesthesiol.*, **23**, 81–93.

31. Fessler, H.E., Hager, D.N. and Brower, R.G. (2008) Feasibility of very high frequency ventilation in adults with acute respiratorydistress syndrome. *Crit. Care Med.*, **36**, 1043–1048.

32. Standiford, T.J. and Morganroth, M.L. (1989) High-frequency ventilation. *Chest*, **96**, 1380–1389.

33. Fessler, H.E., Derdak, S., Ferguson, N.D. *et al.* (2007) A protocol for high-frequency oscillatory ventilation in adults: results from a round table discussion. *Crit. Care Med.*, **35**, 1649–1654.

34. Amato, M.B., Barbas, C.S., Medeiros, D.M. *et al.* (1995) Beneficial effects of the "open lung approach" with low distending pressures in acute respiratory distress syndrome. *Am. J. Respir. Crit. Care Med.*, **152**, 1835–1846.

2.5 Assessing lung physiology

Daniel C. Grinnan[1] and Jonathon D. Truwit[2]

[1] *Division of Pulmonary and Critical Care Medicine, Virginia Commonwealth University, Richmond, VA, USA*
[2] *Division of Pulmonary and Critical Care Medicine, University of Virginia, Charlottesville, VA, USA*

2.5.1 Case presentation

A 47-year-old with history of asthma presents to the emergency department with status asthmaticus and requires intubation for progressive respiratory acidosis despite intravenous corticosteroids and continuous nebulized bronchodilators. Deep sedation is used to decrease his work of breathing and to decrease his respiratory rate. Permissive hypercapnia is the result, and his auto-PEEP decreases. Several days later, you are suddenly called to the bedside to evaluate an acute change noticed by the nurse. He has new onset tachycardia and his peak airway pressure has increased from 40 mm Hg to 60 mm Hg. You evaluate the ventilator and notice that his settings have not changed. You check his plateau pressure, and it is unchanged at 25 mm Hg. What might have happened and what should you do?

2.5.2 Introduction

The topic of lung physiology is vast and complex. However, the basic understanding of lung physiology is vital to managing a patient on mechanical ventilation. While mechanical ventilators have become increasingly complex in this age of combined modes and competition between ventilator manufacturers, the underlying principles have changed little. This chapter is titled "assessing lung physiology,"

A Practical Guide to Mechanical Ventilation, First Edition.
Edited by Jonathon D. Truwit and Scott K. Epstein.
© 2011 John Wiley & Sons, Ltd. Published 2011 by John Wiley & Sons, Ltd.

as it is hoped to provide the tools needed to derive important information from the ventilator and to use this information to help patients. In addition, it is hoped that an understanding of lung physiology will help the reader to understand the goals of mechanical ventilation in different states of pulmonary pathology.

2.5.3   Overview of oxygenation and ventilation in lung physiology

Oxygenation refers to the ability of oxygen to enter the alveoli and to diffuse into the pulmonary circulation. Abnormal oxygenation can result from various phenomena. The general causes of hypoxemia are important to review, as ventilator management can change based on the underlying cause. The most common cause of hypoxemia in lung disease is the mismatching of ventilation and blood flow (VQ mismatch). Normally, the V:Q ratio should be 0.8–1.0 [1]. In a patient with pulmonary embolism, the lung is well ventilated, but perfusion is altered to the affected section of the pulmonary vascular tree, leading to a high V:Q ratio. In a patient with lobar pneumonia, the affected lung is poorly ventilated but is perfused (in fact, inflammation related to the pneumonia commonly causes vasodilatation in the affected region), leading to a low V:Q ratio. Both instances are examples of VQ mismatch, but management of high ratio mismatch and low ratio mismatch can be different. A shunt refers to the passage of blood directly to the systemic circulation without going through a ventilated lung. A shunt represents an extreme of low ratio VQ mismatch (ratio of zero in the affected regions). Causes of shunt include profound atelectasis, right to left cardiac shunts (Eisenmenger's), hepatopulmonary syndrome, and other causes. A hallmark of shunt physiology is the inability to increase arterial PaO_2 on 100% oxygen [2].

Oxygenation also depends on diffusion from the alveoli to the pulmonary capillary. Fick's law of diffusion (V) reads: $V = A/T * D (P1 - P2)$, where A is the area of the vessel wall, T is the thickness of the vessel wall, P1 is the partial pressure of gas in the capillary, and P2 is the partial pressure of gas in the alveolus. D is a constant which reflects the solubility of the gas. A second step to diffusion is the attachment of oxygen to the hemoglobin molecule once it enters the capillary. This is important in understanding the hypoxemia from methemoglobinemia, a state caused by transition of the heme molecule to the ferric state (a transition which prevents oxygen from binding to hemoglobin). Methemoglobinemia can be caused by various medications used in the intensive care unit, including cetacaine, lidocaine, and inhaled nitric oxide. Clinically, a patient will have very low PaO_2 on arterial blood gas, although the arterial saturation will be partially preserved (as methemoglobin registers a saturation of 85% and is interpreted as an oxygenated molecule by pulse oximeter).

Lastly, the effect of hypoventilation on oxygenation is usually mild in comparison to its effect on carbon dioxide tension. Decreasing the minute ventilation produces a comparable increase in carbon dioxide levels. If the minute ventilation is cut in half, the $PaCO_2$ should double. The effect of hypoventilation on oxygenation is related to its effect on carbon dioxide through the alveolar gas equation. The simplified alveolar gas equation is: $PaO_2 = PiO_2 - (PaCO_2/R)$, where PiO_2 is the partial pressure of inspired oxygen, also impacted by altitude, and R is the respiratory exchange ratio (a marker of the difference in metabolism between oxygen and carbon dioxide in the body). In other words, the effect of hypoventilation on arterial carbon dioxide will lead to a predictable decrease on the arterial oxygen level. Again, hypoventilation typically produces a small decrease in oxygen levels compared to the relative increase in carbon dioxide levels.

2.5.4 Control of oxygenation and ventilation with mechanical ventilation

One of the common dilemmas facing a clinician is how to manipulate the ventilator to improve an abnormal blood gas. In this section, the differences between correcting hypoxemia and correcting hypercapnia or hypocapnia are explained.

Changes in ventilation (hypoventilation) produce a large change in $PaCO_2$ with a relatively small change in PaO_2. Therefore, carbon dioxide levels can be manipulated with a mechanical ventilator by changing the rate of ventilation. Minute ventilation (V_E) is defined as: $V_E = V_T * RR$, where V_T is tidal volume and RR is respiratory rate. Many patients on mechanical ventilation have VQ mismatch. Dead space (V_D) reflects areas of the lung which are ventilated, but not perfused. As dead space limits the area of capillary blood in contact with alveoli, it will affect the diffusion of carbon dioxide. Therefore, V_D/V_T is another important variable in understanding the control of $PaCO_2$. In a given patient, if the minute ventilation and the $PaCO_2$ are known, the V_D/V_T can be estimated. The estimation of V_D/V_T can then be used to predict how much minute ventilation should be changed in order to produce a marked effect on $PaCO_2$ (Figure 2.5.1). This can be particularly helpful clinically, as maintenance of $PaCO_2$ and pH through manipulation of minute ventilation is a common requirement when caring for the patient on mechanical ventilation.

In clinical practice, manipulations of tidal volume and respiratory rate to correct abnormal ventilation are common. For example, in patients with severe acute respiratory distress syndrome (ARDS), the ventilator settings may be adjusted to result in permissive hypercapnia. The goal of permissive hypercapnia in the ARDS patient is to allow (or permit) low tidal volumes and low respiratory rates in order to prevent volume and pressure induced trauma to the ventilated alveoli. Lowering tidal volume (to 6 ml/kg of predicted body weight) without increasing respiratory rate will decrease minute ventilation and raise carbon dioxide. Permissive hypercapnia is also used in patients with severe obstructive lung disease (status asthmaticus), but the ventilator manipulation is different. In this case, the intention is to

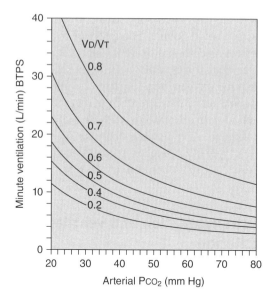

Figure 2.5.1   The relationship between minute ventilation (Ve), arterial $PaCO_2$, and the ratio of dead space to tidal volume is shown. (Reproduced with permission [18].)

decrease the respiratory rate, so that the expiratory phase can be as long as possible (and air trapping, or auto-PEEP, may be avoided). Knowledge of the physiology of governing ventilation is crucial to the proper management of the patient in acute respiratory failure.

Oxygenation can also be manipulated by the ventilator through several mechanisms. First, the fractional intake of oxygen (FiO_2) can be changed to correct hypoxemia. A patient's response at a given FiO_2 can be assessed by calculating the ratio of the PaO_2 to the FiO_2 (P/F). For example, a patient with a PaO_2 of 150 mm Hg on 50% FiO_2 will have a P/F of 300. A P/F of less than 200 is part of the clinical definition of ARDS, while a P/F less than 300 is a criterion for Acute Lung Injury (ALI) [3]. As some degree of shunt is seen in all people, the P/F will become lower as the FiO_2 is increased. Caution should be used when increasing the FiO_2 above 60%. While this is often necessary and is the proper action to take in order to preserve oxygenation, the FiO_2 should not be left at high levels with supraphysiologic oxygenation. High FiO_2 oxygen can increase the formation of free oxygen radicals and has the potential to lead to progressive lung injury. Furthermore, patients with a prior exposure to bleomycin [4] or with pre-existing idiopathic pulmonary fibrosis [5] are at risk for oxygen toxicity.

Positive end-expiratory pressure (PEEP) also influences oxygenation and can be manipulated on the ventilator. PEEP maintains alveoli open at the end of expiration, preventing alveolar collapse and resultant atelectasis. Regional atelectasis is a manifestation of many pulmonary disease processes. This atelectasis results in regions of the lung receiving perfusion but not ventilation (abnormally low VQ). The addition of PEEP "recruits" these atelectatic alveoli, thus decreasing VQ mismatch and improving oxygenation. An extreme example of this is the recruitment maneuver, in which PEEP is maintained at very high levels (often over 35 mm Hg) for a short period (less than 2 min). Both recruitment maneuvers and less dramatic increases in PEEP are well established methods of improving oxygenation in mechanically ventilated patients with ALI or ARDS (among other conditions). Unfortunately, this improvement in oxygenation has not translated into improved clinical outcomes in ALI/ARDS patients in large clinical trials. In fact, recruitment maneuvers were found to have increased risk of barotrauma without improving clinical outcomes [6].

Within a delivered breath, the ratio of inspiratory time to expiratory time (I:E) can be manipulated on the ventilator. Changing the I:E is a third way to effect oxygenation. The rationale is similar to that of PEEP. Given a constant respiratory rate, prolongation of the inspiratory time leads to shortening of the expiratory time. Alveoli will have less time to collapse, leading to less regional atelectasis and improved VQ matching. In normal conditions (spontaneous breathing), the inspiratory phase consists of 40% of the respiratory cycle. Extreme manipulation of the I:E occurs with inverse ratio ventilation, during which the inspiratory phase is made longer than the expiratory phase. Inverse ratio ventilation is commonly employed with a BiLevel mode of ventilation, during which the higher level of PEEP is applied longer than the lower level of PEEP. The patient often requires sedation to accommodate inverse ration ventilation as I:E is the reverse of spontaneous ventilation. Therefore, manipulation of the I:E to improve oxygenation is often limited to those patients who have not responded to increases in FiO_2 and PEEP.

2.5.5 Respiratory mechanics

The understanding of respiratory mechanics is also vital in managing a patient on mechanical ventilation. Understanding respiratory mechanics while caring for a patient on mechanical ventilation can assist with diagnoses of mucous plugging, acute tension pneumothorax, respiratory muscle fatigue, air trapping, and ARDS. Without knowledge of respiratory mechanics, airway emergencies may be more difficult to identify and treat. Airway compliance, resistance, and work of breathing are discussed in this section.

2.5.5.1 Compliance

Compliance describes the willingness of a structure (in this case, the lungs and chest wall) to distend and can be calculated as follows: $C = \Delta V/\Delta P$, where C is compliance, ΔV is change in volume, and ΔP is change in pressure. To eliminate airway resistance from confounding the results of this calculation, compliance must be determined under conditions of zero flow [7]. Therefore, compliance is a static measurement. It must also be obtained under passive conditions. The patient cannot actively be using his/her respiratory muscles at the time of measurement, as the measured pressure will be affected by respiratory efforts. In patients on mechanical ventilation, this commonly requires deep sedation. Therefore, compliance is most commonly calculated on patients receiving most of their work of breathing from the ventilator and is passive, either from sedation or high ventilator tidal volume delivery frequency.

Static conditions create an environment where the alveolar pressure equilibrates with the measured ventilator pressure and are created by occluding the airway, most commonly before and after tidal volume. This allows for measurement of end expiratory alveolar pressure (Pex) and end inspiratory alveolar pressure (plateau pressure, of Ppl). By measuring Pex and Ppl, and knowing the tidal volume (V_T) delivered, compliance may be solved. It should be noted that Pex is the sum of both intrinsic PEEP (auto-PEEP) and extrinsic PEEP (ventilator delivered PEEP). Therefore, in a patient with intrinsic PEEP of 5 cm H_2O, extrinsic PEEP of 5 cm H_2O, plateau pressure of 30 cm H_2O, and tidal volume of 500 ml: C = 500/[30 − (5 + 5)] = 500/20 = 25 ml/cm H_2O. In a normal subject on mechanical ventilation, compliance should be 100 ml/cm H_2O [8]. While most modern ventilators will provide a calculated value of compliance, understanding how to calculate compliance is important when trying to interpret abnormal compliance results. Following compliance over time not only provides information regarding disease progression or resolution, it also can help to narrow the differential diagnosis (Table 2.5.1). The distinction between chest wall compliance and lung compliance requires the placement of an esophageal manometer, which is rarely done in clinical practice.

Table 2.5.1 Causes of decreased intrathoracic compliance. (Reproduced with permission [19].)

Causes of decreased measured chest wall compliance	Causes of decreased measured lung compliance
Obesity	Tension pneumothorax
Ascites	Mainstem intubation
Neuromuscular weakness (Guillain–Barre, steroid myopathy, etc.)	Dynamic hyperinflation
Flail chest (mediastinal removal)	Pulmonary edema
Kyphoscoliosis	Pulmonary fibrosis
Fibrothorax	Acute respiratory distress syndrome
Pectus excavatum	Langerhans cell histiocytosis
Chest wall tumor	Hypersensitivity pneumonitis
Paralysis	Connective tissue disorders
Scleroderma	Sarcoidosis
	Cryptogenic organizing pneumonitis
	Lymphangitic spread of tumor

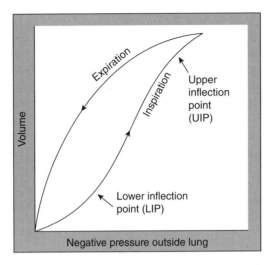

Figure 2.5.2 A pressure–volume curve developed from measurements in isolated lung during inflation (inspiration) and deflation (expiration). The slope of each curve is the compliance. The difference in the curves is hysteresis. (Reproduced with permission [16].)

If static pressure is measured at differing tidal volumes and at differing points within a respiratory cycle, a pressure–volume curve (Figure 2.5.2) can be constructed. The inspiratory curve differs from the expiratory as there is hysteresis. While the slope of either curve represents compliance, convention is to draw a line between the two curves from end-expiration to end-inspiration for a given tidal volume.

The slope of the PV curve is equal to compliance. The inspiratory limb of the pressure–volume curve will normally have a lower inflection point (LIP) and an upper inflection point (UIP). The region between the two points represents the region of greatest compliance. It has been believed that the UIP represents a point of increased alveolar distension, so that inflating the lungs past this point will provide increased risk of barotrauma with little clinical benefit [9]. In patients with ARDS, targeting tidal volumes of 6 ml/kg predicted body weight and maintaining end-inspiratory pressures below 30 cm H_2O leads to improved survival [10]. It also appears that with smaller tidal volume ventilation the lower the end-inspiratory pressure the lower the mortality, even when restricting analysis to those patients with pressures <30 cm H_2O [11].

The LIP was thought to represent the pressure required to overcome alveolar surface tension and open the alveoli that had collapsed during expiration. It was first proven over 50 years ago that the addition of PEEP in patients with profound hypoxemia resulted in rapid improvement of their hypoxemia, presumably by assisting with alveolar recruitment [12]. It has been much more difficult to show that increasing PEEP leads to improved clinical outcomes in patients with ALI or ARDS. The ARDS Network performed a multicenter study designed to answer this question. The results did not reveal that increased PEEP provided clinical benefit compared with lower levels of PEEP in patients with ARDS [6]. Two other large randomized controlled trials also demonstrated similar results [13a, 13b].

However, the methodology has been criticized as being a "one size fits all" approach to a clinical scenario with great individual differences. Indeed, the variability in recruitable alveoli is great among patients with ARDS. A recent study noted that pleural pressures vary widely among critically ill patients, and they placed esophageal balloon catheters in patients to accurately measure the transpulmonary pressure (airway pressure minus pleural pressure) [14]. The study showed that oxygenation was improved compared to the conventional manipulation of PEEP used in the ARDS Network study. Additional studies assessing clinical outcomes in those with esophageal balloon catheters are needed.

2.5.5.2   Resistance

As mentioned above, the presence of airway resistance (R) is dependent on airflow (Q). Resistance is determined by the equation: $R = \Delta P/Q$. In the trachea, flow normally has a turbulent component [15]. However, in the smaller airways, flow generally follows laminar properties. In airways with laminar flow, resistance is related to radius (r), airway length (l), and gas viscosity (η) through Poiseuille's equation ($R = 8\eta l/\pi r^4$). This equation reveals the strong relationship between airway radius and resistance. If the radius is reduced by half, the resistance is increased 16-fold! Because the airway branches lie in parallel, the total resistance (Rt) is less than the individual resistances ($1/Rt = 1/R1 + 1/R2 + \ldots.$). In a normal person, the medium sized bronchi are the site of greatest resistance [16].

In mechanically ventilated patients, knowledge of airway resistance can be vital to helping a patient recover. The pressure gradient that drives flow can be easily approximated by subtracting the plateau (end-inspiratory) pressure (P_s) from the peak dynamic airway pressure (P_D). Therefore, $R = [P_D - P_S]/V$, where V is airflow in l/s. In a normal individual, inspiratory resistance rarely exceeds 15 cm $H_2O/l/s$ [8]. In mechanically ventilated patients, a sudden increase in peak pressure without a corresponding increase in plateau pressure indicates a sudden increase in resistance. This always should prompt an evaluation into the patient's changing condition, and helps to shape the differential diagnosis. For example, in a patient with status asthmaticus, a sudden increase in peak airway pressure could indicate several things. Firstly, the patient may be experiencing bronchospasm of the medium sized bronchi, as this is a major site of inflammation in asthmatics. Secondly, the patient may have developed secretions in the endotracheal tube, narrowing the radius of the tube and causing increased resistance. Thirdly, a mucous plug in a major bronchus is common and can cause sudden increase in peak airway pressures. However, unlike the first two examples, atelectasis from the mucus plug will also increase the plateau pressure, as it will effect airway compliance. Fourthly, a tension pneumothorax from barotrauma will cause elevation of peak airway pressures. Again, this increase in peak pressures will be associated with decreased compliance, differentiating a tension pneumothorax from the first two examples.

In addition to identifying the underlying cause of increased airway resistance and treating that condition, it is possible to manipulate airway resistance in extreme cases by using heliox. Heliox, a mixture of helium (60–80%) and oxygen (20–40%) has a substantially lower density then oxygen blended with room air. While clinical results have not been meaningful in studies of patients with status asthmaticus [17], it is commonly used with upper airway obstruction (tracheal stenosis, intratracheal mass, angioedema) with good result.

2.5.6 Summary

Understanding the basic physiology governing pulmonary pathology is vital to the management of a mechanical ventilator. Similarly, understanding how to assess and manipulate physiology with a mechanical ventilator is vital to managing severe pulmonary disease. In this chapter, some basic principles of lung physiology have been reviewed and placed in the context of mechanical ventilation and commonly encountered clinical situations in the intensive care unit.

2.5.7 Case presentation revisited

The case presentation describes an asthmatic with a sudden increase in airway resistance (not a decrease in compliance, since the plateau pressure is unchanged). A chest X-ray was obtained and did not show pneumothorax or massive atelectasis, although a decrease in compliance would have been anticipated in both conditions. His medication record was reviewed; there were no changes in medication delivery that would be associated with acute bronchospasm. It was noted that he had copious, thick secretions earlier in the day, and that it was difficult to pass the in-line suction catheter at times. Secretions adherent to the endotracheal tube were suspected as the cause of his increased resistance and his endotracheal tube was quickly changed. Following placement of his new endotracheal tube, his peak airway pressure was 35 mm Hg, with an unchanged plateau pressure of 25 mm Hg.

References

1. West, J.B. (1977) State of the art: ventilation-perfusion relationships. *Am. Rev. Respir. Dis.*, **116**, 919–943.
2. West, J.B. and Wagner, P.D. (2000) Ventilation, Blood Flow, and Gas Exchange, in *Murray and Nadal's Textbook of Respiratory Medicine*, 3rd edn (eds J.F. Murray, J.A. Nadel, R.J. Mason and H.A. Bouchery), WB Saunders Company, Philadelphia, pp. 55–89.

3. Bernard, G.R.,Artigas, A., Brigham, K.L. *et al.* (1994) The American-European Consensus Conference on ARDS. Definitions, mechanisms, relevant outcomes, and clinical trial coordination. *Am. J. Respir. Crit. Care Med.*, **149** (3), 818–824.

4. Allen, S.C., Riddell, G.S., and Butchart, E.G. (1981) Bleomycin Therapy and Anaesthesia. The possible hazards of oxygen administration to patients after treatment with bleomycin. *Anaesthesia*, **36** (1), 60–63.

5. Daniil, Z.D., Papageorgiou, E., Koutsokera, A. *et al.* (2006) Serum levels of oxidative stress as a marker of disease severity in idiopathic pulmonary fibrosis. *Pulm. Pharmacol. Ther.*, **21** (1), 26–31.

6. Brower, R.G., Lanken, P.N., MacIntyre, N. *et al.* (National Heart, Lung, and Blood Institute ARDS Clinical Trials Network) (2004) Higher versus lower positive end-expiratory pressures in patients with the acute respiratory distress syndrome. *N. Engl. J. Med.*, **351**, 327–336.

7. Truwit, J.D. (1995) Lung mechanics, in *Comprehensive Respiratory Care* (eds D.R. Dantzer, N.R. MacIntyre and E.D. Bakow), WB Saunders Company, Philadelphia, pp. 18–31.

8. MacIntyre, N.R. (2001) Evidence-based guidelines for weaning and discontinuing ventilatory support. *Chest*, **120**, 375S–396S.

9. Marini, J.J. and Gattinoni, L. (2004) Ventilatory management of acute respiratory distress syndrome: a consensus of two. *Crit. Care Med.*, **32**, 250–255.

10. The Acute Respiratory Distress Syndrome Network (2000) Ventilation with lower tidal volumes as compared with traditional tidal volumes for acute lung injury and the acute respiratory distress syndrome. *N. Engl. J. Med.*, **342**, 1301–1308.

11. Hager, D.N. Krishnan, J.A., Hayden, D.L., and Brower, R.G. (ARDS Clinical Trials Network) (2005) Tidal volumes reduction in patients with acute lung injury when plateau pressures are not high. *Am. J. Respir. Crit. Care Med.*, **172**, 1241–1245.

12. Ashbaugh, D.G., Bigelow, D.B., Petty, T.L. and Levine, B.E. (1967) Acute respiratory distress in adults. *Lancet*, **2**, 319–323.

13a. Mercat, A., Richard, J.M., Vielle, B. *et al.* (2008) Positive end-expiratory pressure setting in adults with acute lung injury and acute respiratory distress syndrome (EXPRESS). *JAMA*, **299**, 646–655.

13b. Meade, M.O., Cook, D.J., Guyatt, G.H. *et al.* (2008) Ventilation strategy using low tidal volumes, recruitment maneuvers, and high positive end-expiratory pressure for acute lung injury and acute respiratory distress syndrome: a randomized controlled trial. *JAMA*, **299**, 637–645.

14. Talmor, D., Sarge, T., Malhotra, A. *et al.* (2008) Mechanical ventilation guided by esophageal pressure in acute lung injury. *N. Engl. J. Med.*, **359**, 2095–2104.

15. Bock, K.R., Silver, P., Rom, M. and Sagy, M. (2000) Reduction in tracheal lumen due to endotracheal intubation and its calculated clinical significance. *Chest*, **118**, 468–472.

16. Costanzo, L.S. (2002) *Physiology*, 2nd edn. WB Saunders Co., Philadelphia.

17. Rodrigo, G., Pollack, C., Rodrigo, C. and Rowe, B.H. (2003) Heliox for nonintubated acute asthma patients. *Cochrane Database Syst. Rev.* 4 (Art. No.: CD002884). doi: 10.1002/14651858.CD002884.pub2

18. Effros, R.M. and Widell, J.L. (2000) Acid-base balance, in *Murray and Nadal's Textbook of Respiratory Medicine*, 3rd edn (eds J.F. Murray, J.A. Nadel, R.J. Mason and H.A. Bouchery), WB Saunders Company, Philadelphia, pp. 163–170.

19. Grinnan, D.C. and Truwit, J.D. (2005) Clinical review: respiratory mechanics in spontaneous and assisted ventilation. *Critical Care*, **9** (5), 472–484.

2.6 Mechanical ventilation in restrictive lung disease

R. Duncan Hite

Pulmonary, Critical Care, Allergy, and Immunology, Wake Forest University, Winston-Salem, NC, USA

2.6.1 Case presentation

A 54-year-old woman was admitted to an outside hospital two days earlier with septic shock from pyelonephritis and perinephric abscess. Despite appropriate antibiotic therapy and percutaneous drainage of her abscess, her septic shock persisted requiring moderate doses of norepinephrine and fluid boluses to maintain a MAP > 65 mm Hg. As a result of her persistent critical illness, she was just transferred to your tertiary care center for further management. She was intubated a few hours after admission to the outside intensive care unit and her requirements for ventilator support have slowly increased throughout her hospital course. Although her initial chest X-ray at the outside hospital did not demonstrate any abnormalities, her subsequent X-rays, including one obtained after arrival at your hospital, reveal bilateral infiltrates consistent with progressive acute lung injury (ALI). On arrival to your intensive care unit, she is on assist control mode with a set rate of 20 breaths per minute, tidal volume of 550 ml, PEEP = 12 cm H_2O and $FiO_2 = 0.90$. Your initial arterial blood gas (ABG) reveals the following: pH = 7.18, $PaCO_2 = 57$ mm Hg and $PaO_2 = 63$ mm Hg.

A Practical Guide to Mechanical Ventilation, First Edition.
Edited by Jonathon D. Truwit and Scott K. Epstein.
© 2011 John Wiley & Sons, Ltd. Published 2011 by John Wiley & Sons, Ltd.

- What adjustments to her mechanical ventilation would you make at this point?
- What additional information would it be helpful to know to optimally titrate her ventilator support?
- Is assist control the best mode of ventilation for this patient now?

2.6.2 Introduction

The list of diseases that can lead to restrictive lung physiology and, when sufficiently severe, can lead to respiratory failure requiring mechanical ventilation is extensive. It is not possible within the scope of this chapter to address in detail this complete disease list. The goals of this chapter are to review the general categories of diseases that lead to restrictive physiology and, using illustrative examples of each, provide general guidelines for optimizing mechanical ventilation in these populations.

Generally, restrictive lung diseases can be defined as any condition that results in reduced lung volume regardless of mechanism. In strict physiological terms, restrictive lung diseases are typically characterized by reduced total lung capacity (TLC) and/or forced vital capacity (FVC) along with normal airway resistance [1]. These diseases can be generally separated into three major categories including:

- Intrapulmonary
  - Intra-alveolar filling processes
  - Alterations in lung interstitium.
- Extrapulmonary
  - Pleural diseases
  - Chest wall abnormalities.
- Neuromuscular diseases
  - Neuropathic
  - Myopathic.

A list of common representative disorders within each category is provided in Table 2.6.1. To further illustrate the different mechanisms by which intrapulmonary diseases versus extrapulmonary diseases lead to restrictive physiology, Figure 2.6.1 provides representative CT scans of patients with both acute respiratory distress syndrome (ARDS) (Figure 2.6.1a) and morbid obesity (Figure 2.6.1b). These differences frequently present different challenges to providing optimal mechanical ventilation and, therefore, often require different approaches. It is important to note some of these diseases can develop a mixed (restrictive and obstructive) physiology at different disease stages, and that patients with restrictive lung problems can have secondary obstructive lung problems that will similarly complicate their presentation and efforts to deliver effective mechanical ventilation.

Naturally, in the management of mechanical ventilation for patients with restrictive lung diseases, the most important variable contributing to mortality and duration of mechanical ventilation is appropriate recognition and treatment of the underlying disease process (e.g., pneumonia, pulmonary edema). Although this

Table 2.6.1 Restrictive lung diseases.

Intrapulmonary	Intra-alveolar filling defects	Pulmonary Edema: cardiogenic and non-cardiogenic (ALI/ARDS)
		Pneumonia: infectious, eosinophilic, cryptogenic (BOOP)
		Diffuse alveolar hemorrhage
		Near drowning
	Alterations of the lung interstitium	Idiopathic pulmonary fibrosis
		Sarcoidosis
		Asbestosis
		Hypersensitivity pneumonitis
Extrapulmonary	Pleural diseases	Pleural effusion: loculated or large (causing lobar collapse)
		Hemothorax
		Pneumothorax
		Mesothelioma
	Chest wall abnormalities	Kyphoscoliosis
		Morbid obesity
		Patient–ventilator dyssynchrony
Neuromuscular	Neuropathies	Myasthenia gravis
		Amyotrophic lateral sclerosis
		Phrenic nerve injury/palsy
		Critical illness neuropathy
	Myopathies	Dermatomyositis
		Muscular dystrophies
		Steroid-induced myopathy
		Critical illness myopathy
		Mitochondrial myopathies

(a)   (b)

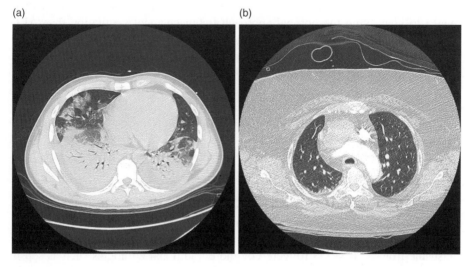

Figure 2.6.1 Representative chest CT images of a patient with ALI/ARDS (a) and a patient with morbid obesity (b).

point cannot be overemphasized, a review of the diagnostic studies and treatment options appropriate for this broad variety of disease processes is well beyond the scope of this chapter and is not be addressed herein. Using representative specific disease processes from within each of the major disease categories, this chapter focuseson the specific management aspects of mechanical ventilation, including mode, tidal volume, positive end-expiratory pressure (PEEP), airflow and more.

2.6.3   Intrapulmonary restrictive disease

2.6.3.1   Alveolar filling defects

To review goals of mechanical ventilation in this category of disease processes, the example of acute lung injury/acute respiratory distress syndrome (ALI/ARDS) is used. Since the hallmark of ALI/ARDS is non-cardiogenic edema from disruption of the alveolar–capillary barrier, this disease process serves as a good example for any lung process which involves alveolar filling from either type of edema, hemorrhage or infection [2]. However, it should also be noted that the restrictive pathophysiology of ALI/ARDS is not limited to alveolar filling defects. Interstitial abnormalities are also common with acute inflammation and edema in the acute phase of the disease, while fibroproliferative changes can develop as early as within several days and worsen as disease duration increases. Also, abnormalities of the chest wall can contribute due to prolonged immobility, patient–ventilator dyssynchrony or concomitant medications that might impair the chest wall musculature. Although obstruction of the airways has been reported in patients with ALI/ARDS, it is typically related to an underlying obstructive lung disease that was present prior to the event that initially triggered ALI/ARDS.

There is likely no disease process on which more has been studied and written related to identifying the optimal approach for mechanical ventilation than ALI/ARDS. This chapter aims to review and distill those extensive studies into general principles that can be applied to the majority of patients with ALI/ARDS. Although some discussion related to "rescue" or "salvage" therapies for patients with severe, refractory ARDS is included, these approaches are more thoroughly addressed in other chapters. Additional details regarding specific modes of mechanical ventilation that can be considered in ALI/ARDS can be found in dedicated chapter on Ventilator Modes (Chapter 2.4).

The recommended approach to mechanical ventilation in patients with ALI/ARDS is the "lung protective ventilation strategy" (LPVS) or "low tidal volume ventilation strategy", which serves to avoid excessive tidal volumes which can directly result in alveolar injury [3, 4]. Numerous experimental models have confirmed that tidal volumes previously recommended and utilized (12–15 ml/kg) prior to the mid to late 1990s can cause non-cardiogenic edema that is largely indistinguishable from ALI/ARDS triggered by more traditional etiologies such as sepsis and trauma. This process is now referred to as "ventilator-induced lung injury"

(VILI) [5, 6]. Prevention of this process is now commonly believed to be an important contributor to the improved outcomes (reduced duration of mechanical ventilation and reduced mortality) demonstrated in the large randomized trial of lung protective ventilation completed by the National Heart, Lung, and Blood Institute (NHLBI)-sponsored ARDS Network (ARDSNet) [3]. Further details regarding this trial and application of the ventilation protocol can be obtained on the ARDS Network website (http://www.ardsnet.org). Although weaknesses to the ARDSNet ventilation protocol do exist and critics of the trial persist, no study over the ensuing 10 years since its publication has provided conclusive findings to suggest an alternative approach that provides superior outcomes.

2.6.3.1.1 Volume

The most well established component of LPVS is the selection of a tidal volume of sufficient size to reduce the risk of VILI. The concept is based on the reduction in available alveolar volume that results from the pulmonary capillary-alveolar leak and subsequent non-cardiogenic pulmonary edema, as demonstrated in the chest CT image in Figure 2.6.1a. Based on the ARDS Network data, a tidal volume of 6 ml/kg of predicted body weight (PBW) is recommended. The importance of utilizing PBW and not actual body weight cannot be overemphasized, so the equations to calculate are the following:

Males (per kg):

$$50 + 2.3 \times (\text{height in inches} - 60) \text{ OR } 50 + 0.91 \times (\text{height in cm} - 152.4)$$

Females (per kg):

$$45.5 + 2.3 \times (\text{height in inches} - 60) \text{ OR } 45.5 + 0.91 \times (\text{height in cm} - 152.4)$$

Determination of PBW can also be achieved by referring to numerous online web sites which provide the equations or actual PBW tables. Clinicians and investigators who raise doubt regarding this size argue on either side, including that slightly larger tidal volumes may still be acceptable and that even smaller tidal volumes may be superior, but provide no clinical trial data to support these arguments [7]. A characteristic pressure–volume (P–V) curve of an ALI/ARDS patient is depicted in Figure 2.6.2 [4]. In this model, the ideal tidal volume (Low V_T) leads to a change in pressure that corresponds to the steepest (most compliant) portion of the P–V curve. Tidal volumes in excess of this that extend beyond the upper inflection point of this curve are likely to result in alveolar overdistension and injury, a process which is frequently referred to as "volutrauma [5]."

Despite the positive impact on key clinical outcomes of mortality and ventilator free days (Table 2.6.2), implementation and adherence to the ARDS Network LPVS remains somewhat difficult for many clinicians [8]. A common explanation for the reluctance of bedside providers (physicians and respiratory therapists) to

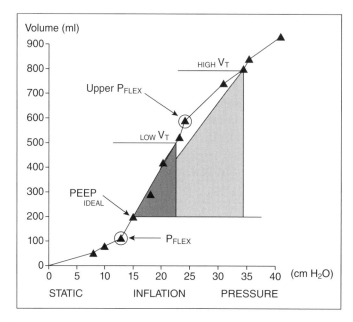

Figure 2.6.2   Model P–V curve for patients with ALI/ARDS. (Reprinted with permission [4].)

Table 2.6.2   Clinical outcomes from the ARDS Network Low Tidal Volume Ventilation Study.* (Reproduced with permission [3].)

Variable	Group Receiving Lower Tidal Volumes	Group Receiving Traditional Tidal Volumes	P Value
Death before discharge home and breathing without assistance (%)	31.0	39.8	**0.007**
Breathing without assistance by day 28 (%)	65.7	55.0	**<0.001**
No. of ventilator-free days, days 1 to 28	12 ± 11	10 ± 11	**0.007**
Barotrauma, days 1 to 28 (%)	10	11	**0.43**
No. of days without failure of nonpulmonary organs or systems, days 1 to 28	15 ± 11	12 ± 11	**0.006**

*Plus–minus values are means ±SD. The number of ventilator-free days is the mean number of days from day 1 to day 28 on which the patient had been breathing without assistance for at least 48 consecutive hours. Barotrauma was defined as any new pneumothorax, pneumomediastinum, or subcutaneous emphysema, or a pneumatocele that was more than 2 cm in diameter. Organ and system failures were defined as described in the Methods section.

consistently utilize LPVS is its frequent deleterious effects on gas exchange when arterial blood gas samples are obtained. It is well established that patients receiving LPVS during the ARDS Network trial exhibited lower P/F ratios and higher $PaCO_2$ levels [3]. These endpoints are measures that commonly drive bedside decision making and are hard habits to modify. However, these discordant results indicate that striving to maintain an optimal ABG can lead to levels of ventilation that may be excessive and deleterious to more important clinical outcomes. Another common issue that may arise during delivery of low tidal volumes is the presence of "air hunger" and patient–ventilator dyssynchrony when patients attempt to generate a greater tidal volume and/or inspiratory flow than targeted. In this setting, the clinician should use their discretion to either allow a larger tidal volume (7–8 ml/kg of ideal body weight) to be used or to increase sedation to improve patient–ventilator synchrony. The relative safety of these approaches when compared to the other is unknown.

2.6.3.1.2 Pressure/PEEP

In addition to a focus on tidal volume, LPVS includes attention to the impact of pressures generated during mechanical ventilation. In general, pressure goals are to minimize airway pressures with a greater emphasis on plateau or static pressure (P_S) than peak inspiratory or dynamic pressure (P_D). In the ARDS Network LPVS protocol, the goal is to maintain P_S <30 cm H_2O, including further reduction of V_T to less than 6 ml/kg if necessary [3]. This additional mandate within the ARDS Network protocol has led some clinicians to conclude that the actual goal of LPVS is to maintain P_S in this range and to put less emphasis on the tidal volume goals. Since the majority of patients managed with less severe ALI/ARDS have P_S pressures that are well below the maximum P_S limit, many patients could tolerate larger tidal volumes and remain within this parameter. However, during the ARDS Network clinical trial, those patients were managed with the study mandated tidal volume (6 ml/kg) and the study results represent the benefits of this approach, not an alternative approach which emphasizes P_S more than tidal volume. However, the safety of ventilating with larger tidal volumes, provided P_S < 30 cm H_2O, has not been demonstrated. Furthermore, Figure 2.6.3 demonstrates that LPVS with a low V_T target was beneficial in all four quartiles of the range of P_S from all patients enrolled in the ARDS Network trial [9]. The results in this figure also suggest that goals for management of airway pressures should be to reduce P_S to as low as can be tolerated, since there is no well established lower limit of P_S below which the risk of VILI is removed. The potential for further reduction in VILI by even lower P_S targets is a hypothesis shared by many investigators but no clinical trial data are currently available.

Although the effectiveness of positive end-expiratory pressure (PEEP) in ALI/ARDS has been established for over 40 years [10], the most effective approach by which PEEP should be titrated remains somewhat unknown and controversial. Many investigators who have carefully examined the intricacies of LPVS, have

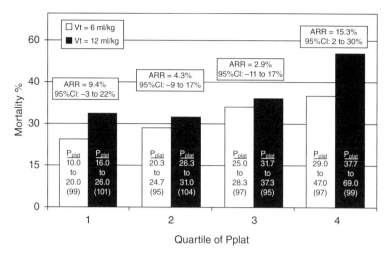

Figure 2.6.3   Impact of low tidal volume on all patients in the ARDS Network study when divided into four quartiles from low to high plateau pressure (Pplat) (Reproduced with permission [9].) Pplat = P_S.

suggested the careful titration of PEEP to a point just above the lower inflection point (Pflex) of the P–V curve (Figure 2.6.2) provides optimal results and results in less repetitive alveolar injury by reducing repetitive closure and reopening of alveolar units during tidal ventilation. For some this approach includes (if not requires) a daily bedside creation of the patient's P–V curve to establish the appropriate PEEP at that time point. In a subsequent ARDS Network trial (ALVEOLI) examining an approach utilizing higher PEEP (lower FiO_2) versus lower PEEP (higher FiO_2), no superiority for either approach could be established, suggesting both are acceptable [11]. The details for titration of PEEP and FiO_2 for both approaches are provided in Figure 2.6.4 (http://www.ardsnet.org) [3]. Critics of this trial suggest that its methodological approach was not sufficiently detailed to identify the benefit for either higher (or more carefully titrated) levels of PEEP. At present, no randomized control trial data are available to suggest that, within an LPVS approach, higher levels of PEEP provide any additional outcome benefit beyond that reached with utilizing smaller tidal volumes.

2.6.3.1.3   Flow/I:E ratio

Although expiratory airflow is a passive process and cannot be manipulated with mechanical ventilation, inspiratory airflow can be regulated and is the principal means by which I:E ratio can be controlled. The reduced lung compliance characteristic of restrictive lung diseases results in higher airway pressures for any given level of inspiratory flow. In addition, restrictive lung diseases are characterized by and differentiated from obstructive lung diseases by no limitation of (or even

Lower PEEP/higher FiO$_2$

FiO$_2$	0.3	0.4	0.4	0.5	0.5	0.6	0.7	0.7
PEEP	5	5	8	8	10	10	10	12

FiO$_2$	0.7	0.8	0.9	0.9	0.9	1.0
PEEP	14	14	14	16	18	18-24

Higher PEEP/lower FiO$_2$

FiO$_2$	0.3	0.3	0.3	0.3	0.3	0.4	0.4	0.5
PEEP	5	8	10	12	14	14	16	16

FiO$_2$	0.5	0.5-0.8	0.8	0.9	1.0	1.0
PEEP	14	20	22	22	22	24

Figure 2.6.4 Parameters for titration of PEEP and FiO$_2$ in the ARDS Network protocol using either a Lower or Higher PEEP approach. (Reprinted with permission from the ARDS Network, http://www.ardsnet.org/system/files/Ventilator%20Protocol%20Card.pdf)

increased) expiratory airflow. Enhanced recoil and expiratory airflow is more typically a component of diseases associated with abnormalities of the lung interstitium than diseases associated with only abnormalities of alveolar filling.

Using these concepts, inspiratory flows should generally be reduced in ALI/ ARDS to help minimize airway pressures and facilitate safer delivery of appropriate tidal volumes with a goal to maintain I:E ratios between 1:1 and 1:1.5 [12]. Prolonged inspiratory times may also lead to improved oxygenation. Figure 2.6.5 demonstrates the potential impact of prolonged inspiration to optimize alveolar patency during each respiratory cycle (Figure 2.6.5b) as compared to a normal I:E ratio (Figure 2.6.5a). Although popular in years past, reduction of inspiratory flows to achieve inspiratory times greater than expiratory times (Figure 2.6.5c), which is known as inverse ratio ventilation, is generally no longer recommended [13]. The benefits of this approach result primarily from the creation of intrinsic (auto) PEEP, which has no greater clinical benefit than extrinsic PEEP, and more difficult to measure and maintain.

2.6.3.1.4   Mode

As a result of the emphasis on lower tidal volumes, the most commonly utilized mode of mechanical ventilation in ALI/ARDS has become a volume-cycled approach with assist control (AC) [14]. In this mode, patients are able to consistently receive the targeted tidal volume and to utilize their own endogenous respiratory drive to establish the respiratory rate required to achieve the required minute ventilation. This simple approach is generally sufficient for the majority of ALI/ ARDS, particularly those with mild to moderate disease. Although less commonly utilized, pressure-cycled modes of ventilation (PCV and PSV) can be used with efficacy equivalent to AC, but require greater attention from bedside providers to

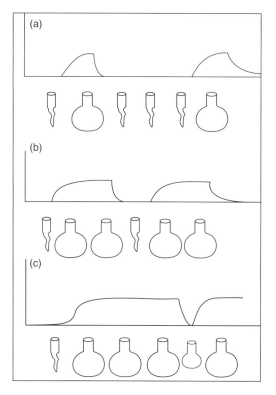

Figure 2.6.5   Prolonged inspiration. Pressure–time curves for normal ventilation (a), which includes an I:E ratio of approximately 1:3; (b) describes prolonged inspiration with sufficient time between breaths to fully exhale; and (c) prolonged inspiration with insufficient exhalation to permit clearance of full tidal volume prior to initiation of the next breath leading to air trapping (i.e., auto-PEEP or intrinsic PEEP). (Reprinted with permission [12].)

achieve and maintain tidal volume and minute ventilation goals [15]. Some centers routinely utilize other modes for all patients with ALI/ARDS, including airway pressure release ventilation (APRV) and pressure-regulated volume control (PRVC) [16–18]. Neither approach has been demonstrated to provide equivalent or superior patient outcomes in large randomized multicenter trials, and require greater experience to deliver effectively. Although not outlined in the ARDS Network LPVS, conversion of patients from AC mode to PSV mode during the recovery phase from ALI/ARDS is commonly performed.

In the small subset of patients with severe ALI/ARDS who require sustained levels of FiO_2 and PEEP at or near their respective limits, numerous alternative modes of mechanical ventilation have been utilized including: PCV, APRV, high frequency ventilation (HFV) and extracorporeal support (ECMO) [17–21]. There are currently no established protocols or triggers for when these alternative modes should be implemented, but many clinicians will begin to consider them once high levels of FiO_2 (≥ 0.80) and PEEP (>15 cm H_2O) are required or when airway pressures remain high ($P_S > 30$ cm H_2O) for a prolonged period (>12–24 h). Although the temptation to change to these alternative strategies earlier may be hard to resist, it is important to realize that the impact of PEEP on alveolar recruitment and the lung's endogenous ability to regulate pulmonary blood flow away from the most severely injured lung through hypoxic pulmonary vasoconstriction can take many hours to achieve. For patients with severe sustained hypoxemia, APRV has become a commonly utilized mode due to its ability to expose patients to higher levels of sustained pressure and lead to greater alveolar recruitment. In cases for which gas exchange goals are relatively well achieved, but airway pressures remain high, PCV mode may often provide an effective alternative. Utilization of HFV and ECMO remains controversial and these are generally considered forms of "salvage" or "rescue" therapy for patients with very severe disease. Decisions on whether to utilize HFV or ECMO in these uncommon instances are more frequently dictated by the availability of local expertise and resources, since guidelines for the appropriate utilization and efficacy of these modes remains limited.

2.6.3.2 Other alveolar filling diseases

Studies examining direct application of an LPVS strategy to patients with other forms of alveolar filling defects are far more limited than in ALI/ARDS. Despite these limitations, it is commonly the approach utilized by a majority of clinicians. For example, pneumonia is a common etiology for the development of ALI/ARDS (including those patients enrolled in ARDSNet studies), and it is generally considered to be a preferred approach in patients with pneumonia, even when radiographic and other clinical parameters do not indicate the presence of ALI/ARDS [22]. Likewise, in patients with alveolar hemorrhage or congestive heart failure, it is generally recommended that an LPVS approach be utilized until additional clinical trial data that identify a superior approach become available.

Many of the principles that drive the recommended approach for mechanical ventilation in ALI/ARDS also serve as the basis for ventilation in the other forms of restrictive lung diseases. For the sake of brevity and to minimize repetition, the remaining discussion in this chapter related to other forms of restrictive diseases refers to and, when appropriate, provides contrast to the points that have already been outlined for ALI/ARDS in this section.

2.6.3.3 Alterations of the lung interstitium

Idiopathic pulmonary fibrosis (IPF) is the most well recognized disease within the large category of idiopathic interstitial pneumonias (IIPs), which are a subset of the even larger category of diffuse parenchymal lung diseases (DPLDs) [23]. For this section, IPF serves as the most pure model for unique considerations of mechanical ventilation for interstitial abnormalities in the absence of corresponding alveolar filling defects, particularly when disease severity is more advanced and more extensive interstitial fibrosis ("honeycombing") is present. For other IIP variants (e.g., non-specific interstitial pneumonitis, desquamative interstitial pneumonitis, etc.) or patients with IPF at less advanced disease stages which might include an acute exacerbation involving acute inflammation and/or ground glass opacifications, concomitant alveolar filling abnormalities are likely to be present.

In general, guidelines and recommendations regarding the most effective approach to mechanical ventilation in patients with IPF do not exist. Most available data represent modestly sized case series collected at a single institution over a period of several years. Fortunately, for patients and clinicians, the prevalence of respiratory failure requiring mechanical ventilation is far lower than for ALI/ARDS. Unfortunately, particularly for patients and their families, the benefits of mechanical ventilation in IPF are highly limited, which is largely related to the absence of a proven therapy capable of consistently slowing or reversing the underlying disease process. In several small studies, intensive care unit mortality for patients with usual interstitial pneumonitis who undergo invasive mechanical ventilation are 80–100%, and for patients fortunate enough to achieve extubation and hospital discharge, long term survival is typically 2–6 months [24, 25]. Noninvasive ventilation (NIV) has also been utilized in IPF, but has not proven to improve these dismal clinical outcomes. These grim statistics also highlight the need to avoid mechanical ventilation in patients with IPF whenever possible thru optimal outpatient follow up, including appropriate end-of-life discussions with patients and their families.

When patients with IPF are intubated and placed on mechanical ventilation, it is frequently due to either the lack of an established diagnosis or the presence of an acute exacerbation of their disease. In the latter setting, some greater potential for response to immunosuppressive therapy is possible and, as mentioned, is more likely to be associated with acute inflammation that may also result in an alveolar filling abnormality. The goals of mechanical ventilation in these situations are generally very similar to those for ALI/ARDS, as outlined above with few exceptions.

2.6.3.3.1   Volume

Low tidal volume ventilation has been a standard approach in patients with IPF for longer than ALI/ARDS, but was historically not based on the concept of reducing VILI. Instead, it was simply the means by which to keep airway pressures below unacceptably high levels (>40 cm H_2O). Recent case series suggest tidal volumes of 6–7 ml/kg of ideal body weight are typically used but some have suggested that volumes as low as 4 ml/kg might be preferred when possible [24]. This approach may further exacerbate the baseline level of tachypnea, which is common and often difficult to manage during mechanical ventilation in IPF due to stimulation of alveolar stretch receptors.

2.6.3.3.2   Pressure/PEEP

Providing sufficient minute ventilation while minimizing airway pressures is challenging in IPF sufficiently severe to require mechanical ventilation, and the goals for P_D and P_S should generally be similar to those in ALI/ARDS or lower. Since airway resistance is typically not a component of IPF, the difference between P_D and P_S tends to be very low. Goals for PEEP in IPF are likewise similar to ALI/ARDS LPVS goals, but recruitment of alveoli in pure interstitial lung abnormalities is typically of less value than in ALI/ARDS or other diseases with predominantly alveolar filling defects. For this same reason, the titration of PEEP to a level slightly above the lower inflection point of the P–V curve (Pflex) has less theoretical value than in ALI/ARDS.

2.6.3.3.3   Flow/I:E ratio

Given the marked increase in elastic recoil typical of IPF, inspiratory flow can be significantly reduced in IPF to help maintain goals for P_D and P_S. As compared to ALI/ARDS, somewhat more inverted I:E ratios (I > E) can often be tolerated without the development of intrinsic PEEP.

2.6.3.3.4   Mode

Given the relatively low prevalence of IPF patients receiving mechanical ventilation and the associated poor outcomes, there are no studies comparing modes of ventilation in IPF. Most published series indicate volume-cycled AC mode is the most commonly utilized for initial management of the intensive care unit admission. This approach theoretically provides greater ability to control and maintain the volume and pressure targets outlined above. However, there is no major theoretical disadvantage to utilizing pressure-cycled modes (PSV or PCV), and PSV is commonly utilized during prolonged weaning phases. Other newer modes of ventilation such as pressure-regulated volume control ventilation or adaptive support ventilation (ASV) might have some yet unproven potential [16, 26]. However, modes designed to optimize delivery of higher levels of PEEP or mean airway pressure, such as APRV or HFV, are likely of little value and typically should not considered in IPF. Given the poor clinical outcomes and lack of proven therapies to directly address the underlying disease process of IPF, ECMO is not appropriate.

2.6.4   Extrapulmonary restrictive lung disease

2.6.4.1   Pleural diseases

In general, pleural diseases lead to restrictive lung physiology through extrinsic compression or constriction of a lobe or entire hemithorax, regardless of whether the pleural space is filled with fluid (exudative or transudative), blood, air or soft tissue in the pleura [27]. In the setting of mechanical ventilation, pleural diseases lead to changes in compliance (dynamic and static) through alterations of chest wall compliance rather than lung compliance, even though the pleural space may not be strictly viewed as a component of the chest wall. Although pleural diseases can lead to bilateral restriction, they can frequently be unilateral, which distinguishes them from the typically bilateral alveolar and interstitial diseases discussed previously. In cases of unilateral disease, the severity of the pleural process often needs to be much more advanced to cause respiratory failure sufficient to require mechanical ventilation, since the corresponding hemithorax is unaffected and able to maintain sufficient ventilation. In the presence of other underlying lung diseases (obstructive or restrictive), unilateral pleural diseases are far more likely to play a major role in acute respiratory failure and need consideration during mechanical ventilation.

Pleural effusions will be used as the disease model for this section, since they are common in critically ill patients, and their impact on lung function and appropriate indications for management/drainage remain confusing and controversial [28, 29]. The relative impact of any pleural effusion in the critically ill depends principally on its composition (e.g., transudative, malignant, empyema and hemothorax) and size, but the scope of this section does not permit more than a brief review of these variables. Although many pleural effusions can cause mild reduction in oxygenation through an intrapulmonary shunt, only pleural effusions sufficiently large or viscous to cause lobar collapse or constriction ("trapped lung") will be enough to need for or impact decisions related to mechanical ventilation [30, 31]. Thus, small to moderate transudative effusions (even when bilateral) caused by generalized edema, which is common in critically ill patients, typically do not have major physiologic significance and do not require drainage other than for the purpose of diagnosis. Figure 2.6.6 provides a helpful example of bilateral pleural effusions in a patient requiring mechanical ventilation in which the left sided effusion has reached sufficient complexity (malignant in this case) and size to warrant therapeutic drainage and the right sided effusion is simple (transudate) and small enough to not cause significant compromise of the adjacent lung parenchyma. Of note, massive effusions (even transudative effusions in the absence of volume loss of the lung parenchyma) may impede ventilation due to a sufficient loss of thoracic volume to impair the delivery of even a normal tidal volume during mechanical ventilation. Increased utilization of bedside ultrasonography in the intensive care unit has positively impacted the ability to accurately evaluate pleural effusions when used in conjunction with radiographic studies, in particular thoracic CT [32, 33].

No specific guidelines regarding goals for mechanical ventilation in the setting of pleural effusions are currently available but, given their typically restrictive effect, the goals should generally follow those outlined for ALI/ARDS with the following considerations:

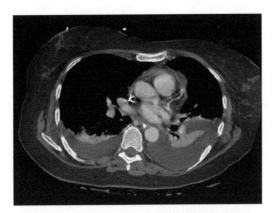

Figure 2.6.6 Chest CT image of a patient with bilateral pleural effusions. The left sided effusion is causing significant volume loss of the left lower lobe and more likely to impact overall lung function and delivery of mechanical ventilation than the right side effusion.

2.6.4.1.1 Volume

Since pleural diseases typically do not alter actual lung compliance, the importance of low tidal volume ventilation in patients with pleural and no coexisting parenchymal disease is unknown. Even in this setting, utilization of tidal volumes larger than 8–10 ml/kg of PBW should be used cautiously.

2.6.4.1.2 Pressure/PEEP

Management of airway pressures for pleural diseases may be significantly different than alveolar filling defects and interstitial abnormalities, since the higher pressures associated with any volume are not associated with an increase in transpleural pressure gradient, which many have speculated is the key variable associated with barotrauma and possibly volutrauma. As a result, the limits for P_D and P_S outlined for ALI/ARDS may not be as appropriate in the setting of significant pleural effusions. The impact of PEEP in pleural diseases is highly variable and balances the lack of effect on alveolar recruitment as seen in alveolar filling defects but may maintain patency of small distal airways and alveoli when constricting pleural pressures are present. The frequent unilateral and focal nature of many complex pleural pressures serves only to increase the variability of PEEP effects.

2.6.4.1.3 Flow/I:E ratio

Although the impact of significant pleural effusions on flow can frequently limit inspiratory flow and enhance expiratory flow as seen in intrapulmonary abnormalities, the relative importance of this effect is much more variable. In some complex pleural effusions, expiratory flow might even be impacted and reduced similar to obstructive lung diseases due to enhanced dynamic compression of large airways from the increased pleural pressures.

2.6.4.1.4   Mode

No specific considerations related to mode are recommended for pleural effusions with both volume-cycled and pressure-cycled modes likely to be effective after being appropriately adjusted for the volume and pressure issues mentioned. For the uncommon pleural disease of bronchopleural fistulas, high frequency jet ventilation is a mode that is commonly considered to be advantageous [34].

2.6.4.2   Chest wall abnormalities

As described for pleural diseases, the impact of chest wall abnormalities differs from intrapulmonary abnormalities through their direct impact on chest wall compliance rather than lung compliance [35]. Unlike pleural diseases, which are often unilateral, most diseases of the chest wall are circumferential and therefore impact bilateral lung function. As a result, when these abnormalities are present they are much more likely to require consideration and adjustment by clinicians when trying to optimize delivery of mechanical ventilation. A very common chest wall abnormality, which is frequently unrecognized and can manifest both intermittently and inconsistently, is anxiety and agitation leading to dyssynchrony with the delivery of the volume or pressure targets of the ventilator [36].

For the purposes of reviewing specific adjustments in mechanical ventilation for chest wall abnormalities, this chapter focuses on morbid obesity. As in the example provided in Figure 2.6.2, morbid obesity can substantially impact the P–V relationship. This image further highlights that the size of the lungs correlates far more closely with predicted body weight, and why LPVS is not based on actual body weight. In addition to the impact of chest wall compliance, obesity also worsens oxygenation through basilar atelectasis and increases work of breathing, often by as much as twofold. Furthermore, the effects of obesity are typically further exacerbated by lying in a supine position, as is the case for critically ill patients on mechanical ventilation [37, 38].

Although no clear guidelines exist regarding specific adjustments in mechanical ventilation that should be used to compensate for obesity, the following general rules should be considered:

2.6.4.2.1   Volume

As already stated on multiple occasions during this chapter, tidal volumes should be based on predicted body weight. Using actual body weight in the morbidly obese can readily lead to volumes that have been well established to cause volutrauma and VILI.

2.6.4.2.2 Pressure/PEEP

As discussed for pleural effusions, the impact of reduced chest wall compliance should be considered during management of airway pressures in the morbidly obese. This problem can often be most problematic in the setting of weaning from mechanical ventilation when using PSV mode and during the performance of spontaneous breathing trials (SBTs) using low levels of PSV (0–5 cm H_2O). In these settings, higher pressures are often required, but do not have the same reflection of lung compliance and/or lung function as compared to non-obese patients. Specifically, some clinicians consider extubation of the obese patient after the patient demonstrates adequate ventilation at levels of PSV as high as 10 cm H_2O. Although possibly effective, this practice has not been formally studied and its effectiveness and reliability are unknown. For these same general reasons, the impact of PEEP on alveolar recruitment is generally less predictable and effective in the obese patient than the non-obese [39].

2.6.4.2.3 Flow/I:E ratio

In obesity, the reduced chest wall compliance will lead to higher P_D and P_S, so reduction of inspiratory flow to minimize airway pressures may be appropriate. However, obstructive lung diseases are often seen as a comorbid condition in obesity, which will need to be considered, as lowering inspiratory flows may be more likely to lead to intrinsic (auto) PEEP or air trapping.

2.6.4.2.4 Mode

There are no recommendations for modification or adjustment of mode to compensate for obesity. Effective ventilation can be achieved with either volume-cycled or pressure-cycled modes assuming appropriate correction for the volume and pressure issues already outlined is performed [40]. Of note, morbid obesity is a relative contra-indication to the delivery of HFV, with certain devices having strict weight limits above which the machine is not certified.

2.6.4.3 Neuromuscular diseases

For this section, both the neuropathies and myopathies are considered together, since the respiratory failure and subsequent need for mechanical ventilation in each is very similar [41]. Weakness of the neuromuscular complex of the thorax, which includes the thoracic and abdominal muscles as well as the accessory muscles of the neck, leads to reduced lung volumes during pulmonary function testing such as spirometry and lung volumes. However, unlike the intrapulmonary and extrapulmonary diseases outlined thus far, there is no pathologic abnormality of the actual lung parenchyma or anatomic structures that make up the chest wall. As a result, when a patient's neuromuscular disease (NMD) is sufficiently severe to require mechanical ventilation, once intubated their dynamic and static compliance is typically normal, and achieving ventilation goals while they remain intubated and on mechanical ventilation is relatively easy as compared to most of the other restrictive diseases. It should be noted that for many patients with NMDs, their need for mechanical ventilation often is the result of a secondary acute event (e.g., pneumonia, sepsis, pulmonary embolism), which when combined leads to respiratory decompensation. In the setting of NMDs, the severity of the secondary event sufficient to cause respiratory failure is frequently much less than in patients without NMD. The biggest challenge in NMDs is whether options for correction of the underlying neuromuscular abnormality or treatment of the secondary event will be sufficient to permit liberation from mechanical ventilation.

The disease that will be used as a model in this section is myasthenia gravis (MG) [42]. As stated above, many patients with MG require mechanical ventilation as a result of a secondary event leading to further impairment of respiratory function; but MG also has two unique mechanisms by which patients might develop respiratory failure and require mechanical ventilation. Patients with MG may have acute respiratory events or crises that can be driven by either an acute exacerbation of the disease itself (myasthenic crisis) or from an excess of therapy with cholinesterase inhibitors (cholinergic crisis). The scope of this chapter does not permit a detailed discussion of the management of these two different types of acute respiratory failure, but it is important for an intensivist to know that these can be discriminated using a Tensilon (edrophonium) Test [43].

Similar to many other restrictive conditions other than ALI/ARDS, there are no established guidelines for the ventilator management of patients with MG. The general application and adjustments that clinicians should consider in these patients are as follows:

2.6.4.3.1 Volume

Since the lung parenchyma and compliance of both the lungs and chest wall in patients with MG are normal, attention to low tidal volumes and strict LPVS is less important. In fact, many patients with MG may desire a normal tidal volume (8–10 ml/kg), as they might otherwise have inadequate triggering of airway stretch receptors and air hunger.

2.6.4.3.2 Pressure/PEEP

Few, if any, issues related to management of pressure are unique for patients with MG. However, adjustment of pressures during pressure-cycled modes of ventilation should be monitored closely, as these can be indirect surrogate markers of the patient's underlying weakness, with less pressure required as the patient's weakness begins to improve. PEEP is typically not required for patients with MG alone, but may often be needed to address a secondary respiratory event such as acute pneumonia.

2.6.4.3.3 Flow/I:E ratio

There are no issues unique to MG that warrant adjustment of I:E ratios from normal values (i.e., $1:2.0\text{--}4.0$).

2.6.4.3.4 Mode

Effective ventilation can be provided in MG using virtually all modes of ventilation given the underlying normal lung function post intubation. Pressure-cycled modes are often favored over volume-cycled modes, as they can be used to monitor the improvement of the patient's underlying weakness with less pressure required as weakness improves. For this same reason, many patients with MG and other NMDs are managed with noninvasive ventilation (NIV), particularly BiPAP, in efforts to avoid intubation and potentially long-term periods of mechanical ventilation [44]. This topic is discussed in much more detail in the NIV chapters.

2.6.5 Summary

There are many varieties of diseases which can lead to restrictive lung function abnormalities that, when sufficiently severe, can result in the need for mechanical ventilation. Depending on the type of restrictive disease process (intrapulmonary, extrapulmonary or neuromuscular), guidelines and bedside management of mechanical ventilation may be different. Since the typical hallmark of restrictive lung diseases is reduced dynamic and static compliance, and that ventilation of the lungs with excessive volume or pressure can lead to direct VILI, avoidance of excessively large tidal volumes is a key component of LPVS in many of these diseases. The LPVS protocol published by the ARDS Network for the management of patients with ALI/ARDS is currently the most validated approach. Although deviations from the ARDSnet protocol should be pursued when necessary, deviations should be minimized when only driven by nothing more than clinician preference, since the safety of such deviations is unproven. For conditions with no or less alveolar filling abnormalities than ALI/ARDS, deviations from the LPVS protocol are more appropriate and the specific adjustments appropriate for each of those unique situations are outlined herein.

2.6.6 Case presentation revisited

Although this patient's oxygenation is extremely poor (P/F ratio = 70), the first adjustment to the patient's mechanical ventilation should be to reassess her tidal volume, which is likely too large. To complete this step, obtain or measure the patient's height (66 inches in this case), calculate her PBW (~59 kg), which should result in a target tidal volume of ~350 ml (6 ml/kg), which is substantially less than originally set. Although this reduction in tidal volume may lead to further decline in oxygenation, this patient has only been on PEEP for a short time and is likely to have improved recruitment of involved alveoli over the next 6–12 h. An oxygen level of 60 mm Hg or greater is typically sufficient as it generally translates into a level of SaO$_2$ of ≥90%, which is sufficient to provide adequate oxygen delivery. In addition to knowing the patient's height, it will also be very helpful to know the corresponding airway pressures (P$_D$ and P$_S$). These values will help further define the safe limits of PEEP titration, which, if increased further, could help counterbalance any negative impact of tidal volume reduction. As for mode, assist control is likely the best mode for this patient at this early stage of their intensive care unit management, since it provides a guaranteed tidal volume and as many breaths as needed or requested by the patient. Additional information that would be helpful is the patient's total respiratory rate. It is likely higher than the set rate of 20 bpm and, if so, represents the maximum minute ventilation that can likely be delivered at this time. If the patient is not breathing above the set rate, a higher rate could be considered if airway pressures and/or concomitant obstructive lung disease and reduced expiratory airflow are not limitations. Although quite low, the patient's pH does not mandate an adjustment in ventilation. If a higher pH is desired, the clinician could consider addition of intravenous bicarbonate. It is too early in this patient's intensive care unit course to consider deviation from LPVS, but should the patient's severe oxygenation abnormalities persist over the next 12–24 h despite further adjustments up to the maximum of LPVS, then consideration of other ventilation strategies such as APRV, HFV and ECMO would be appropriate.

References

1. Pellegrino, R., Viegi, G., Brusasco, V. *et al.* (2005) Interpretative strategies for lung function tests. *Eur. Respir. J.*, **26**, 948–968.
2. Artigas, A., Bernard, G.R., Carlet, J. *et al.* (1998) The American-European Consensus Conference on ARDS, part 2: Ventilatory, pharmacologic, supportive therapy, study design strategies, and issues related to recovery and remodeling. *Am. J. Respir. Crit. Care Med.*, **157**, 1332–1347.
3. The Acute Respiratory Distress Syndrome Network (2000) Ventilation with lower tidal volumes as compared with traditional tidal volumes for acute lung injury and the acute respiratory distress syndrome. *N. Engl. J. Med.*, **342**, 1301–1308.
4. Amato, M.B., Barbas, C.S., Medeiros, D.M. *et al.* (1995) Beneficial effects of the "open lung approach" with low distending pressures in acute respiratory distress syndrome. *Am. J. Respir. Crit. Care Med.*, **152**, 1835–1846.
5. Dreyfuss, D. and Saumon, G. (1998) Ventilator-induced lung injury. *Am. J. Respir. Crit. Care Med.*, **157**, 293–323.
6. Tremblay, L.N. and Slutsky, A.S. (2005) Pathogenesis of ventilator-induced lung inury: trials and tribulations. *Am. J. Physiol. Lung Cell Mol. Physiol.*, **288**, L596–L598.
7. Eichacker, P.Q., Gerstenberger, E.P., Banks, S.M. *et al.* (2002) Meta analysis of acute lung injury and acute respiratory distress syndrome trials testing low tidal volumes. *Am. J. Respir. Crit. Care Med.*, **166**, 1510–1514.

8. Cooke, C.R., Kahn, J.M., Watkins, T.R. *et al.* (2009) Cost-effectiveness of implementing low-tidal volume ventilation in patients with acute lung injury. *Chest*, **136**, 79–88.

9. Hager, D.N., Krishnan, J.A., Hayden, D.L. *et al.* (2005) Tidal volume reduction in patients with acute lung injury when plateau pressures are not high. *Am. J. Respir. Crit. Care Med.*, **172**, 1241–1245.

10. Ashbaugh, D.G., Bigelow, D.B., Petty, T.L. and Levine, B.E. (1967) Acute respiratory distress in adults. *Lancet*, **12**, 319–323.

11. Brower, R.G., Lanken, P.N., MacIntyre, N. *et al.* (2004) National Heart, Lung, and Blood Institute ARDS Clinical Trials Network. Higher versus lower positive end-expiratory pressures in patients with the acute respiratory distress syndrome. *N. Engl. J. Med.*, **351**(4), 327–336.

12. Armstrong, B.W. and MacIntyre, N.R. (1995) Pressure-controlled, inverse ratio ventilation that avoids air trapping in the adult respiratory distress syndrome. *Crit. Care Med.*, **23**, 279–285.

13. Shanholtz, C. and Brower, R. (1994) Should inverse ratio ventilation be used in adult respiratory distress syndrome? *Am. J. Respir. Crit. Care Med.*, **149**, 1354–1358.

14. Esteban, A., Ferguson, N.D., Meade, M.O. *et al.* (2008) Evolution of mechanical ventilation in response to clinical research. *Am. J. Respir. Crit. Care Med.*, **177**, 170–177.

15. Esteban, A., Alia, I., Gordo, F. *et al.* (2000) Prospective randomized trial comparing pressure-controlled ventilation and volume-controlled ventilation in ARDS. *Chest*, **117**, 1690–1696.

16. Guldager, H., Nielsen, S.L., Carl, P. and Soerensen, M.B. (1997) A comparison of volume control and pressure-regulated volume control ventilation in acute respiratory failure. *Crit. Care*, **1**, 75–77.

17. Varpula, T., Valta, P., Niemi, R. *et al.* (2004) Airway pressure release ventilation as a primary ventilatory mode in acute respiratory distress syndrome. *Acta Anaesthesiol. Scand.*, **48**, 722–731.

18. Seymour, C.W., Frazer, M., Reilly, P.M. and Fuchs, B.D. (2007) Airway pressure release and biphasic intermittent positive airway pressure ventilation: are they ready for prime time? *J. Trauma*, **62**, 1298–1308.

19. Fessler, H.E., Hager, D.N. and Brower, R.G. (2008) Feasibility of very high frequency ventilation in adults with acute respiratory distress syndrome. *Crit. Care Med.*, **36**, 1043–1048.

20. Fessler, H.E., Derdak, S., Ferguson, N.D. *et al.* (2007) A protocol for high-frequency oscillatory ventilation in adults: results from a roundtable discussion. *Crit. Care Med.*, **35**, 1649–1654.

21. Peek, G.J., Mugford, M., Tiruvoipati, R. *et al.* (2009) Efficacy and economic assessment of conventional ventilatory support versus extracorporeal membrane oxygenation for severe adult respiratory failure (CESAR): a multicentre randomised controlled trial. *Lancet*, **374**, 1351–1363.

22. Kurahashi, K., Ota, S., Nakamura, K. *et al.* (2004) Effect of lung-protective ventilation on severe *Pseudomonas aeruginosa* pneumonia and sepsis in rats. *Am. J. Physiol. Lung Cell Mol. Physiol.*, **287**, L402–L410.

23. ATS/ERS (2002) International multidisciplinary consensus classification of the idiopathic interstitial pneumonias. *Am. J. Respir. Crit. Care Med.*, **165**, 277–304.

24. Mollica, C., Paone, G., Conti, V. *et al.* (2010) Mechanical ventilation in patients with end-stage idiopathic pulmonary fibrosis. *Respiration*, **79**, 209–215.

25. Saydain, G., Islam, A., Afessa, B. *et al.* (2002) Outcome of patients with idiopathic pulmonary fibrosis admitted to the intensive care unit. *Am. J. Respir. Crit. Care Med.*, **166**, 839–842.

26. Jaber, S., Sebbane, M., Verzilli, D. *et al.* (2009) Adaptive support and pressure support ventilation behavior in response to increased ventilatory demand. *Anesthesiology*, **110**, 620–627.

27. Light, R.W. (1995) *Pleural Diseases*, Williams & Wilkins, Baltimore, MD.

28. Agusti, A.G.N., Cardus, J., Roca, J. *et al.* (1997) Ventilation-perfusion mismatch in patients with pleural effusion: effects of thoracentesis. *Am. J. Respir. Crit. Care Med.*, **156**, 1206–1209.

29. Graf, J. (2009) Pleural effusion in the mechanically ventilated patient. *Curr. Opin. Crit. Care*, **15**, 10–17.

30. Pneumatikos, I. and Bouros, D. (2008) Pleural effusions in critically ill patients. *Respiration*, **76**, 241–248.

31. Doelken, P., Abreu, R., Sahn, S.A. and Mayo, P.H. (2006) Effect of thoracocentesis on respiratory mechanics and gas exchange in patients receiving mechanical ventilation. *Chest*, **130**, 1354–1361.

32. Yang, P.C., Luh, K.T., Chang, D.B. *et al.* (1992) Value of sonography in determining the nature of pleural effusion: analysis of 320 cases. *Am. J. Roentgenol.*, **159**, 29–33.

33. Balik, M., Plasil, P., Waldauf, P. *et al.* (2006) Ultrasound estimation of volume of pleural fluid in mechanically ventilated patients. *Intensive Care Med.*, **32**, 318–321.

34. Spinale, F.G., Linker, R.W., Crawford, F.A. and Reines, H.D. (1989) Conventional versus high frequency jet ventilation with a bronchopleural fistula. *J. Surg. Res.*, **46**, 147–151.

35. Verschakelen, J. and Vock, P. (2007) Diseases of the chest wall, pleura and diaphragm, in *Diseases of the Heart, Chest and Breast* (eds J. Hodler, G.K. Zollikofer and C.L. von Schulthess), Springer, New York, pp. 99–103.

36. Epstein, S.K. (2001) Optimizing patient-ventilator synchrony. *Semin. Respir. Crit. Care Med.*, **22**, 137–152.

37. Pelosi, P., Croci, M., Ravagnan, I. *et al.* (1996) Total respiratory system, lung, and chest wall mechanics in sedated-paralyzed postoperative morbidly obese patients. *Chest*, **109**, 144–151.

38. Kress, J.P., Pohlman, A.S., Alverdy, J. and Hall, J.B. (1999) The impact of morbid obesity on oxygen cost of breathing (VO_2resp) at rest. *Am. J. Respir. Crit. Care Med.*, **160**, 883–886.

39. Bohm, S.H., Thamm, O.C., von Sandersleben, A. *et al.* (2009) Alveolar recruitment strategy and high positive end-expiratory pressure levels do not affect hemodynamics in morbidly obese intravascular volume-loaded patients. *Anesth. Analg.*, **109**, 160–163.

40. De Baerdemaeker, L.E., Van der Herten, C., Gillardin, J.M. *et al.* (2008) Comparison of volume-controlled and pressure-controlled ventilation during laparoscopic gastric banding in morbidly obese patients. *Obes. Surg.*, **18**, 680–685.

41. Hutchinson, D. and Whyte, K. (2008) Neuromuscular disease and respiratory failure. *Pract. Neurol.*, **8**, 229–237.

42. Gracey, D.R., Divertie, M.B. and Howard, F.M. (1983) Mechanical ventilation for respiratory failure in myasthenia gravis. Two-year experience with 22 patients. *Mayo Clin. Proc.*, **58**, 597–602.

43. Berrouschot, J., Baumann, I., Kalischewski, P. *et al.* (1997) Therapy of myasthenic crisis. *Crit. Care Med.*, **25**, 1228–1235.

44. Agarwal, R., Reddy, C. and Gupta, D. (2006) Noninvasive ventilation in acute neuromuscular respiratory failure due to myasthenic crisis: case report and review of literature. *Emerg. Med. J.*, **23**, e6.

2.7 Mechanical ventilation in obstructive lung disease

Rodolfo M. Pascual and Jeremy S. Breit

Pulmonary, Critical Care, Allergy and Immunology, Wake Forest University, Winston-Salem, NC, USA

2.7.1 Case presentation

You are called by a nurse to see a patient with respiratory distress and hypotension. He is a thin male who required intubation after failing a trial of noninvasive ventilation for a chronic obstructive pulmonary disease (COPD) exacerbation. He is diaphoretic and appears anxious with intercostal and scalene muscle contractions; his respiratory frequency appears to be 24. The chest is quiet with distant, continuous wheezes and distant heart tones. The trachea is palpated in the midline. The vital signs include respiratory rate 12 on the monitor; blood pressure 86/70 mm Hg, pulse 130, pulse oximetry 88%. The ventilator settings are frequency 12, tidal volume 420 ml (6 ml/kg PBW), fraction of inspired oxygen 0.6, positive end-expiratory pressure (PEEP) 5 cm H_2O, square waveform inspiratory flow at 60 l/min. He is receiving albuterol that was nebulized by high flow oxygen in-line with the ventilator circuit. Why does he have hypotension and distress? What should be done next?

2.7.2 Indications for invasive mechanical ventilation

Invasive mechanical ventilation for obstructive lung disease is indicated for severe or worsening respiratory failure whenever noninvasive positive pressure ventilation

A Practical Guide to Mechanical Ventilation, First Edition.
Edited by Jonathon D. Truwit and Scott K. Epstein.
© 2011 John Wiley & Sons, Ltd. Published 2011 by John Wiley & Sons, Ltd.

(NIPPV) [1, 2] cannot be used or has been attempted unsuccessfully. Invasive mechanical ventilation is initiated immediately for full or near respiratory arrest, cardiovascular collapse or cardiac arrest, when severe delirium is present, when ventilation via mask is not possible, or when the patient is unable to protect the airway from aspiration or handle airway secretions. Invasive ventilation should also be used promptly for severe respiratory failure if there is not a prompt response to NIPPV. However, invasive mechanical ventilation should not be used nonchalantly, especially in the severe asthma patient because of the potential for barotrauma [3]. This problem can be greatly mitigated by using "lung protective" strategies [4]. Most patients that die from asthma die prior to reaching the health care system but a significant number of those who die during hospitalization die from complications of mechanical ventilation.

2.7.3   Peak inspiratory pressure and plateau pressure

Patients on mechanical ventilation with obstructive lung disease often have air trapping and hyperinflation which leads to higher than normal measured pressure at the proximal airway (P_{ao}). Two commonly recorded ventilator pressures are peak or dynamic pressure (P_D) and the plateau or static pressure (P_S). The P_D is a function of tidal volume (V_T), PEEP, resistance to airflow, the elastic recoil of lungs and chest wall (compliance of the respiratory system), and inspiratory flow rate. P_S is a function of the tidal volume, PEEP, and elastic recoil of the lungs and the chest wall (compliance of the respiratory system) and is a zero flow measurement.

Determination of plateau pressure requires occlusion of the airway at end-inspiration so that flow ceases and airway pressure (P_{ao}) equilibrates with alveolar pressure (P_{alv}); the inspired breath is held in until the pressure reaches a plateau, generally 0.5 s. As shown in Figure 2.7.1, the difference between P_D and P_S can be examined to see if there is significant resistance in the respiratory system, such would be the case with COPD and especially with asthma. Changes in airway resistance would be expected with bronchospasm, reduced lung volumes, and bronchial or endotracheal tube obstruction with secretions. Examining the peak-plateau gradient can help differentiate those causes of high P_D from those that elevate both P_D and P_S, namely those that reduce respiratory system compliance like pneumothorax, pleural effusion, or pulmonary edema.

2.7.4   Auto-PEEP in obstructive lung disease

Auto-PEEP or intrinsic PEEP occurs with dynamic hyperinflation or air trapping; it reflects increased alveolar pressure. Dynamic hyperinflation results from airflow obstruction, early airway closure, and air trapping. One clue to the presence of auto-PEEP is a failure of expiratory flow to cease prior to the initiation of the next

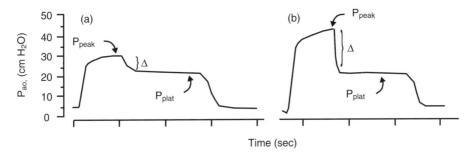

Figure 2.7.1   Airway pressure (P_{ao}) tracings from normal subjects and patients with obstructive lung disease during volume-targeted square wave flow mechanical ventilation. (a) Peak-plateau pressure gradient (Δ) is small in normal subjects as resistance is low. (b) Peak-plateau pressure gradient (Δ) widens with increased airways or ventilator circuit resistance.

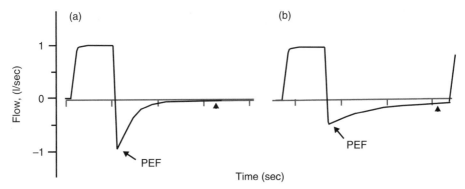

Figure 2.7.2   Inspiratory and expiratory flow from normal subjects and patients with obstructive lung disease during volume-targeted square wave flow mechanical ventilation. (a) Peak expiratory flow (PEF) rate is high initially and expiratory flow falls to zero prior to the next inspiration in normal subjects as expiratory resistance is low. (b) PEF is reduced and expiratory flow does not return to zero prior to the next inspiration in patients with obstructive lung disease and associated auto-PEEP.

inspiration as illustrated in Figure 2.7.2. As shown in Figure 2.7.3, auto-PEEP can be measured by allowing for a prolonged expiration against a closed expiratory port and, hence, equilibration of pressures along the respiratory tree so that P_{ao} approximates P_{alv}. This measurement is made most accurately in the relaxed patient. In the presence of dynamic hyperinflation, P_{ao} rises during airway occlusion to equilibrate with P_{alv}. The post occlusion P_{ao} represents the summation of PEEP and auto-PEEP. The difference between P_{ao} pre and post occlusion is auto-PEEP. External PEEP can be raised without impacting post occlusion P_{ao} up until it exceeds the associated auto-PEEP. This becomes important when trying to reduce triggering pressures (see below).

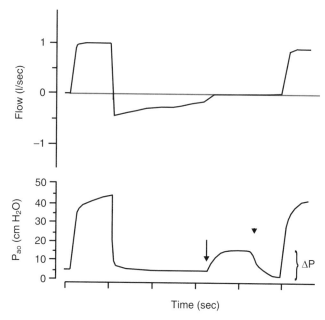

Figure 2.7.3   Measuring AutoPEEP. The expiratory port is closed during expiration (arrow) and a rise in P_{ao} is seen reflecting P_{alv}. The patient is not relaxed and initiates a breath (arrowhead), note that a relatively high ΔP is needed for triggering.

It is important to recognize that P_{alv} is not a single pressure but rather results from the pressure exerted by the population of the millions of alveoli which are distended to varying extents. When auto-PEEP, and by extension high P_{alv} and high transpulmonary pressure, are present, hypoxemia because of poor ventilation/ perfusion (V/Q) matching, hypotension because of reduced preload, and baro-trauma because of high transpulmonary pressure may result. Additionally auto-PEEP will lead to reduced ΔP (P_D minus PEEP or driving pressure) and, by extension, reduced delivered volumes in pressure-targeted modes, whereas in volume-targeted modes there will be resultant alveolar over-distension.

Moreover, autoPEEP can cause ineffective ventilator triggering, ventilator–patient dyssynchrony and increased work of breathing. Ventilator–patient dyssyn-chrony may lead to worse outcomes, such as prolonged mechanical ventilation and increased length of stay [5]. Ventilators will be triggered when the patient makes an inspiratory effort sufficient to cause a pressure or flow change beyond a pre-set threshold value. This value is usually relative to the extrinsic PEEP or zero flow, respectively. Hence, if auto-PEEP is present the patient must generate a pressure greater than the sum of the auto-PEEP and threshold pressure in order to trigger an inspiration. Similarly, in a flow-triggered mode when auto-PEEP is present (hence air trapping) the patient must generate a flow greater than the sum of the expiratory flow and threshold flow in order to trigger an inspiration.

Extrinsic or applied PEEP is a value set on the ventilator and is used to prevent atelectasis or alveolar closure during exhalation. A common PEEP setting is 5 cm H_2O that is often considered "physiologic PEEP." The ventilator is programmed to maintain positive airway pressure at the end of expiration and if applied PEEP is not transmitted to the alveolus, provided it is less than end-expiratory alveolar pressure. Modern ventilators are engineered to permit excess expiratory flow, for example during coughing, even as PEEP is maintained. However, auto-PEEP can and often does exceed extrinsic PEEP because it is measured when the expiratory port is closed, thus reflecting the pressure "trapped" in slowly emptying alveoli (P_{alv}). Alveolar pressure may not be sensed at the airway opening in a non-equilibrium state. The judicious application of extrinsic PEEP at a level closer to but not exceeding the auto-PEEP can reduce the inspiratory force (hence pressure or flow) change demanded of the patient to trigger the ventilator. It is recommended that applied PEEP be set at < 80% of the measured auto-PEEP or lower if it allows the patient to trigger the ventilator relatively easily.

2.7.5   Management of I:E ratio

In the relaxed, normal, patient receiving mechanical ventilation the expiratory phase is typically mostly passive. The force required for exhalation is derived from the elastic recoil of the expanded lung (stored work done by the ventilator during the duty cycle) and active muscle contraction of the abdominal or the chest wall muscles is not required. However, when airflow obstruction is present, expiratory flow rates are reduced and more time is needed to completely exhale and deflate the lungs. Airflow obstruction will be exclusively of the intrathoracic variety in the patient that has a translaryngeal airway whereas this assumption may not be valid in the case of the patient ventilated via a mask. Moreover, the stored elastic recoil pressure of the lung that is often reduced in COPD may not be sufficient to overcome the increased total resistance from bronchospasm and early small airway closure [6]. Expressed in another way, the respiratory system time constant or the product of resistance and compliance is reduced in obstructive lung disease, hence lung emptying is delayed. When the time constant is markedly reduced, air trapping results because complete expiration may not be achieved before the next inspiration or duty cycle is due or before the patient makes another inspiratory effort. The patient will sense air trapping and hyperinflation and may attempt to augment exhalation with active muscle contraction; this is a situation that unfortunately increases the work of breathing and may lead to patient–ventilator dyssynchrony.

Several possible remedies for hyperinflation or auto-PEEP are shown in Figure 2.7.4. All will allow for more complete emptying of the lungs during the expiratory phase. Firstly, reducing tidal volume given a constant frequency reduces the volume of gas that needs to be exhaled. Also, at a given inspiratory flow rate, smaller tidal volume will reduce the inspiratory time or duty cycle while reducing the inspiratory:expiratory (I:E) ratio. Secondly, reducing respiratory frequency will

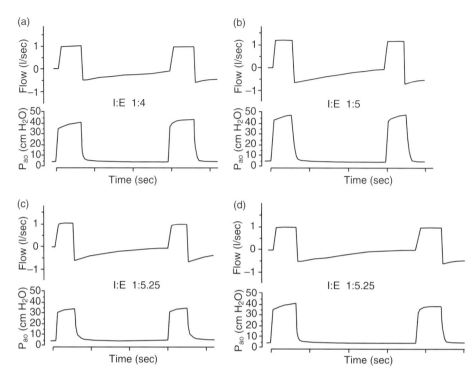

Figure 2.7.4 Adjusting I:E ratio. (a) Baseline, V_T 600 ml, f 20/min, flow 1 l/s, T_i 0.6 s, I:E 1:4. (b) Increasing flow by 20% reduces T_i and increases expiratory time. I:E is improved but P_D is increased. (c) Reducing tidal volume (V_T) by 20% reduces T_i, increases expiratory time and reduces P_D. (d) Reducing frequency (f) by 20% increases expiratory time.

reduce the number of duty cycles, reduce minute ventilation, and will similarly reduce the I:E ratio. Finally, reducing the length of the duty cycle by increasing inspiratory flow rates, hence reducing inspiratory time, will also reduce the I:E ratio. It can be seen from Figure 2.7.4 that measures that reduce minute ventilation (reducing frequency or V_T) are most efficient at reducing the I:E ratio. Moreover, lower V_T means less gas needs to be exhaled, further improving lung emptying.

The main disadvantage to reduced minute ventilation is hypercapnia, however this is well tolerated by most patients. The primary goals of mechanical ventilation during a COPD or asthma exacerbation are to permit the patient to rest, to prevent barotrauma, and to maintain an adequate arterial pH but not necessarily a normal pH while allowing for anti-inflammatory and bronchodilator medications to take effect. It should be noted that reductions in V_E also reduce mean airway pressure and P_{alv}, and hence should reduce barotrauma. Increasing inspiratory flow rates will increase peak airway pressures and this may be an issue if the ventilator is set up to limit peak pressures, because typically the cycled volume will be truncated once the peak pressure is reached. Importantly, it cannot be assumed that changes in V_T, frequency, or flow rates do not result in changes in the patient's respiratory drive. For example Laghi *et al.* observed that increases in inspiratory flow administered to COPD patients resulted in increased patient-initiated respiratory frequency [7]. Therefore, when a ventilator parameter is changed the patient should be reassessed to ensure that the desired effect is achieved.

2.7.6 Delivery of nebulized/aerosolized medications

The optimal delivery of aerosols to mechanically ventilated patients is reviewed elsewhere [8]. The efficiency of aerosol delivery or the percentage of dosed drug that actually reaches the target tissue is greatly reduced by the presence of an artificial airway [9]. Aerosol delivery is reduced in a ventilator circuit in which the air is conditioned (warmed and humidified) when compared to ambient conditions. However, manipulation of the ventilator circuit increases the risk of pneumonia. Nevertheless, bronchodilation can be achieved in patients receiving mechanical ventilation if several factors are accounted for. Things that should be considered when delivering aerosols to mechanically ventilated patients include the position of the patient, the type of aerosol generator, the position and configuration of the aerosol generator in the circuit, aerosol particle size, timing of aerosol delivery; conditions of the ventilator circuit such as temperature and humidity; and ventilator parameters such as tidal volume and inspiratory flow rate. Other issues to consider include drug dosage and half-life, and patient airway characteristics like the degree of obstruction and hyperinflation [8].

Aerosol delivery systems were designed to deliver drugs to non-intubated patients. Yet many of the same principles for effective drug delivery apply to mechanically ventilated patients. When giving aerosol medication the patient should be placed in a seated, standing or semi-recumbent position. Particles dispersed from the nebulizers with a mass median aerodynamic diameter (MMAD) between one and five μm reach the lower respiratory tract whereas larger particles are impacted upon the circuit.

Alternatively, bronchodilating medications can be delivered from a pressurized metered dose inhaler (pMDI). Efficiency of delivery is enhanced when a spacer device is utilized and pMDIs should be actuated early in inspiration during a relatively slow inspiration. Additionally, it is important to recognize that pMDI-HFA (hydrofluoroalkane) devices do not have the same drug delivery when used with pMDI-CFC (chlorofluorocarbon) adapters and vice versa. Unfortunately, those factors that increase drug delivery, namely higher V_T or slower inspiration, can increase air trapping. However, this air trapping can be tolerated, as time required for dosage delivery from a pMDI is much less than that needed for a nebulizer.

All other things being equal, pMDIs deliver medication much more efficiently than jet or ultrasonic nebulizers, require lower drug doses, and also, because they

Table 2.7.1 Key points when using aerosols in mechanically ventilated patients.

Issue or measure	Comment
1. pMDIs are preferred to nebulizers	pMDIs are cheaper, more efficient, faster
2. Reduce inspiratory flow rate	Improves efficiency, may worsen air trapping
3. Set V_T greater than dead space (≥ 500 ml)	Can be set higher temporarily for dosing, may worsen air trapping
4. Less efficient delivery compared to non-intubated patients	Increase dose to compensate, four puffs of pMDI is generally effective
5. Space dose out by at least 15 s for pMDI	For nebulizers intermittent dosing during inspiration is also better
6. Shortened drug half-life	Dose more often, every 3–4 h as needed
7. Minimize manipulation of ventilator circuit	More manipulation increases risk of ventilator-associated pneumonia
8. Use drug-specific adapters and spacers	Improves efficiency
9. Assess for efficacy of treatment	Use physical examination and waveform analysis

can be given more quickly, are much cheaper (Table 2.7.1) [10]. For example, it will take from 15 to 30 minutes to deliver medication via a nebulizer but less than two minutes for a pMDI. Four puffs of albuterol from a pMDI (400 μg) will provide similar bronchodilation to 2.5 mg (2500 μg) of albuterol delivered via a nebulizer. Similar to non-intubated patients, there is little evidence that bronchodilators have effects on clinically relevant outcomes like hospital- or long-term mortality, intensive care unit or hospital length of stay, or duration of mechanical ventilation. They have been shown to reduce work of breathing, airway resistance, and dyspnea while improving mucus clearance and pulmonary edema. Because the therapeutic index is much greater when these agents are delivered by aerosol than when they are given orally or parenterally, the aerosol route is highly preferred. There is little known about the optimal dosing of long-acting inhaled beta-adrenergic agonists like formoterol or salmeterol in mechanically ventilated patients, and higher than usual doses are not recommended because of potential toxicity, so they are not recommended for use in mechanically ventilated patients.

In contrast to bronchodilators, parenteral steroids are effective in exacerbations of asthma or COPD. There is little evidence that inhaled corticosteroids (ICS) are effective in mechanically ventilated patients, and little is known about the delivery of inhaled steroids during mechanical ventilation. Moreover, higher dose ICS have been associated with pneumonia in COPD [11]. Because of lack of evidence of efficacy and the risk of increased ventilator-associated pneumonia, the use of ICS alone or in combination inhalers for mechanically ventilated patients is not recommended.

2.7.7 Case presentation solution

The patient developed respiratory distress and hypotension because of air trapping from over-ventilation. The nebulizer set up resulted in extra minute ventilation administered to the patient and resultant auto-PEEP. This problem could have been avoided by using a pressurized metered dose inhaler to deliver albuterol. The patient's current problem can be addressed by disconnecting the ventilator from the ET tube allowing for emptying of the lungs, using an metered dose inhaler, and by further reducing minute ventilation if respiratory distress persists.

References

1. Keenan, S.P. and Mehta, S. (2009) Noninvasive ventilation for patients presenting with acute respiratory failure: the randomized controlled trials. *Respir. Care*, **54** (1), 116–126.
2. Nowak, R., Corbridge, T. and Brenner, B. (2009) Noninvasive ventilation. *Proc. Am. Thorac. Soc.*, **6** (4), 367–370.
3. Shapiro, J.M. (2001) Intensive care management of status asthmaticus. *Chest*, **120** (5), 1439–1441.
4. Oddo, M., Feihl, F., Schaller, M.D. and Perret, C. (2006) Management of mechanical ventilation in acute severe asthma: practical aspects. *Intensive Care Med.*, **32** (4), 501–510.
5. de Wit, M., Miller, K.B., Green, D.A. *et al.* (2009) Ineffective triggering predicts increased duration of mechanical ventilation. *Crit. Care Med.*, **37** (10), 2740–2745.
6. West, J.B. and West, J.B. (2008) Pulmonary Pathophysiology the Essentials, 7th edn. Wolters Kluwer/Lippincott Williams & Wilkins, Philadelphia.
7. Laghi, F., Segal, J., Choe, W.K. and Tobin, M.J. (2001) Effect of imposed inflation time on respiratory frequency and hyperinflation in patients with chronic obstructive pulmonary disease. *Am. J. Respir. Crit. Care Med.*, **163** (6), 1365–1370.
8. Dhand, R. and Guntur, V.P. (2008) How best to deliver aerosol medications to mechanically ventilated patients. *Clin. Chest Med.*, **29** (2), 277–296.
9. MacIntyre, N.R., Silver, R.M., Miller, C.W. *et al.* (1985) Aerosol delivery in intubated, mechanically ventilated patients. *Crit. Care Med.*, **13** (2), 81–84.
10. Bowton, D.L., Goldsmith, W.M. and Haponik, E.F. (1992) Substitution of metered-dose inhalers for hand-held nebulizers. Success and cost savings in a large, acute-care hospital. *Chest*, **101** (2), 305–308.
11. Nannini, L., Cates, C.J., Lasserson, T.J. and Poole, P. (2007) Combined corticosteroid and long acting beta-agonist in one inhaler for chronic obstructive pulmonary disease. *Cochrane Database Syst. Rev.* 3 (Art. No.: CD003794). doi: 10.1002/14651858.CD003794.pub3.

2.8 Ancillary methods to mechanical ventilation

Kyle B. Enfield and Jonathon D. Truwit

Division of Pulmonary and Critical Care Medicine, University of Virginia, Charlottesville, VA, USA

2.8.1 Case presentation

A 45-year-old man s/p renal transplant on chronic Mycophenolate Mofetil (MMF) and prednisone is transferred to the intensive care unit for hypoxemic respiratory failure early in the fall of 2009. He arrives intubated from a referring facility on volume control ventilation, TV 360 (6 ml/kg) with a positive end-expiratory pressure (PEEP) of 10 and FiO_2 of 1.0. On arrival, he is found to have bilateral pulmonary infiltrates with a PaO_2/FiO_2 of 75 (PaO_2 75). Following arrival he develops progressive hypoxia, without change in his chest X-ray and unresponsive to further increases in PEEP or recruitment maneuvers.

2.8.2 Introduction

A subsegment of patients with acute and chronic respiratory failure will need adjunctive or ancillary methods of ventilation during the course of their treatment. These methods, reviewed here, are challenging for the clinician due to their novelty and often relative lack of clinical research support. While the potential list is long, this chapter reviews neuromuscular blocking agents (NMBAs), high frequency oscillatory ventilation, inhalational therapies including heliox, and tracheal gas

A Practical Guide to Mechanical Ventilation, First Edition.
Edited by Jonathon D. Truwit and Scott K. Epstein.
© 2011 John Wiley & Sons, Ltd. Published 2011 by John Wiley & Sons, Ltd.

Table 2.8.1 Randomized controlled trials of NMBAs in patients with acute respiratory distress syndrome.

Source	n	Setting	Type of respiratory failure	NMBA	Duration of infusion (h)	Effect on oxygenation
Lagneau [1]	102	ICU	ARF P/F <200	Cisatracurium	2	Improvement
Gainnier [2]	56	ICU	ARF P/F <150	Cisatracurium	48	Improvement
Forel [3]	36	ICU	ARF P/F <200	Cisatracurium	48	Improvement

insufflation. As shown in Table 2.8.1, there have been three prospective randomized controlled trials that showed that short duration paralytic use is associated with improvement in oxygenation.

2.8.3 Neuromuscular blocking agents

Neuromuscular blocking agents are commonly used in patients with hypoxic respiratory failure. Surveys in the United States and Europe show that their use ranges from 18 to 20% of patients in the intensive care unit [4]. In the ARMA study conducted by the ARDSnet, they were used in 25% of the 861 patients in the study at the time of enrollment [5]. At the same time, the recent focus for decreased sedation in critically ill patients, which has been shown to improve outcomes, has called into question the utility of NMBAs in the critically ill patient.

These studies lack the ability to be combined in a meta-analysis, for while they each showed improvement in oxygenation, they are heterogeneous in design. Lagneau *et al.* [1] showed improvement in oxygenation, but randomized patients to deep paralysis (Train of Four 0/4) compared to lighter paralysis (Train of Four 2/4). Gainnier *et al.* [2] and Forel *et al.* [3] randomized patients to NMBA or no NMBA but used different inclusion criteria.

Understanding of how NMBAs improve oxygenation is not complete, and is difficult to study independent of the effects of sedation. Several hypotheses exist, including reduction in oxygen consumption, reduction in patient–ventilator dyssynchrony, improvement in chest wall compliance, and a anti-inflammatory effect of NMBas [4]. Gainnier *et al.* [2] showed that the improvement in P/F ratio came at the end of the infusion (Figure 2.8.1), suggesting that a reduction in oxygen consumption may not be responsible, but perhaps facilitates low tidal volume ventilation.

Supporting this are findings that paralytics facilitate precise control of volume and pressure, helping to prevent alveolar collapse and reducing both volu- and barotraumas [6]. These benefits must be weighed against the potential negative effects of NMBAs that have linked the use of NMBAs to critical illness myopathy. Additionally, the evidence, based on three heterogeneous randomized controlled

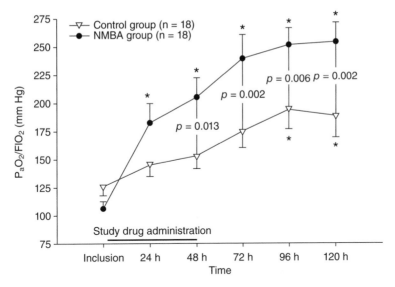

Figure 2.8.1   Evolution of the PaO_2 to FiO_2 ratio over 120 h in 56 acute respiratory distress syndrome (ARDS) patients randomized to receive or not a 48-h cisatracurium perfusion. Results are expressed as mean ± SEM. *$p < 0.001$ vs. baseline by Tukey test. FiO_2, inspired oxygen fraction; NMBA, neuromuscular blocking agent; PaO_2, partial pressure of oxygen in arterial blood. (Reproduced with permission [2].)

trials, is insufficient to recommend their automatic use for all patients with hypoxic respiratory failure. A multicenter randomized controlled trial, NMBA vs placebo, demonstrates a reduction in 90 day mortality after adjustment for baseline differences (CI:0.68 (0.48–0.98, $p = 0.04$) [4].   Crude 28 day mortality was reduced (23.7% vs. 33.3%, $p = 0.05$), and a trend at 90 days favoring NMBA (31.6% vs. 40.7%, $p = 0/08$) was noted.   While the data needs to be confirmed in another RCT, it does suggest benefit from early use of NMBA in severe ARDS.

2.8.4   High frequency oscillatory ventilation

The clinical utility of high frequency oscillatory ventilation (HFOV) is well established in neonatology. It has been proposed as an alternative mode of ventilation in acute respiratory distress syndrome (ARDS) to improve oxygenation without further injuring the lung. A retrospective study of 28 patients with burns treated with HFOV supported it as a safe mode of ventilating these patients [7]. Building on previous observational studies, a randomized controlled trial of 148 patients with ARDS showed the HFOV improved oxygenation index initially; however, this did not persist past 24 hours and was not associated with a statistically significant difference in mortality [8].

Theoretically, HFOV ventilates patients at low tidal volumes and avoids volutrauma by maintaining an "open lung" approach on the deflation limb of the

Table 2.8.2 Suggested initial settings for HFOV[10].

Frequency	
pH <7.1	4 Hz
pH 7.1–7.19	5 Hz
pH 7.2–7.35	6 Hz
pH >7.35	7 Hz
Amplitude (power)	70–90 cm H_2O
Paw	5 cm H_2O >plateau pressure on CV to max of 35 cm H_2O
Bias flow	40 l/min
Inspiratory time	33%
FiO_2	100%

pressure–volume curve at a relatively constant airway pressure [9]. This may result in improvement by preventing atelectotrauma in alveoli with long and variable filling times and in less fibrotic segments of the lung by decreasing preferential airflow to those regions resulting in volutrauma. Given the lack of outcomes data to support HFOV, a consensus guideline suggests its use when conventional ventilator settings are greater than an FiO_2 of 70% and PEEP greater than 14 cm H_2O, or when arterial pH is less than 7.25 with a tidal volume that is greater than 6 ml/kg PBW and a plateau pressure that is greater than 30 cm H_2O [10]. The guideline also suggests initial settings for HFOV control respiratory frequency, amplitude of ventilation, mean airway pressure, bias flow, percentage of inspiratory time, and FiO_2 (Table 2.8.2). One Hertz is equal to one breath per second. It is important to remember as well that given a fixed inspiratory and expiratory time, tidal volume (amplitude) is inversely proportional to frequency. Adjustments in FiO_2, Paw, and bias flow improve oxygenation, while frequency, power, and introduction of an endotracheal cuff leak will improve $PaCO_2$ [10].

2.8.5 Inhaled pulmonary vasodilators

Respiratory failure that is predominantly V/Q mismatch can be refractory to changes in FiO_2 and increased levels of PEEP [11]. Inhaled nitric oxide (INO) and inhaled prostacyclin target pulmonary vessels supplying ventilated lung, theoretically improving V/Q mismatch by "opening" segments of the pulmonary architecture. Both INO and inhaled prostacyclin have been shown to improve oxygenation in a variety of clinical conditions; however, more meaningful outcomes are controversial [12].

The biologic effects of nitric oxide (NO) were first described in 1987. NO was first described as the endothelium-derived relaxing factor [13]. Inhaled nitric oxide has two potential theoretic benefits: [4] reducing right heart strain [5], improving V/Q mismatch by "opening" segments of the pulmonary vasculature. The clinical use of this agent surrounds this. Post-cardiac and lung transplant, INO has been used to reduce right heart strain. The primary goal in this setting is to decrease pulmonary vascular resistance (PVR), resulting in right heart afterload reduction and theoretically increased augmented cardiac output. However, there is a lack of outcome studies supporting this. In 2006 a retrospective non-controlled study was published by George *et al.* [14] showing improved mortality and lower cost for patients treated with INO compared to historic controls undergoing orthotopic heart transplantation and orthotopic lung transplantation. A 2007 meta-analysis including 12 trials and 1237 patients of INO for ARDS showed that there were improved physiologic outcomes, but this failed to translate into improved clinical outcomes (risk ratio for hospital mortality 1.10, 95% CI 0.94–1.30). In this same group there was a 1.50 increased risk for developing acute renal failure in the patients receiving INO (95% CI 1.11–2.02) [15].

In patients with pulmonary hypertension and New York Heart Association (NYHA) Class III or IV symptoms, inhaled prostacyclin, is clearly shown to improve exercise tolerance and improve pulmonary artery pressure [16]. Inhaled prostacyclin has advantages over intravenous: [4] it is not associated with rebound pulmonary hypertension with cessation of use [5]; there is no associated tachyphy-laxis; and [1], there is selective dilation of the pulmonary vasculature [17]. Inhaled aerosolized prostacyclin (IAP) is known to improve PaO_2/FiO_2 and $P(A–a)O_2$ in a dose response fashion [18]. Similar to INO, IAP has not been shown to improve clinical outcome. A randomized control study is needed. Given that their mecha-nism of action is similar, their application and clinical usefulness are likely related. The lower cost associated with IAP may favor its use clinically [12, 19]. Arguably, the lack of evidence for clinical outcomes may reflect sample size or patient section, and preventing significant hypoxia may be important in an undefined patient population.

2.8.6 Inhaled carbon monoxide (ICO)

The idea of using a substance traditionally seen as toxic is counterintuitive given its known toxicity at high doses. In contrast to high doses, low doses of inhaled carbon monoxide (ICO) may offer a degree of cytoprotection during ischemia/reperfusion. Endogenous carbon monoxide, produced through heme degradation, is known to alter intracellular signaling pathways that regulate vasoregulatory, anti-inflammatory, anti-apoptotic, and anti-proliferative effects. There are ongoing trials looking at inhaled low dose carbon monoxide in the prevention of inflammation and rejection following solid organ transplant. There is some suggestion from the early results that there may be a role for ICO in the intensive care unit in the near future [20, 21].

2.8.7 Heliox

The replacement of nitrogen with helium (heliox), takes advantage of the unique physical properties of helium (low density, high thermal conductivity, and inertness) to create an inhalational mixture that is three times less dense than air. In regions of turbulent airflow (upper airways) where flow is density dependent, this lower density mixture can have clinical importance.

Heliox has been used in diseases characterized by increased airway resistance (e.g., upper airway obstruction, upper airway narrowing (croup), asthma). Most of this work has been anecdotal [12]. Early evidence in children with post-extubation stridor supported this, with the heliox patients reporting a 38% reduction in respiratory distress scores [22]. However, in the two controlled trials published studying the application of heliox for croup, there were no differences in clinical outcomes despite improved croup scores. Neither trial compared heliox against placebo; further trials are needed [23].

The use of heliox for obstructive lung disease (asthma and COPD) has been explored as well. In both spontaneous breathing and mechanically ventilated patients there are physiologic improvements that may have clinical importance. In the spontaneous breathing asthma patients, heliox improved peak flow and decreased both pulsus paradoxus and $PaCO_2$ [24]. A meta-analysis has shown that this improvement in peak flow may be as much as 30% (95% CI 16.6–42.6) [25]. In the intubated asthmatic there is a reduction in the peak airway pressure and $PaCO_2$ as well [26]. For patients with chronic obstructive pulmonary disease (COPD), the pooled data for the spontaneously breathing or noninvasively ventilated patient would not favor heliox. There are some data that indicate that, in the intubated patient in both asthma and COPD, heliox may help to lower iPEEP [25]. However, outcomes data for these patients is not available.

While in theory there are attractive reasons for the use of heliox, there remain little clinical benefits except in the patients with post-extubation stridor. Additionally, heliox has significant associated costs and technical limitations associated with its use.

2.8.8   Tracheal gas insufflation

Administration of oxygen directly into the trachea has been used in both stable chronic respiratory failure and in the patients with severe acute respiratory failure [27]. Recognition that apneic patients provided with 100% oxygenation maintained adequate PaO_2 was shown in 1959 by Frumin *et al.* [28]. In 1985, Slutsky *et al.* showed similar data in 10 anesthetized, paralyzed dogs, providing continuous oxygen at flow rates of 2.0–3.0 l/min through a small catheter positioned 1 cm from the carina [29]. Slutsky went on to show that catheters placed further into the lung, up to 3.5 cm into each mainstem, could provide effective ventilation in paralyzed dogs [30]. These early studies have led to investigations of Tracheal Gas Insufflation (TGI) as an adjuvant to mechanical ventilation, as a stand-alone mode of ventilator support, and as an aid to weaning from mechanical ventilation [27].

As an adjuvant to traditional mechanical ventilation, there is a large number of animal studies with experimental lung injury, which has recently been summarized by Nahum [31]. These data show that TGI during expiration flushes the anatomic dead space, improving carbon dioxide clearance, increasing to a plateau as the flow rate increases. These models have been supported by small clinical studies in patients with ARDS managed with a strategy of permissive hypercapnia. The conclusion of these trials is that TGI can be used on volume- and pressured-cycled ventilation, allowing for further reductions in tidal volume without raising $PaCO_2$ [32–36], or to lower $PaCO_2$ in severe metabolic acidosis or intracranial hypertension [37]. When compared to optimization of mechanical ventilation, TGI has similar efficacy [36]; outcome studies are lacking.

While experimental models to study the use of TGI in weaning trials suggested it would increase the work of breathing [38], outcome studies have been more promising. Early work by Nakos et al. [33] in 12 spontaneously breathing patients with COPD showed a decrease in the V_D/V_T ratio. Similar results were shown by Schönhofer et al. when TGI was applied immediately after liberation from mechanical ventilation. A follow-up study by the same group showed a 28% reduction in inspiratory work in COPD patients who had experienced long-term mechanical ventilation [39]. This early work suggested that TGI may be beneficial in other patients with prolonged mechanical ventilation. A small study suggests that some patients may benefit; however, more work is needed [40].

In chronic respiratory failure, the use of TGI was first described by Heimlich in 1982 [41]. Compared to nasal oxygen therapy, transtracheal provides adequate oxygenation at lower flow rates while remaining safe, efficacious, and convenient for patients with chronic respiratory failure [42–45]. Hoffman et al. [45] studied 20 patients (14 men and six women) before and after placement of TGI, showing that post-TGI they required 45% less oxygen at rest and 39% less during exercise. Exercise tolerance, measured by a 12-min walk test, also improved. There were adverse events associated with the placement of the catheter, most resolving after the track had matured. These studies were all carried out in low flow states; recently high flow TGI has been introduced. In a study of 14 patients, high flow TGI decreased minute ventilation by 20%. This group showed an increase in expiratory time with a decrease in end-expiratory volume. This trial is limited by the short duration the patients were exposed to the therapy (1 h), but is promising for future therapy [46].

2.8.9 Summary

While there are several promising ancillary methods of support for acute and chronic respiratory failure, there remains a paucity of clinical outcomes data for many of these novel and traditional therapies. These therapies rely, therefore, on strong clinical skills as well as frank discussions with the patient or their surrogate of the relative risk and benefits of the therapy in the absence of an ongoing research protocol.

2.8.10   Case presentation revisited

The patient was paralyzed and started on inhaled flolan early in his intensive care unit stay. Despite initial concerns for Novel 2009 H1N1, rhinovirus was isolated from the respiratory secretions. The patient's oxygenation index slowly improved, and both NMBAs and flolan were discontinued. Ultimately, the patient was discharged from the intensive care unit and hospital without further sequela of his disease. This case illustrates that while important hard end points are missing to evaluate these ancillary methods for mechanical ventilation, there may be important patient level benefits that are derived. In this patient's care, supporting their worsening hypoxemia supported them during the recovery phase of their illness. Caution must be exercised, however, in interpreting this case, as it is not fully know what the natural history would have been if flolan and NMBAs were not used.

References

1. Lagneau, F., D'honneur, G., Plaud, B. *et al.* (2002) A comparison of two depths of prolonged neuromuscular blockade induced by cisatracurium in mechanically ventilated critically ill patients. *Intensive Care Med.*, **28** (12), 1735–1741.
2. Gainnier, M., Roch, A., Forel, J. *et al.* (2004) Effect of neuromuscular blocking agents on gas exchange in patients presenting with acute respiratory distress syndrome. *Crit. Care Med.*, **32** (1), 113–119.
3. Forel, J., Roch, A., Marin, V. *et al.* (2006) Neuromuscular blocking agents decrease inflammatory response in patients presenting with acute respiratory distress syndrome. *Crit. Care Med.*, **34** (11), 2749–2757.
4. Papazian, L., Forel, J., Gacouin, A. *et al.* (2010) Neuromuscular blockers in early acute respiratory distress syndrome. *N. Engl. J. Med.*, **363** (12), 1107–1116.
5. The Acute Respiratory Distress Syndrome Network (2000) Ventilation with lower tidal volumes as compared with traditional tidal volumes for acute lung injury and the acute respiratory distress syndrome. *N. Engl. J. Med.*, **342** (18), 1301–1308.
6. Murray, M.J., Cowen, J., DeBlock, H. *et al.* (2002) Clinical practice guidelines for sustained neuromuscular blockade in the adult critically ill patient. *Crit. Care Med.*, **30** (1), 142–156.
7. Cartotto, R., Ellis, S., Gomez, M. *et al.* (2004) High frequency oscillatory ventilation in burn patients with the acute respiratory distress syndrome. *Burns*, **30** (5), 453–463.
8. Derdak, S., Mehta, S., Stewart, T.E. *et al.* (2002) High-frequency oscillatory ventilation for acute respiratory distress syndrome in adults: a randomized, controlled trial. *Am. J. Respir. Crit. Care Med.*, **166** (6), 801–808.
9. Fort, P., Farmer, C., Westerman, J. *et al.* (1997) High-frequency oscillatory ventilation for adult respiratory distress syndrome–a pilot study. *Crit. Care Med.*, **25** (6), 937–947.
10. Fessler, H.E., Derdak, S., Ferguson, N.D. *et al.* (2007) A protocol for high-frequency oscillatory ventilation in adults: results from a roundtable discussion. *Crit. Care Med.*, **35** (7), 1649–1654.
11. Hall, J., Schmidt, G. and Wood, L. (2005) *Principles of Critical Care*, 3rd edn. McGraw-Hill, New York.
12. Robinson, B.R., Athota, K.P. and Branson, R.D. (2009) Inhalational therapies for the ICU. *Curr. Opin. Crit. Care*, **15** (1), 1–9.

13. Moncada, S., Palmer, R.M. and Higgs, E.A. (1989) Biosynthesis of nitric oxide from L-arginine. A pathway for the regulation of cell function and communication. *Biochem. Pharmacol.*, **38** (11), 1709–1715.

14. George, I., Xydas, S., Topkara, V.K. *et al.* (2006) Clinical indication for use and outcomes after inhaled nitric oxide therapy. *Ann. Thorac. Surg.*, **82** (6), 2161–2169.

15. Adhikari, N.K.J., Burns, K.E.A., Friedrich, J.O. *et al.* (2007) Effect of nitric oxide on oxygenation and mortality in acute lung injury: systematic review and meta-analysis. *BMJ*, **334** (7597), 779.

16. Chen, Y., Jowett, S., Barton, P. *et al.* (2009) Clinical and cost-effectiveness of epoprostenol, iloprost, bosentan, sitaxentan and sildenafil for pulmonary arterial hypertension within their licensed indications: a systematic review and economic evaluation. *Health Technol. Assess.*, **13** (49), 1–320.

17. Voswinckel, R., Enke, B., Reichenberger, F. *et al.* (2006) Favorable effects of inhaled treprostinil in severe pulmonary hypertension: results from randomized controlled pilot studies. *J. Am. Coll. Cardiol.*, **48** (8), 1672–1681.

18. van Heerden, P.V., Barden, A., Michalopoulos, N. *et al.* (2000) Dose-response to inhaled aerosolized prostacyclin for hypoxemia due to ARDS. *Chest*, **117** (3), 819–827.

19. Siobal, M.S. and Hess, D.R. (2010) Are inhaled vasodilators useful in acute lung injury and acute respiratory distress syndrome? *Respir. Care*, **55** (2), 144–157; discussion 157–161.

20. Bilban, M., Haschemi, A., Wegiel, B. *et al.* (2008) Heme oxygenase and carbon monoxide initiate homeostatic signaling. *J. Mol. Med.*, **86** (3), 267–279.

21. Piantadosi, C.A. (2008) Carbon monoxide, reactive oxygen signaling, and oxidative stress. *Free Radic. Biol. Med.*, **45** (5), 562–569.

22. Kemper, K.J., Ritz, R.H., Benson, M.S. and Bishop, M.S. (1991) Helium-oxygen mixture in the treatment of postextubation stridor in pediatric trauma patients. *Crit. Care Med.*, **19** (3), 356–359.

23. Vorwerk, C. and Coats, T. (2010) Heliox for croup in children. *Cochrane Database Syst. Rev.* 2 (Art. No.: CD006822). doi: 10.1002/14651858.CD006822.pub2.

24. Manthous, C.A., Hall, J.B., Caputo, M.A. *et al.* (1995) Heliox improves pulsus paradoxus and peak expiratory flow in nonintubated patients with severe asthma. *Am. J. Respir. Crit. Care Med.*, **151** (2 Pt 1), 310–314.

25. Colebourn, C.L., Barber, V. and Young, J.D. (2007) Use of helium-oxygen mixture in adult patients presenting with exacerbations of asthma and chronic obstructive pulmonary disease: a systematic review. *Anaesthesia*, **62** (1), 34–42.

26. Gluck, E.H., Onorato, D.J. and Castriotta, R. (1990) Helium-oxygen mixtures in intubated patients with status asthmaticus and respiratory acidosis. *Chest*, **98** (3), 693–698.

27. Epstein, S.K. (2002) TGIF: tracheal gas insufflation. *Chest*, **122** (5), 1515–1517.

28. Frumin, M.J., Epstein, R.M. and Cohen, G. (1959) Apneic oxygenation in man. *Anesthesiology*, **20**, 789–798.

29. Slutsky, A.S., Watson, J., Leith, D.E. and Brown, R. (1985) Tracheal insufflation of O_2 (TRIO) at low flow rates sustains life for several hours. *Anesthesiology*, **63** (3), 278–286.

30. Slutsky, A.S. and Menon, A.S. (1987) Catheter position and blood gases during constant-flow ventilation. *J. Appl. Physiol.*, **62** (2), 513–519.

31. Nahum, A. (2001) Animal and lung model studies of tracheal gas insufflation. *Respir. Care*, **46** (2), 149–157.

32. Nakos, G., Lachana, A., Prekates, A. *et al.* (1995) Respiratory effects of tracheal gas insufflation in spontaneously breathing COPD patients. *Intensive Care Med.*, **21** (11), 904–912.

33. Ravenscraft, S.A., Burke, W.C., Nahum, A. *et al.* (1993) Tracheal gas insufflation augments CO_2 clearance during mechanical ventilation. *Am. Rev. Respir. Dis.*, **148** (2), 345–351.

34. Kalfon, P., Rao, G.S., Gallart, L. *et al.* (1997) Permissive hypercapnia with and without expiratory washout in patients with severe acute respiratory distress syndrome. *Anesthesiology*, **87** (1), 6–17; discussion 25A–26A.

35. Kuo, P., Wu, H., Yu, C. *et al.* (1996) Efficacy of tracheal gas insufflation in acute respiratory distress syndrome with permissive hypercapnia. *Am. J. Respir. Crit. Care Med.*, **154** (3), 612–616.

36. Richecoeur, J., Lu, Q., Vieira, S.R.R. *et al.* (1999) Expiratory washout versus optimization of mechanical ventilation during permissive hypercapnia in patients with severe acute respiratory distress syndrome. *Am. J. Respir. Crit. Care Med.*, **160** (1), 77–85.

37. Levy, B., Bollaert, P.E., Nace, L. and Larcan, A. (1995) Intracranial hypertension and adult respiratory distress syndrome: usefulness of tracheal gas insufflation. *J. Trauma*, **39** (4), 799–801.

38. Hoyt, J.D., Marini, J.J. and Nahum, A. (1996) Effect of tracheal gas insufflation on demand valve triggering and total work during continuous positive airway pressure ventilation. *Chest*, **110** (3), 775–783.

39. Schönhofer, B., Wenzel, M., Wiemann, J. and Köhler, D. (1995) [Value of transtracheal oxygen insufflation in the weaning period after long-term ventilation]. *Med. Klin. (Munich)*, **90** (1 Suppl. 1), 9–12.

40. Hoffman, L.A., Tasota, F.J., Delgado, E. *et al.* (2003) Effect of tracheal gas insufflation during weaning from prolonged mechanical ventilation: a preliminary study. *Am. J. Crit. Care*, **12** (1), 31–39.

41. Heimlich, H.J. (1982) Respiratory rehabilitation with transtracheal oxygen system. *Ann. Otol. Rhinol. Laryngol.*, **91** (6 Pt 1), 643–647.

42. Christopher, K.L., Spofford, B.T., Brannin, P.K. and Petty, T.L. (1986) Transtracheal oxygen therapy for refractory hypoxemia. *JAMA*, **256** (4), 494–497.

43. Christopher, K.L., Spofford, B.T., Petrun, M.D. *et al.* (1987) A program for transtracheal oxygen delivery. *Ann. Intern. Med.*, **107** (6), 802–808.

44. Banner, N.R. and Govan, J.R. (1986) Long term transtracheal oxygen delivery through microcatheter in patients with hypoxaemia due to chronic obstructive airways disease. *Br. Med. J. (Clin. Res. Ed.)*, **293** (6539), 111–114.

45. Hoffman, L.A., Wesmiller, S.W., Sciurba, F.C. *et al.* (1992) Nasal cannula and transtracheal oxygen delivery. A comparison of patient response after 6 months of each technique. *Am. Rev. Respir. Dis.*, **145** (4 Pt 1), 827–831.

46. Brack, T., Senn, O., Russi, E.W. and Bloch, K.E. (2005) Transtracheal high-flow insufflation supports spontaneous respiration in chronic respiratory failure*. *Chest*, **127** (1), 98–104.

2.9 Mechanical ventilator outcomes

Ali S. Wahla[1] and Edward F. Haponik[2]

[1] *Shaukat Khanum Memorial Cancer Hospital and Research Center, Lahore, Pakistan*
[2] *Pulmonary, Critical Care, Allergy, and Immunologic Medicine, Wake Forest University, Winston-Salem, NC, USA*

2.9.1 Case presentation

A 52-year-old man admitted with severe dyspnea and hypoxemia. He had been well until two days ago, when he developed a fever and cough. He subsequently had shaking chills, diarrhea and muscle aches. In the emergency department his vital signs were blood pressure 100/50 mm Hg, heart rate 140 beats/min, respiratory rate 30 breaths/min, temperature 102 °F and oxygen saturation 83% RA. He was able to communicate with single words and was oriented ×3. His oropharynx was dry, bilateral rales appreciated, tachycardic without murmur rub or gallop, abdomen was soft with hypoactive bowel sounds, and extremities were cyanotic without edema or clubbing. Chest X-ray revealed bilateral infiltrates. Laboratory results included WBC of 19 000/mm^3, Creatinine of 2.0 mg/dl, AST and ALT of 250 and 350 IU/l, CK of 2000 IU/l and a room air arterial blood sample pH 7.30, $PaCO_2$ 25 mm Hg and PaO_2 52 mm Hg. Neither his O_2Sats, nor his dyspnea responded to supplemental oxygen. He was intubated, after blood cultures obtained antibiotics for community-acquired pneumonia were initiated, as was Oseltamivir for H1N1 infection. Patient was transferred to the intensive care unit.

A Practical Guide to Mechanical Ventilation, First Edition.
Edited by Jonathon D. Truwit and Scott K. Epstein.
© 2011 John Wiley & Sons, Ltd. Published 2011 by John Wiley & Sons, Ltd.

2.9.2   Introduction

This chapter focuses on factors effecting survival among mechanically ventilated (MV) patients as well as outcomes among patients with different underlying disease states.

2.9.3   Outcomes for all patients mechanically ventilated after an acute event

2.9.3.1   Mortality

Once patients have been placed on a mechanical ventilator their outcomes are determined by a number of factors, which include the underlying cause of respiratory failure, their comorbid conditions and their pre-admission functional status. Various studies have reported hospital mortality rates in mechanically ventilated patients to be between 35 and 39% [1, 2]. To determine the survival rates of mechanically ventilated patients Esteban *et al.* designed a prospective cohort of adult patients admitted to 361 intensive care units (ICUs) over a one-month period between 1 March 1998 and 31 March 1998 [1]. Data were collected on each patient from the time of initiation of mechanical ventilation for up to 28 days. Of the 5183 patients they looked at, the ICU mortality rate was 30.7%, while the overall hospital mortality was 39.2%.These survival numbers are similar to those reported by Behrendt [2] in a retrospective review of 61 223 hospital discharge records during 1994. She reported in hospital mortality rate of 35.9%.

Estaban *et al.* [1] found these factor to be independently associated with increased mortality: age, SAPS II score at ICU admission, prior functional status, initiation of mechanical ventilation because of coma, acute respiratory distress syndrome (ARDS) or sepsis before or after initiation of mechanical ventilation, use of vasoactive drugs, use of neuromuscular blockers, peak ventilator pressures greater than 50 cm H_2O or plateau pressures of >35 cm H_2O, barotraumas, PaO_2/FiO_2 ratio less than 200 and the development of organ failure. The latter included: cardiovascular shock, renal failure, hepatic failure, coagulopathy and metabolic acidosis.

2.9.3.2   Short-term complications among survivors of MV

Complication rates are quite high in this critically ill population. Esteban *et al.* noted that various complications in patients receiving mechanical ventilation ranged from 3 to 22%, (Table 2.9.1). De Jonghe *et al.* [3] noted an incidence of ICU acquired paresis (ICUAP) of 25.3%. Patients with ICUAP had a significantly longer duration of mechanical complication when compared to patients without ICUAP (18.2 vs. 7.6, $p = 0.03$).

Patients who required mechanical ventilation and survived hospitalization are at risk for readmissions. Disease management programs have been used in an effort

Table 2.9.1 Complications during mechanical ventilation.

Complication	Incidence
Barotrauma	154 (3%)
ARDS	218 (4.4%)
Pneumonia	439 (9.8%)
Sepsis	457 (9.7%)
Shock	1145 (22.1%)
Acute renal failure	971 (18.7%)
Hepatic failure	326 (6.3%)
Coagulopathy	552 (10.6%)
Respiratory acidosis	228 (5.6%)
Metabolic acidosis	311 (6%)

to decrease readmission rates, improve survival and decrease mean days of rehospitalization. Daly *et al.* [4] looked at 334 patients who had been intubated for more than 72 hours and were discharged alive from the hospital. 231 patients were included in the experimental group and 103 in the control group. The intervention group received care coordination, family support, teaching and monitoring of therapies by a team of advanced-practice nurses, a geriatrician and a pulmonologist for two months post discharge. There was no difference between the two groups over 60 days with regards to survival or hospital readmission. Although patients who received Disease Management (DM) had significantly fewer mean days of rehospitalization (11.4 days, 95% CI 9.3–12.6) compared to the control group (16.7 days, 95% CI 12.5–21, $p = 0.01$). Total cost savings associated with the intervention were approximately \$481,811 for the 93 subjects who were readmitted to the hospital.

2.9.3.3 Long-term complications among survivors of MV

The majority of the studies exploring long-term outcomes in MV patients have followed patients who were admitted for ARDS. Herridge *et al.* [5] studied the one-year outcomes of 109 survivors of ARDS. Patients tended to be young (median age, 45 years) and had long lengths of ICU stay (median, 25 days). They noted that at the time of discharge, patients had lost an average of 18% of their baseline body weight. Of these, 71% had returned to their baseline weight one year after discharge. Lung volumes and spirometric measurements were normal by six months, DLCO remained low (72% predicted at 12 months). No patients required supplemental oxygen at 12 months. However, six minute walk distance remained lower than predicted and at one year only 49% of patients were working. They concluded that at one year most patients have extrapulmonary conditions, with muscle wasting and weakness being most prominent.

Orme and coworkers [6] demonstrated that approximately 80% of ARDS survivors had reduced diffusion capacity (most often mild 46%, or moderate 23%), whereas obstructive and restrictive defects were equally present (20% for each). More importantly they noted decreased health-related quality of life one year after hospital discharge.

In recent years, there has been increasing awareness of neurocognitive dysfunction in long-term survivors of ARDS, directly impacting health care quality of life (HCQL) [7–11]. Hopkins *et al.* [7] showed that 30% of ARDS survivors continued to have impaired intellectual functioning one year after discharge and 78% of the survivors had impairment of memory and concentration. They correlated these deficits with increased severity of hypoxemia as recorded during the ICU, suggesting that CNS hypoxia was a potential mechanism.

Psychiatric abnormalities are common in ARDS survivors, and have significant impact on quality of life (QOL). The incidence of depression is significant in survivors of ARDS, with ARDS survivors reporting moderate to severe depression (16% and 23%) and anxiety (24% and 23%) at one and two years, respectively [12]. Post-traumatic stress disorder (PTSD) also has significant impact on QOL, with reported prevalence rates of varying from 5 to 63% [8]. The highest prevalence estimates occurred in studies with fewer than 30 patients. Recently, Girard and coworkers [13] have identified female gender and use of high doses of Lorazepam as risk factors for the development of PTSD. Although PTSD may be a serious problem among MV survivors, at this time the magnitude of the problem is unclear and further research into this matter is needed.

2.9.4   Outcomes for patients with prolonged mechanical ventilation (PMV) after an acute event

2.9.4.1   Definition

The National Association for Medical Direction of Respiratory Care (NAMDRC) in its consensus statement has defined prolonged mechanical ventilation (PMV) as the need for >21 consecutive days of MV for >6h/day [14]. Multicenter studies using this strict definition of PMV have not been performed; however, single-center studies [15, 16] indicate that approximately 3–7% of patients receiving MV meet such criteria. This group of patients has acquired increasing importance because it constitutes <10% of all patients requiring MV but accounts for 40% of ICU bed days, thus consuming substantial resources [17, 18].

2.9.4.2   Mortality

Patients with PMV cared for in short-term acute care (STAC) hospitals have mortality rates ranging between 25 and 61%. This wide variation is, in part, due to differing patient populations and definitions of PMV [15, 19–21]. Martin *et al.* [22]

Table 2.9.2 Causes of LTAC admission.

Cause	Percentage
Medical cause	60.8%
Pneumonia	36.5%
COPD exacerbation	21.3%
Aspiration pneumonia	16.0%
Decompensated or new onset heart failure	15.0%
Sepsis with shock	12.2%
Surgical cause	39.2%
Coronary artery bypass grafting	30.0%
Hart valve replacement	13.7%
GI surgery	15.9%

examined 331 patients who met their criteria of prolonged stay, defined as >21 days at a teaching hospital or >10 days at a community hospital. ICU and hospital mortality for prolonged stay patients were 24.4 and 35.2%, respectively, compared to 11 and 15.9% for short stay patients ($p < 0.001$). Among prolonged stay patients the hospital mortality was highest in the group with multiple organ failure (53%). One-year survival of PMV patients may be more meaningful from a clinical perspective and has been reported to range from 23 to 76% [23–25].

Scheinhorn and colleagues [26] collected data from 23 long-term acute care (LTAC) hospitals over a two year period between March 2002 and February 2003. They evaluated 1419 MV patients (median age 71.8 years) and found that 54.1% of patients were weaned, 20.9% remained ventilator dependent, and 25.0% deceased. Table 2.9.2 summarizes the cause of LTAC admission within this cohort. Their study demonstrated that a majority of PMV patients were indeed weanable with median time to wean ($n = 766$) being 15 days.

In a cohort of 133 patients admitted to a single LTAC hospital, age, functional status prior to acute illness and diabetes were independent predictors of death one year after LTAC admission [23]. Combining the two strongest predictors, age and prior functional status, produced a model that identified a group of patients at very high risk of death in one year. Patients who were >75 years of age or 65–75 years of age with prior poor functional status had only a 5% likelihood of being alive after one year. All other patients had a 56% chance of surviving one year. This model has yet to be validated in other settings.

2.9.4.3 Long-term outcomes

Patients discharged after PMV carry a high burden of comorbidities and are at high risk of hospital readmission or permanent functional impairment. Carson *et al.* demonstrated only 10% of PMV patients managed in post-ICU settings were functionally independent at one year [27]. Similar results were reported in another study looking at 186 PMV patients managed in an LTAC hospital: 71% survived to discharge; 23% were discharged home but only half of these (8% of total PMV admissions) reported good functional status [28].

Combes *et al.* [29] looked at the health care quality of life (HCQL) in 87 patients receiving more than 14 days of mechanical ventilation. HCQL Questionnaires were completed an average of three years after discharge with all but one patient living at home (average age 62 ± 16 years). Compared with those of a general French population, their scores were significantly worse for each of the Nottingham Health Profile domains, with the exception of social isolation.

Prolonged mechanical ventilation is associated with impaired health-related quality of life compared with that of a matched general population. Despite these handicaps, 99% of long-term survivors evaluated were independent and living at home three years after ICU discharge. While acute physiology is the primary risk factor for death in the initial ICU period within the first 14 days, age, a pre-admission immunocompromised status, and duration of mechanical ventilation for >35 days are the primary risk factors for death after ICU discharge.

2.9.5   Outcomes in geriatric patients

2.9.5.1   Mortality

Elderly patients, those >65 years of age, account for 26–51% of patients admitted to ICUs [30]. With an aging population, an increasing proportion of MV patients will be elderly. Studies examining ICU or hospital survival in elderly patients have had conflicting results with some studies demonstrating that elderly patients had increased mortality rates [31, 32], with others [30, 33–35] concluding that age in of itself is not an important independent predictor of worse outcomes.

Esteban and colleagues [36] looked at 5183 patients in the three age groups. 1612 patients were older than 70 (31%), 2506 patients between 43 and 70 (48%) and 1057 patients less than 43 years of age (20%). The survival in the ICU patients older than 70 years was 63% [37–41] compared to 69% [42–45] in the middle age group ($p < 0.001$). Hospital survival was 45% [6, 10, 11, 46–48] in older age patients compared to 55% [49–53] for patients in middle age group ($p < 0.001$).

The older group had limited prior functional status, 50% [11, 49, 54–57], compared to 38% [58–61] in the middle age group ($p < 0.001$). Older patients were more likely to be ventilated because of cardiac disease as compared to patients in the middle group, who were more likely to be ventilated because of coma, ARDS and trauma ($p < 0.001$). SAPS II scores were not significantly different. Older patients had a higher incidence of shock and acute renal failure. The older group had a similar duration of mechanical ventilation, weaning, length of stay in the ICU and length of stay in the hospital. Patients in older age group had survival of less than 30% if they developed acute renal failure and shock while on mechanical ventilation. Survival of patients with severe hypoxemia was 45% versus 84% for patients without it. Severe hypoxemia was defined as PaO_2/FiO_2 of <150.

In another study, Ely and colleagues [62] examined the ARDSnet database and noted that older patients attained certain important milestones of physiologic measurements (e.g., spontaneous breathing trials, SBTs) at a pace similar to that of younger patients. However after passing SBTs older patients required a longer period to achieve unassisted breathing and be discharged from the ICU. In addition, median duration of MV, ICU length of stay and mortality rates increased with increasing age.

Somme *et al.* [63] also looked at long-term outcomes in 412 patients elderly patients admitted to the ICU. They were classified in three subgroups: old (75–79 years, $n = 184$, 54% on MV), very old (80–84 years, $n = 137$, 42% on MV) and the oldest (>85 years, $n = 91$, 31% on MV). The mortality rates three months after discharge from the ICU were 21.6%, 26.7% and 28.9% respectively, as opposed to 0.9, 1.6 and 3.7% for the same age group in the general French population. APACHE II score [odds ratio (OR): 1.11] was identified as the only factor associated with ICU mortality, and age (OR: 2.17, for patients ≥85 years old and 1.82, for patients 80–84 years old) and limitation of activity before admission (OR: 1.74) as factors associated with long-term mortality.

2.9.5.2 Long-term outcomes

Similar results were noted by Chelluri and colleagues [64], who examined the two-month mortality rate of 817 MV patients and found that older age, in addition to functional status and comorbidities, was associated with increased mortality at two months. They noted that for every additional comorbidity the odds of dying at two months increased by 24%.

In summary, increasing age of the MV patient is likely an independent risk factor for short-term and long-term mortality among MV patients, especially in the setting of ARDS, with survival markedly worsened with the onset of multisystem organ failure.

2.9.6 Disease specific outcomes

2.9.6.1 ARDS/ALI and mechanical ventilation

Management of mechanically ventilated patients with acute respiratory distress syndrome/ acute lung injury (ALI) has traditionally required increased resource utilization with poor outcomes. As a consequence, in the past three decades this group of patients has been the focus of much research effort to better understand this disease process and improve survival. When ARDS was originally described by Ashbaugh *et al.* [58] in 1967, case fatality approached 60% and remained at this level through the early 1980s [59–61]. Montgomery *et al.* [61] in 1982 found that sepsis was the commonest cause of death among ARDS patients with only 16% dying due to insupportable respiratory failure. Stapleton and coworkers [65], from the same institute, compared mortality from ARDS during the years 1990, 1994 and 1998. They noted that ARDS case fatality had decreased from 55 to 65% in the early 1980s to 29–35% by the late 1990s. This in spite of an increase in the age and APACHE II scores of ARDS patients. They noted no decrease in the distribution of causes of death, with the sepsis still being the commonest cause of death. However there was a significant increase in the percentage of deaths in ARDS patients occurring in the setting of withdrawal of care (40% to 67%, $p = 0.03$).

Recently, Zambon and Vincent [66] performed a meta-analysis of 72 ARDS studies between 1994 and 2006. They noted that the pooled mortality rate for all studies was 43% (95% CI, 40–46%). Meta regression analysis suggested a significant decrease in overall mortality rates of approximately 1.11% per year over the period (Figure 2.9.1). Since sepsis and multisystem organ failure remain the commonest cause of death within this group, it is likely that advances in supportive care have decreased extrapulmonary organ failures. In addition, the adoption of low tidal volume ventilation (6 ml/kg predicted body weight, PBW) has also been shown to reduce in hospital mortality (31% vs. 39.8%, $p = 0.007$) when compared with tidal volumes of 12 ml/kg PBW [46].

Among ARDS patients, trauma patients have the best outcomes [47, 62]. Persistent hypoxemia has good predictive value, whereas the initial degree of hypoxemia is a poor predictor of outcomes, unless it is severe ($PaO_2/FiO_2 < 50$)

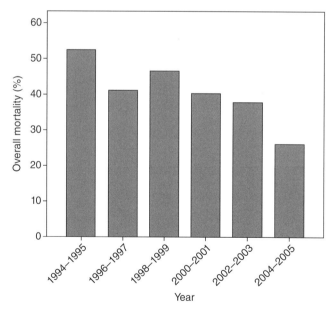

Figure 2.9.1 Variation in overall pooled mortality rates over time in the 72 ALI/ARDS studies.

[48, 61]. For details regarding the long-term outcomes of ARDS patients please refer above to the section on long-term complications among survivors of MV.

2.9.6.2 COPD and mechanical ventilation

An Acute Exacerbation of Chronic Obstructive Pulmonary Disease (AECOPD) may range from self-limited disease to acute respiratory failure requiring invasive mechanical ventilation. Menzies *et al.* [54] looked at survival among COPD patients undergoing invasive mechanical ventilation in the 1980s. They studied a cohort of 95 COPD patients requiring invasive mechanical ventilation, of whom half had an FEV1 < 30%. They noted that 20 of these patients (21%) could not be weaned and died on the ventilator. Although 76% were successfully weaned off the ventilator, only 42% of those weaned were alive at one year, so the overall survival was only 32%. These figures were similar to one-year COPD survival figures of 32–49% published in the previous three decades [55–57].

In the 1990s Seneff and colleagues [49] examined hospital and one-year survival among 362 COPD patients admitted to the ICU with an acute exacerbation. 170 (47%) of these patients required invasive MV. COPD hospital mortality rate was noted to be 24%. Although ventilated patients had twice the hospital mortality of non-ventilated patients, multivariate analysis did not show use of MV to be predictor of 180-day mortality. In addition, this study revealed that the hospital and one-year mortality rates of patients over the age of 65 years were 30% and 59% respectively.

Major advancements in the care of COPD patients with acute respiratory failure (ARF) came with the introduction of noninvasive ventilation (NIV). In 1995, Brochard and coworkers [114] demonstrated that the use of NIV in AECOPD patients reduced the need for intubation (26% vs. 74%) when compared to standard therapy. Subsequent clinical trials of NIV versus conventional therapy showed improvements in one-year survival when compared to conventional therapy (Table 2.9.3). A meta-analysis by Peter and Moran [67] showed that patients with a serum pH < 7.37 or a $PaCO_2$ > 55 mm Hg were likely to benefit from NIV, implying a benefit with respiratory failure. In addition to preventing intubation in COPD

Table 2.9.3 Noninvasive ventilation in COPD.

Controlled clinical trials of noninvasive ventilation (NIV) versus conventional therapy: one-year survival

	n	Conventional (%)	NIV (%)
Plant *et al.* [50]	236	54	62
Bardi *et al.* [51]	30	53	87
Confalonieri *et al.* [52]	48	50	71
Vitacca *et al.* [53]	57	37	70

patients, NIV has also been successfully used to aid in weaning COPD patients off the ventilator.

In conclusion, the biggest advancement in the management of COPD patients over the past two decades has been the use of NIV to prevent intubations in patients with AECOPD. Once invasive mechanical ventilation is instituted, however, mortality rates remain high, with a recent study reporting a one-year mortality rate of 40.5% [68]. Nevins and Epstein [69] reported in-hospital mortality rates of 28% for their entire cohort of COPD patients requiring invasive mechanical ventilation, but 12% for patients with a COPD exacerbation requiring invasive mechanical ventilation without a comorbid illness. Therefore, it appears that mortality rates are worse with comorbid illnesses.

2.9.6.3   Pulmonary fibrosis and mechanical ventilation

Traditionally the use of mechanical ventilation in patients with pulmonary fibrosis, secondary to Idiopathic Pulmonary Fibrosis (IPF) or interstitial lung diseases (ILDs) has proven futile. The limited body of evidence suggests very high hospital mortality rates, ranging from 53 to 100% (Table 2.9.4). Of those who do survive, long-term survival rates have been dismal. Blivet *et al.* [37] retrospectively reviewed the outcomes of 15 patients admitted to their ICU for acute respiratory failure. Eleven patients died on the ventilator. Of the four that were discharged alive from the hospital only two were alive six months after discharge. These findings were also demonstrated by Saydain and coworkers [38] who found that 92% of hospital survivors died two months after being discharged from the hospital.

The largest study of patients with pulmonary fibrosis requiring MV was recently published by Fernández-Pérez *et al.* [39] who retrospectively reviewed the outcomes of 94 patients with ILD admitted to their institution for respiratory failure. Their cohort included 53 medical and 41 post-surgical ICU admissions. The overall mortality rate for their cohort was 53%, and 69% for non-surgical ICU admissions.

Table 2.9.4   MV outcomes among patients with pulmonary fibrosis.

Study	*n*	Mean age (years)	Mean duration between diagnosis of fibrosis and ICU admission (months)	Mortality (%)
Blivet *et al.* [37]	15	64	26.5	73
Stern *et al.* [40]	23	52.9	31	91
Fumeaux *et al.* [41]	14	72	68	100
Saydain *et al.* [38]	19	68.3	24 (median)	68
Al-Hameed and Sharma [70]	25	69	n/a	96
Fernández-Pérez *et al.* [39]	94	70 (median)	6.3 (median)	53

An important finding from this study was the fact that patients in this cohort had moderate PFT abnormalities and no specific cause of respiratory failure could be identified in 76% of patients. Therefore, it very difficult for the clinician to predict which ILD patients will develop an exacerbation leading to acute respiratory failure.

In a multivariate regression analysis, hospital mortality was predicted by severe hypoxemia (lower PaO_2/FiO_2), higher PEEP during the first 24 hours of MV, older age and higher severity if illness on the day of ICU admission. Of note they found that the median one-year survival time of patients ventilated with a PEEP of >10 cm H_2O was 5.8 days compared to >350 days for PEEP of <5 cm H_2O. This finding highlighted the fact that high PEEP settings failed to improve oxygenation and were associated with lung over-distention with no improvement in respiratory efficiency.

In conclusion, the overall prognosis for pulmonary fibrosis patients on MV remains poor, with high PEEP requirements within the first 24 hours predicting poorer outcomes.

2.9.6.4 HIV and mechanical ventilation

There has been a significant improvement in care of HIV patients over the past two decades. This has largely been due to the introduction of highly active antiretroviral therapy (HAART), which has significantly reduced the morbidity and mortality associated with HIV infection [71]. A similar improvement in outcomes has also been noted in MV HIV patients, with in-hospital mortality rates declining from 79% in the early 1990s to 55–63% in the current decade (Table 2.9.5). 4–12% of HIV patients admitted to the hospital will end up requiring ICU level of care.

Multiple studies have shown that the need for MV is an independent predictor of poor short and long-term outcomes in HIV patients. Nickas and Wachter [45], in a study done in the 1990s, noted only 11% of patients who survived ICU hospitalizations were alive four years after discharge. Although this study was done in the HAART era, they noted that only half of the patients admitted to the ICU were on HAART therapy at the time of hospital admission and were presumably noncompliant even after discharge. Vincent et al. [74] compared outcomes in HIV patients admitted during the pre-HAART era with ICU outcomes in the HAART era. 44% of patients had no history of antiretroviral (ARV) medications and 35% failed to respond to ARV. They did not find a difference in ICU mortality but did note that three-month mortality was decreased in the HAART era group. Morris et al. [73] noted that patients on HAART therapy had a higher mean CD4 count; they were more likely to be admitted with a non-AIDS associated diagnosis and higher serum albumin levels. The use of HAART was associated with improved survival in univariate analysis but not in multivariate analysis. However, use of HAART likely plays an important role in multivariate modeling through its impact on ICU admission diagnosis (i.e., AIDS or non-AIDS associated diagnosis, diagnosis of PCP) and serum albumin levels.

Table 2.9.5 MV outcomes among patients with HIV.

Study	Period of study	% of all HIV admissions, admitted to the ICU	N (number of admissions)	Number of mechanically ventilated patients (%)	In-hospital mortality, for all patients [%] (for MV patients [%])	Factors associated with increased in-hospital mortality
De Palo et al. [42]	1991–1992	4.2	65	23 (35)	55 (79)	Low CD4 cell count, high APACHE II score, low serum albumin, <90% ideal body weight
Rosen et al. [43]	1988–1990	5.1	63 (68)	28 (44)	40 (57)	n/a
Casalino et al. [44]	1990–1992	n/a	354 (354)	171 (48)	39 (n/a)	Functional status, time since AIDS diagnosis, HIV disease stage, SAPS I, need for and duration of MV
Nickas and Wachter [45]	1992–1995	7	394 (443)	217 (55)	37 (50)	High APS, MV, PCP infection, low serum albumin
Afessa and Green [72]	1995–1999	12	141 (169)	91 (54)	29.6 (48)	High APACHE II Score
Morris et al. [73]	1995–1999	n/a	295 (354)	191 (54)	29 (38.5)	
Vincent et al. [74]	1995–2000	5.2	425	160 (37.6)	26[a] (55)[a]	Low CD4 cell count, inotropic support, PCP infection, SAPS-II, Kaposi's sarcoma
Dickson et al. [75]	1999–2005	n/a	102 (113)	63 (62)	68 (63)	Low CD4 cell count, high APACHE II score, low hemoglobin, MV
Davis et al. [76]	1996–2004	n/a	148	148 (100)	(57)	High tidal volume

[a]These data refer to ICU mortality rather than Hospital Mortality. PCP = Pneumocystis Carinii, APS = Acute Physiology Score.

In conclusion, most studies have shown that low CD4 cell count, high APACHE II score and poor baseline nutritional status are all predictors of poor outcomes in MV HIV patients. Use of HAART therapy, through multivariate analysis, does not predict ICU or hospital mortality but there is some evidence to suggest that these patients may have improved survival once discharged from the hospital.

2.9.6.5 Cancer and mechanical ventilation

For many years it has been assumed that the outcomes of cancer patients requiring MV for any reason other than post-operative support are very poor [77]. This has been because factors specific to cancer patients influence the management of ARF, including a distinctive pattern of lung diseases and a specific profile of immunosuppression. This led many physicians to advocate avoidance of MV in cancer patients given the enormous cost involved in carding for these patients in the ICU in the face limited resources [78].

Among patients receiving anti-cancer treatments, ARF remains a common and life threatening complication with ARF occurring in nearly 5% of patients with solid tumors and up to 50% in those with hematological malignancy [79]. In hospital mortality rates among MV cancer patients have been 53–87.5% (Table 2.9.6), with outcomes being generally worse in patients with hematological malignancies rather than solid tumors [83]. As understanding and care of critically ill cancer patients has progressed there has been a gradual improvement in hospital mortality among MV cancer patients (Table 2.9.6). Another factor resulting in improved overall ICU survival has been the introduction and adoption of noninvasive mechanical ventilation (NIMV) [98]. Tables 2.9.7 and 2.9.8 list risk factors that have been shown to be associated with increased mortality and survival.

The two largest studies, done by Groeger et al. [83] and Soares et al. [94], revealed age, evidence of progression or recurrence of malignancy and development of multi-organ system failure (MOSF) to be independently associated with poor outcomes. Importantly, Soares and colleagues [93] also demonstrated that survival was similar among cancer patients who required prolonged mechanical ventilation (PMV) and those who were intubated for less than 21 days, thus arguing against withdrawal of care based on length of MV alone. Long-term survival data on patients discharged alive from the hospital have not been well studied and are likely influenced by the patients underlying malignancy.

2.9.6.6 Bone marrow transplantation (BMT) and mechanical ventilation

Over fifty years have passed since the first reported case of a successful allogenic bone marrow transplantation (BMT) procedure being performed [99]. Since that time there has been a tremendous increase in the number of patients receiving allogenic as well as autologous BMTs. This has led to a significant number of patients

Table 2.9.6 MV outcomes among patients with HIV.

Study	Study period	Type of study	Sample size (MV patients)	Hospital mortality [%] (MV mortality [%])	Type of tumor solid tumors (ST), Hematological tumors (HT), or HSCT patients.
Azoulay et al. [80]	1990–1997	Retrospective review	120 (65)	59[a] (73)[a]	All STs (27% Lung, 21.5% Breast, 51.5% others)
Azoulay et al.[81].	1997–2002	Prospective observational	203 (114)	47.8 (75.4)	9% STs, 67% HTs, 24% HSCT
Groger et al. [82]	1994–1997	Prospective observational	1483 (377)	42 (69)	54.6% ST, 45.4% HT and HSCT
Groger et al.[83]	1994–1996	Prospective observational	782 (782)	76 (76)	39% ST, 61% HT and HSCT
Darmon et al.[84]	1990–2000	Retrospective review	102 (70)	58 (n/a)	8.8% ST, 91.2% HT and HSCT
Maschmeyer et al. [85]	1998–1999	Prospective observational	189 (94)	65 (72.3)	54.5% ST, 45.5% HT
Azoulay et al. [86]	1990–1995	Retrospective review	237 (237)	72.5 (72.5)	29% ST, 54% HT, 17% HSCT
Groger et al. [87]	1994–1998	Prospective cohort	810 (444)	54.5 (71)	47.5% ST, 40% HT, 17.5% HSCT
Larché et al. [88]	19995–2000	Retrospective review	88 (68)	65.5[a] (n/a)	9% ST, 69% HT, 22% HSCT
Soares et al. [89]	2000–2004	Prospective observational	772 (241)	58[b] (69)[b]	83% ST, 17% HT, 0 % HSCT
Soares et al. [90]	2000–2004	Prospective observational	463 (463)	64 (64)	78% ST, 22% HT
Regazzoni et al. [91]	1994–1999	Prospective observational	73 (45)	53.4 (68)	57.5% ST, 42.5% HT
Darmon et al. [92]	1997–2003	Prospective observational	100 (54)	41 (87.5)	12% ST, 88% HT
Soares et al. [93]	2000–2005	Prospective observational	163 (161)	51 (n/a)	85% ST, 15% HT
Soares et al. [94]	2000–2004	Prospective observational	862 (609)	48 (60)	87% ST, 13% HT
Adam and Soubani [95]	1998–2005	Retrospective review	139 (68)	40 (53)	100% ST (100% Lung Cancer)
Soares et al. [96]	2000–2006	Retrospective review	143 (100)	59 (69)	100% ST (100% Lung Cancer)
Lecuyer et al. [97]	2001–2004	Prospective observational	188 (188)	78.2 (78.2)	30% ST, 70% HT

[a]30-day mortality.
[b]6-month mortality.

Table 2.9.7   Factors associated with increased mortality among ICU cancer patients.

Mechanical ventilation [80–82, 84, 87, 91, 92]
Evidence of progression or recurrence of malignancy [82, 83, 87, 90, 94, 96]
Poor pre-admission performance status [82, 87, 90, 93]
Age [84, 90, 93, 94]
Need for vasopressors [81, 83, 85, 95]
Multi-organ system failure [93–95, 97]
Renal failure requiring hemodialysis [84, 85, 92]
High logistic organ dysfunction (LOD) score [80, 97]
Liver failure [91, 92]
High SAPS II score [86]
High adult comorbidity evaluation (ACE-27) score [89]
High SOFA score [90]
Invasive aspergillosis [81]
Lack of identifiable organism [81]
Late noninvasive mechanical ventilation (NIMV) failure [81]
CPR prior to ICU admission [82]
Intracranial mass [82]
Allogenic HSCT [82]
All HSCT patients [83]
DIC [83]
Cardiac arrhythmias [83]
Coma [84]
Sepsis [85]
Neutropenia [85]
$PaO_2/FiO_2 < 250$ [87]
Airway invasion due to cancer [97]

Table 2.9.8   Factors associated with improved survival among ICU cancer patients.

Surgical treatment of tumor [80, 83]
Cardiogenic pulmonary edema [81]
Use of noninvasive mechanical ventilation (NIMV) [86]

suffering complications necessitating MV and ICU care, with acute respiratory failure occurring in nearly 30% of BMT patients [79].

The first of a series of studies examining outcomes of mechanically ventilated BMT patients was published by Crawford *et al.* [100], who retrospectively evaluated outcomes in BMT patients admitted to their institution from 1981 to 1985. They noted that of 151 adult BMT patients who underwent MV, less than 10% survived one month past hospital discharge. In a subsequent study [101], encompassing the next five years they noted no improvements in survival rates with <3% of 348 MV patients surviving six months past hospital discharge. Subsequent studies throughout the 1990s consistently revealed poor outcomes in BMT patients

Table 2.9.9   MV outcomes among BMT patients.

Publication	Study period	n	Hospital survival (%)	Long-term survival (%)
Crawford *et al.* [100]	1981–1985	232	n/a	9.9 (1 month)
Crawford *et al.* [101]	1986–1990	348	4.3	3% (6 months)
Rubenfeld *et al.* [102]	1980–1992	909	n/a	6.1 (1 month)
Paz *et al.* [103]	1984–1991	36	3.8	n/a
Faber-Langendoen *et al.* [104]	1978–1990	191	9	3 (6 months)
Jackson *et al.* [105]	1988–1993	92	17	n/a
Huaringa *et al.*[106]	1992–1993	60	18	5 (6 months)
Dunagan *et al.* [107]	1990–1994	21	4	n/a
Ewig *et al.* [108]	1984–1993	76	10	n/a
Price *et al.* [109]	1994–1996	115	18	n/a
Afessa *et al.* [110]	1996–2000	112	26	n/a
Khassawneh *et al.* [111]	1991–1999	78	27	17 (6 months)
Soubani *et al.* [112]	1998–2001	51	20	n/a

Table 2.9.10   Factors influencing mortality with BMT patients.

Publication	Median age	% MV of total	APACHE II score	Primary factors associated with mortality
Crawford *et al.* [100]	n/a	21	n/a	Increased age
Crawford *et al.* [101]	30	23	n/a	Not reported
Rubenfield *et al.* [102]	33	100	n/a	MOSF (>2 organ systems)
Paz *et al.* [103]	36	77	19.4	Respiratory failure, MV, shock, length of stay, APACHE II
Faber-Langendoen *et al.* [104]	33	100	n/a	Increasing age, decreased time from BMT to MV
Jackson *et al.* [105]	37	79.3	33	MV, MOSF, APACHE II
Huaringa *et al.* [106]	38.7	100	20.76	MV duration, GVHD
Dunagan *et al.* [107]	n/a	30	n/a	n/a
Ewig *et al.* [108]	36	58.4	n/a	Infectious etiology
Price *et al.* [109]	43	41.7	n/a	MV, infection, GI bleeding, MOSF
Afessa *et al.* [110]	49	55	n/a	MOSF, MV, sepsis, APACHE III
Khawassneh *et al.* [111]	n/a	100	n/a	MOSF
Soubani *et al.* [112]	46.6	60	n/a	MOSF, MV, lactate acidosis

with ARF requiring MV (Table 2.9.9). This led many experts to argue that, given the poor outcomes, BMT patients should not be mechanically ventilated and instead be made DNR/DNI if they experienced respiratory distress. Table 2.9.10 highlights the factors that have been shown to influence mortality with this patient population.

Subsequent studies in the mid to late 1990s however showed significantly improved survival with up to 27% of patients surviving to hospital discharge (Table 2.9.9). The exact reasons for this improvement are not clear but likely involve multiple factors, including an increase in autologous BMTs, better patient selection and improvements in ICU and MV care. Another observation made during this period was the increased use of BiPAP ventilation in an effort to reduce to number of patients requiring MV [113]. This has led to more optimism within the intensivist community when dealing with such patients. However, it should be noted that the majority of survivors had only lung injury or only required vasopressors when mechanically ventilated. Both Afessa *et al.* [110] and Khassawneh *et al.* [111] showed that patients who developed multi-organ system failure continued to fare poorly with less than 5% surviving the hospitalization. Therefore, the development of MOSF should prompt the physician and family members to re-evaluate treatment goals and possibly consider withdrawal of care on such patients.

2.9.7 Case presentation resolution

Upon arrival to the ICU the patient was ventilated with volume mode ventilation of assist control with tidal volume of 6 ml/kg predicted body weight. Antibiotics were continued and fluid resuscitation remained aggressive for the first six hours. Intermittent boluses of lorazepam and fentanyl were used for sedation and analgesia. On the subsequent day his central line was removed as peripheral intravenous lines could not be placed. An oral gastric tube was placed and enteral nutrition was begun, as were oral anxiolytics and analgesics. Over the next five days his oxygen and PEEP levels were reduced and a spontaneous breathing trial (SBT) was initiated. As he was alert and passed his SBT he was extubated. He was subsequently transferred to the acute care ward and on day 11 he was discharged home. His blood cultures were negative, but his influenza type A PCR test result was positive.

References

1. Esteban, A., Anzueto, A., Frutos, F. *et al.* (2002) Characteristics and outcomes in adult patients receiving mechanical ventilation. A 28-day international study. *JAMA*, **287** (3), 345–355.
2. Behrendt, C.E. (2000) Acute respiratory failure in the United States: incidence and 31-day survival. *Chest*, **118** (4), 1100–1105.
3. De Jonghe, B., Sharshar, T. and Lefaucheur, J.P. (2002) Paresis acquired in the intensive care unit: a prospective multicenter study. *JAMA*, **288** (22), 2859–2867.
4. Daly, B.J., Douglas, S.L., Kelley, C.G. *et al.* (2005) Trial of a disease management program to reduce hospital readmissions of the chronically critically ill. *Chest*, **128** (2), 507–517.
5. Herridge, M.S., Cheung, A.M., Tansey, C.M. *et al.* (2003) One year outcomes in survivors of the acute respiratory distress syndrome. *N. Engl. J. Med.*, **348** (8), 683–693.

6. Orme, J. Jr, Romney, J.S., Hopkins, R.O. *et al.* (2003) Pulmonary function and health-related quality of life in survivors of acute respiratory distress syndrome. *Am. J. Respir. Crit. Care Med.*, **167**, 690–694.

7. Hopkins, R.O., Weaver, L.K., Pope, D. *et al.* (1999) Neuropsychological sequelae and impaired health status in survivors of severe acute respiratory distress syndrome. *Am. J. Respir. Crit. Care Med.*, **160** (1), 50–56.

8. Jackson, J.C., Hart, R.P., Gordon, S.M. *et al.* (2007) Post-traumatic stress disorder and post-traumatic stress symptoms following critical illness in medical intensive care unit patients: assessing the magnitude of the problem. *Crit. Care*, **11** (1), 1–11.

9. Jackson, J.C., Hart, R.P., Gordon, S.M. *et al.* (2003) Six-month neuropsychological outcome of medical intensive care unit patients. *Crit. Care Med.*, **31** (4), 1226–1234.

10. Davidson, T.A., Caldwell, E.S., Curtis, J.R. *et al.* (1999) Reduced quality of life in survivors of acute respiratory distress syndrome compared with critically ill control patients. *JAMA*, **281**, 354–360.

11. Weinert, C.R., Goss, C.R., Kangas, J.R. *et al.* (1997) Health related quality of life after acute lung injury. *Am. Rev. Respir. Dis.*, **156**, 1120–1126.

12. Hopkins, R.O., Weaver, L.K., Collingridge, D. *et al.* (2005) Two-year cognitive, emotional, and quality-of-life outcomes in acute respiratory distress syndrome. *Am. J. Respir. Crit. Care Med.*, **171** (4), 340–347.

13. Girard, T.D., Shintani, A.K., Jackson, J.C. *et al.* (2007) Risk factors for post-traumatic stress disorder symptoms following critical illness requiring mechanical ventilation: a prospective cohort study. *Crit. Care*, **11** (1), R28.

14. MacIntyre, N.R., Epstein, S.K., Carson, S. *et al.* (2005) Management of patients requiring prolonged mechanical ventilation: report of a NAMDRC consensus conference. *Chest*, **128** (6), 3937–3954.

15. Gracey, D.R., Viggiano, R.W., Naessens, J.M. *et al.* (1992) Outcomes of patients admitted to a chronic ventilator-dependent unit in an acute-care hospital. *Mayo Clin. Proc.*, **67**, 131–136.

16. Bureau of Data Management and Strategy (1999) 100% MEDPAR Inpatient Hospital Fiscal Year 1998, 6/99 Update. United States Health Care Finance Administration. US Government Printing Office, Washington, DC.

17. Wagner, D.P. (1989) Economics of prolonged mechanical ventilation. *Am. Rev. Respir. Dis.*, **140** (2 Pt 2), S14–S18.

18. Engoren, M., Arslanian-Engoren, C. and Fenn-Buderer, N. (2004) Hospital and long-term outcome after tracheostomy for respiratory failure. *Chest*, **125**, 220–227.

19. Spicher, J.E. and White, D.P. (1987) Outcome and function following prolonged mechanical ventilation. *Arch. Intern. Med.*, **147**, 421–425.

20. Seneff, M.G., Zimmerman, J.E., Knaus, W.A. *et al.* (1996) Predicting the duration of mechanical ventilation: the importance of disease and patient characteristics. *Chest*, **110**, 469–479.

21. Cox, C.E., Carson, S.S., Holmes, G.M. *et al.* (2004) Increase in tracheostomy for prolonged mechanical ventilation in North Carolina, 1993–2002. *Crit. Care Med.*, **32** (11), 2219–2226.

22. Martin, C.M., Hill, A.D., Burns, K. and Chen, L.M. (2005) Characteristics and outcomes for critically ill patients with prolonged intensive care unit stays. *Crit. Care Med.*, **33** (9), 1922–1927.

23. Carson, S.S., Bach, P.B., Brzozowski, L. *et al.* (1999) Outcomes after long-term acute care: an analysis of 133 mechanically ventilated patients. *Am. J. Respir. Crit. Care Med.*, **159**, 1568–1573.

24. Scheinhorn, D.J., Chao, D.C., Stearn-Hassenpflug, M. *et al.* (1997) Post-ICU mechanical ventilation: treatment of 1,123 patients at a regional weaning center. *Chest*, **111**, 1654–1659.

25. Stoller, J.K., Meng, X., Mascha, E. *et al.* (2003) Long-term outcomes for patients discharged from a long-term hospital-based weaning unit. *Chest*, **124**, 1892–1899.

26. Scheinhorn, D.J., Hassenpflug, M.S., Votto, J.J. *et al.* (2007) Post-ICU mechanical ventilation at 23 long-term care hospitals: a multicenter outcomes study. *Chest*, **131** (1), 85–93.

27. Carson, S.S. and Bach, P.B. (2002) The epidemiology and costs of chronic critical illness. *Crit. Care Clin.*, **18**, 461–476.

28. Scheinhorn, D.J., Stearn-Hassenpflug, M., Chao, D.C. *et al.* (2004) Post ICU mechanical ventilation: functional status before and after prolonged mechanical ventilation [abstract]. *Chest*, **126**, 870S.

29. Combes, A., Costa, M.-A. and Trouillet, J.-L. (2003) Morbidity, mortality, and quality-of-life outcomes of patients requiring >14 days of mechanical ventilation. *Crit. Care Med.*, **31** (5), 1378–1381.

30. Rockwood, K., Noseworthy, T.W., Gibney, R.T. *et al.* (1993) One-year outcome of elderly and young patients admitted to intensive care units. *Crit. Care Med.*, **21**, 687–691.

31. Campion, E.W., Mulley, A.G., Goldstein, R.L. *et al.* (1981) Medical intensive care for the elderly: a study of current use, costs, and outcomes. *JAMA*, **246**, 2052–2056.

32. Mahul, P., Perrot, D., Tempelhoff, G. *et al.* (1991) Short- and long-term prognosis, functional outcome following ICU for elderly. *Intensive Care Med.*, **17**, 7–10.

33. Chelluri, L., Pinsky, M.R., Donahoe, M.P. *et al.* (1993) Long-term outcome of critically ill elderly patients requiring intensive care. *JAMA*, **269**, 3119–3123.

34. Kass, J.E., Castriotta, R.J. and Malakoff, F. (1992) Intensive care unit outcome in the very elderly. *Crit. Care Med.*, **20**, 1666–1671.

35. Mayer-Oakes, S.A., Oye, R.K. and Leake, B. (1991) Predictors of mortality in older patients following medical intensive care: the importance of functional status. *J. Am. Geriatr. Soc.*, **39**, 862–868.

36. Esteban, A., Anzueto, A., Frutos-Vivar, F. *et al.* (2004) Outcome of older patients receiving mechanical ventilation. *Intensive Care Med.*, **30** (4), 639–646.

37. Blivet, S., Philit, F. and Sab, J.M. (2001) Outcome of patients with idiopathic pulmonary fibrosis admitted to the ICU for respiratory failure. *Chest*, **120** (1), 209–212.

38. Saydain, G., Islam, A. and Afessa, B. (2002) Outcome of patients with idiopathic pulmonary fibrosis admitted to the intensive care unit. *Am. J. Respir. Crit. Care Med.*, **166** (6), 839–842.

39. Fernández-Pérez, E.R., Yilmaz, M. and Jenad, H. (2008) Ventilator settings and outcome of respiratory failure in chronic interstitial lung disease. *Chest*, **133** (5), 1113–1119.

40. Stern, J.B., Mal, H., Groussard, O. and Brugière, O. (2001) Prognosis of patients with advanced idiopathic pulmonary fibrosis requiring mechanical ventilation for acute respiratory failure. *Chest*, **120** (1), 213–219.

41. Fumeaux, T., Rothmeier, C. and Jolliet, P. (2001) Outcome of mechanical ventilation for acute respiratory failure in patients with pulmonary fibrosis. *Intensive Care Med.*, **27** (12), 1868–1874.

42. De Palo, V.A., Millstein, B.H., Mayo, P.H. *et al.* (1995) Outcome of intensive care in patients with HIV infection. *Chest*, **107** (2), 506–510.

43. Rosen, M.J., Clayton, K., Schneider, R.F. *et al.* (1997) Intensive care of patients with HIV infection: utilization, critical illnesses, and outcomes. Pulmonary Complications of HIV Infection Study Group. *Am. J. Respir. Crit. Care Med.*, **155** (1), 67–71.

44. Casalino, E., Mendoza-Sassi, G., Wolff, M. *et al.* (1998) Predictors of short- and long-term survival in HIV-infected patients admitted to the ICU. 1. *Chest*, **113** (2), 421–429.

45. Nickas, G. and Wachter, R.M. (2000) Outcomes of intensive care for patients with human immunodeficiency virus infection. *Arch. Intern. Med.*, **160** (4), 541–547.

46. Network, A.R.D.S. (2000) Ventilation with lower tidal volumes as compared to traditional tidal volumes for acute lung injury and the acute respiratory distress syndrome. *N. Engl. J. Med.*, **342**, 1301–1308.

47. Milberg, J.A., Davis, D.R., Steinberg, K.P. and Hudson, L.D. (1995) Improved survival of patients with acute respiratory distress syndrome (ARDS) 1983–1993. *JAMA*, **273**, 306–309.

48. Monchi, M., Bellenfant, F., Cariou, A. *et al.* (1998) Early predictive factors of survival in the acute respiratory distress syndrome: a multivariate analysis. *Am. J. Respir. Crit. Care Med.*, **158**, 1076–1081.

49. Seneff, M.G., Wagner, D.P., Wagner, R.P. *et al.* (1995) Hospital and 1-year survival of patients admitted to intensive care units with acute exacerbation of chronic obstructive pulmonary disease. *JAMA*, **274** (23), 1852–1857.

50. Plant, P.K., Owen, J.L. and Elliott, M.W. (2001) Non-invasive ventilation in acute exacerbations of chronic obstructive pulmonary disease: long term survival and predictors of in-hospital outcome. *Thorax*, **56** (9), 708–712.

51. Bardi, G., Pierotello, R. and Desideri, M. (2000) Nasal ventilation in COPD exacerbations: early and late results of a prospective, controlled study. *Eur. Respir. J.*, **15** (1), 98–104.

52. Confalonieri, M., Parigi, P. and Scartabellati, A. (1996) Noninvasive mechanical ventilation improves the immediate and long-term outcome of COPD patients with acute respiratory failure. *Eur. Respir. J.*, **9** (3), 422–430.

53. Vitacca, M., Clini, E. and Rubini, F. (1996) Non-invasive mechanical ventilation in severe chronic obstructive lung disease and acute respiratory failure: short- and long-term prognosis. *Intensive Care Med.*, **22** (2), 94–100.

54. Menzies, R., Gibbons, W. and Goldberg, P. (1989) Determinants of weaning and survival among patients with COPD who require mechanical ventilation for acute respiratory failure. *Chest*, **95** (2), 398–405.

55. Sluiter, H.J., Blokzijl, E.J. and van Dijl, W. (1972) Conservative and respirator treatment of acute respiratory insufficiency in patients with chronic obstructive lung disease. A reappraisal. *Am. Rev. Respir. Dis.*, **105** (6), 932–943.

56. Jessen, O., Kristensen, H.S. and Rasmussen, K. (1967) Tracheostomy and artificial ventilation in chronic lung disease. *Lancet*, **2** (7505), 9–12.

57. Wessel-Aas, T., Vale, J.R. and Hauge, H.E. (1970) Artificial ventilation in chronic pulmonary insufficiency. Indications and prognosis. *Scand. J. Respir. Dis. Suppl.*, **72**, 36–41.

58. Ashbaugh, D.G., Bigelow, D.B., Petty, T.L. *et al.* (1967) Acute respiratory distress in adults. *Lancet*, **2**, 319–323.

59. Fowler, A.A., Hamman, R.F., Good, J.T. *et al.* (1983) Adult respiratory distress syndrome: risk with common predispositions. *Ann. Intern. Med.*, **98**, 593–597.

60. Baumann, W.R., Jung, R.C., Koss, M. *et al.* (1986) Incidence and mortality of adult respiratory distress syndrome: a prospective analysis from a large metropolitan hospital. *Crit. Care Med.*, **14**, 1–4.

61. Montgomery, A.B., Stager, M.A., Carrico, C.J. *et al.* (1985) Causes of mortality in patients with the adult respiratory distress syndrome. *Am. Rev. Respir. Dis.*, **132**, 485–489.

62. Ely, E.W., Wheeler, A.P., Thompson, B.T. *et al.* (2002) Recovery rate and prognosis in older persons who develop acute lung injury and the acute respiratory distress syndrome. *Ann. Intern. Med.*, **136** (1), 25–36.

63. Somme, D., Maillet, J.M., Gisselbrecht, M. *et al.* (2003) Critically ill old and the oldest-old patients in intensive care: short- and long-term outcomes. *Intensive Care Med.*, **29** (12), 2137–2143.

64. Chelluri, L., Rotondi, A.J., Mendelsohn, A.B. *et al.* (2002) 2-month mortality and functional status of critically ill adult patients receiving prolonged mechanical ventilation. *Chest*, **121** (2), 549–558.

65. Stapleton, R.D., Wang, B.M., Hudson, L.D. *et al.* (2005) Causes and timing of death in patients with ARDS. *Chest*, **128** (2), 525–532.

66. Zambon, M. and Vincent, J.L. (2008) Mortality rates for patients with acute lung injury/ ARDS have decreased over time. *Chest*, **133** (5), 1120–1127. Epub 8 February 2008.

67. Peter, J.V. and Moran, J.L. (2004) Noninvasive ventilation in exacerbations of chronic obstructive pulmonary disease; implications of different meta-analytic strategies. *Ann. Intern. Med.*, **141**, W78–W79.

68. Christensen, S., Rasmussen, L., Horváth-Puhó, E. *et al.* (2008) Arterial blood gas derangement and level of comorbidity are not predictors of long-term mortality of COPD patients treated with mechanical ventilation. *Eur. J. Anaesthesiol.*, **25** (7), 550–556.

69. Nevins, M.L. and Epstein, S.K. (2001) Predictors of outcome for patients with COPD requiring invasive mechanical ventilation. *Chest*, **119** (6), 1840–1849.

70. Al-Hameed, F.M. and Sharma, S. (2004) Outcome of patients admitted to the intensive care unit for acute exacerbation of idiopathic pulmonary fibrosis. *Can. Respir. J.*, **11** (2), 117–122.

71. Palella, F.J. Jr., Delaney, K.M., Moorman, A.C. *et al.* (1998) Declining morbidity and mortality among patients with advanced human immunodeficiency virus infection. HIV Outpatient Study Investigators. *N. Engl. J. Med.*, **338** (13), 853–860.

72. Afessa, B. and Green, B. (2000) Clinical course, prognostic factors, and outcome prediction for HIV patients in the ICU. The PIP (Pulmonary complications, ICU support, and prognostic factors in hospitalized patients with HIV) study. *Chest*, **118** (1), 138–145.

73. Morris, A., Creasman, J., Turner, J. *et al.* (2002) Intensive care of human immunodeficiency virus-infected patients during the era of highly active antiretroviral therapy. *Am. J. Respir. Crit. Care Med.*, **166** (3), 262–267.

74. Vincent, B., Timsit, J.F., Auburtin, M. *et al.* (2004) Characteristics and outcomes of HIV-infected patients in the ICU: impact of the highly active antiretroviral treatment era. *Intensive Care Med.*, **30** (5), 859–866.

75. Dickson, S.J., Batson, S., Copas, A.J. *et al.* (2007) Survival of HIV-infected patients in the intensive care unit in the era of highly active antiretroviral therapy. *Thorax*, **62** (11), 964–968.

76. Davis, J.L., Morris, A., Kallet, R.H. *et al.* (2008) Low tidal volume ventilation is associated with reduced mortality in HIV-infected patients with acute lung injury. *Thorax*, **63** (11), 988–993.

77. Shaw, A., Weavind, L. and Feeley, T. (2001) Mechanical ventilation in critically ill cancer patients. *Curr. Opin. Oncol.*, **13** (4), 224–228.

78. Hinds, C.J., Martin, R. and Quinton, P. (1998) Intensive care for patients with medical complications of haematological malignancy: is it worth it? *Schweiz. Med. Wochenschr.*, **128**, 1467–1473.

79. Azoulay, E. and Schlemmer, B. (2006) Diagnostic strategy in cancer patients with acute respiratory failure. *Intensive Care Med.*, **32** (6), 808–822.

80. Azoulay, E., Moreau, D., Alberti, C. *et al.* (2000) Predictors of short-term mortality in critically ill patients with solid malignancies. *Intensive Care Med.*, **26** (12), 1817–1823.

81. Azoulay, E., Thiéry, G., Chevret, S. *et al.* (2004) The prognosis of acute respiratory failure in critically ill cancer patients. *Medicine (Baltimore)*, **83** (6), 360–370.

82. Groeger, J.S., Lemeshow, S., Price, K. *et al.* (1998) Multicenter outcome study of cancer patients admitted to the intensive care unit: a probability of mortality model. *J. Clin. Oncol.*, **16** (2), 761–770.

83. Groeger, J.S., White, P. Jr., Nierman, D.M. *et al.* (1999) Outcome for cancer patients requiring mechanical ventilation. *J. Clin. Oncol.*, **17** (3), 991–997.

84. Darmon, M., Azoulay, E., Alberti, C. *et al.* (2002) Impact of neutropenia duration on short-term mortality in neutropenic critically ill cancer patients. *Intensive Care Med.*, **28** (12), 1775–1780.

85. Maschmeyer, G., Bertschat, F.L., Moesta, K.T. *et al.* (2003) Outcome analysis of 189 consecutive cancer patients referred to the intensive care unit as emergencies during a 2-year period. *Eur. J. Cancer*, **39** (6), 783–792.

86. Azoulay, E., Alberti, C., Bornstain, C. *et al.* (2001) Improved survival in cancer patients requiring mechanical ventilatory support: impact of noninvasive mechanical ventilatory support. *Crit. Care Med.*, **29** (3), 519–525.

87. Groeger, J.S., Glassman, J., Nierman, D.M. *et al.* (2003) Probability of mortality of critically ill cancer patients at 72 h of intensive care unit (ICU) management. *Support. Care Cancer*, **11** (11), 686–695.

88. Larché, J., Azoulay, E., Fieux, F. *et al.* (2003) Improved survival of critically ill cancer patients with septic shock. *Intensive Care Med.*, **29** (10), 1688–1695.

89. Soares, M., Salluh, J.I., Ferreira, C.G. *et al.* (2005) Impact of two different comorbidity measures on the 6-month mortality of critically ill cancer patients. *Intensive Care Med.*, **31** (3), 408–415.

90. Soares, M., Salluh, J.I., Spector, N. and Rocco, J.R. (2005) Characteristics and outcomes of cancer patients requiring mechanical ventilatory support for >24 hrs. *Crit. Care Med.*, **33** (3), 520–526.

91. Regazzoni, C.J., Irrazabal, C., Luna, C.M. and Poderoso, J.J. (2004) Cancer patients with septic shock: mortality predictors and neutropenia. *Support. Care Cancer*, **12** (12), 833–839.

92. Darmon, M., Thiery, G., Ciroldi, M. *et al.* (2005) Intensive care in patients with newly diagnosed malignancies and a need for cancer chemotherapy. *Crit. Care Med.*, **33** (11), 2488–2493.

93. Soares, M., Salluh, J.I., Torres, V.B. *et al.* (2008) Short- and long-term outcomes of critically ill patients with cancer and prolonged ICU length of stay. *Chest*, **134** (3), 520–526.

94. Soares, M., Carvalho, M.S., Salluh, J.I. *et al.* (2006) Effect of age on survival of critically ill patients with cancer. *Crit. Care Med.*, **34** (3), 715–721.

95. Adam, A.K. and Soubani, A.O. (2008) Outcome and prognostic factors of lung cancer patients admitted to the medical intensive care unit. *Eur. Respir. J.*, **31** (1), 47–53.

96. Soares, M., Darmon, M., Salluh, J.I. *et al.* (2007) Prognosis of lung cancer patients with life-threatening complications. *Chest*, **131** (3), 840–846.

97. Lecuyer, L., Chevret, S., Thiery, G. *et al.* (2007) The ICU trial: a new admission policy for cancer patients requiring mechanical ventilation. *Crit. Care Med.*, **35** (3), 808–814.

98. Nava, S. and Cuomo, A.M. (2004) Acute respiratory failure in the cancer patient: the role of non-invasive mechanical ventilation. *Crit. Rev. Oncol. Hematol.*, **51** (2), 91–103.

99. Thomas, E.D., Lochte, J.H.L., Lu, W.C. and Ferrebee, J.W. (1957) Intravenous infusion of bone marrow in patients receiving radiation and chemotherapy. *N. Engl. J. Med.*, **257**, 491–496.

100. Crawford, S.W., Schwartz, D.A., Petersen, F.B. and Clark, J.G. (1988) Mechanical ventilation after marrow transplantation. Risk factors and clinical outcome. *Am. Rev. Respir. Dis.*, **137** (3), 682–687.
101. Crawford, S.W. and Petersen, F.B. (1992) Long-term survival from respiratory failure after marrow transplantation for malignancy. *Am. Rev. Respir. Dis.*, **145** (3), 510–514.
102. Rubenfeld, G.D. and Crawford, S.W. (1996) Withdrawing life support from mechanically ventilated recipients of bone marrow transplants: a case for evidence-based guidelines. *Ann. Intern. Med.*, **125** (8), 625–633.
103. Paz, H.L., Crilley, P., Weinar, M. and Brodsky, I. (1993) Outcome of patients requiring medical ICU admission following bone marrow transplantation. *Chest*, **104** (2), 527–531.
104. Faber-Langendoen, K., Caplan, A.L. and McGlave, P.B. (1993) Survival of adult bone marrow transplant patients receiving mechanical ventilation: a case for restricted use. *Bone Marrow Transplant.*, **12** (5), 501–507.
105. Jackson, S.R., Tweeddale, M.G., Barnett, M.J. *et al.* (1998) Admission of bone marrow transplant recipients to the intensive care unit: outcome, survival and prognostic factors. *Bone Marrow Transplant.*, **21** (7), 697–704.
106. Huaringa, A.J., Leyva, F.J., Giralt, S.A. *et al.* (2000) Outcome of bone marrow transplantation patients requiring mechanical ventilation. *Crit. Care Med.*, **28** (4), 1014–1017.
107. Dunagan, D.P., Baker, A.M., Hurd, D.D. and Haponik, E.F. (1997) Bronchoscopic evaluation of pulmonary infiltrates following bone marrow transplantation. *Chest*, **111** (1), 135–141.
108. Ewig, S., Torres, A., Riquelme, R. *et al.* (1998) Pulmonary complications in patients with haematological malignancies treated at a respiratory ICU. *Eur. Respir. J.*, **12** (1), 116–122.
109. Price, K.J., Thall, P.F., Kish, S.K. *et al.* (1998) Prognostic indicators for blood and marrow transplant patients admitted to an intensive care unit. *Am. J. Respir. Crit. Care Med.*, **158** (3), 876–884.
110. Afessa, B., Tefferi, A., Dunn, W.F. *et al.* (2003) Intensive care unit support and Acute Physiology and Chronic Health Evaluation III performance in hematopoietic stem cell transplant recipients. *Crit. Care Med.*, **31** (6), 1715–1721.
111. Khassawneh, B.Y., White, P. Jr., Anaissie, E.J. *et al.* (2002) Outcome from mechanical ventilation after autologous peripheral blood stem cell transplantation. *Chest*, **121** (1), 185–188.
112. Soubani, A.O., Kseibi, E., Bander, J.J. *et al.* (2004) Outcome and prognostic factors of hematopoietic stem cell transplantation recipients admitted to a medical ICU. *Chest*, **126** (5), 1604–1611.
113. Rabitsch, W., Staudinger, T., Locker, G.J. *et al.* (2005) Respiratory failure after stem cell transplantation: improved outcome with non-invasive ventilation. *Leuk. Lymphoma*, **46** (8), 1151–1157.
114. Brochard, L., Mancebo, J., Wysocki, M. *et al.* (1995) Noninvasive ventilation for acute exacerbations of chronic obstructive pulmonary disease. *N. Engl. J. Med.*, **333**, 817–822.

Part III
Discontinuation from mechanical ventilation

3.1 Definitions

Scott K. Epstein

Office of Educational Affairs, Tufts University School of Medicine, Boston, MA, USA

3.1.1 Introduction

Invasive mechanical ventilation can have beneficial effects on the pathophysiology of acute respiratory failure by increasing delivered FiO_2, re-expanding collapsed or atelectatic lung, and providing adequate alveolar ventilation. In many instances such as pneumonia, acute lung injury, pulmonary edema, exacerbation of chronic obstructive pulmonary disease, drug overdose, and acute neuromuscular disease, the principal goal of mechanical ventilation is to provide support while waiting for the respiratory system to recover. In fact, invasive mechanical ventilation may be considered a classic example of a "double-edged sword." Invasive mechanical ventilation is associated with significant risks and complications, including sinusitis, airway injury, thromboembolism, and gastrointestinal bleeding [1]. The risk for the most serious complication, ventilator-associated pneumonia, increases with the duration of intubation and appears to contribute to excess mortality. These complications of mechanical ventilation increase the duration of intensive care unit and hospital stay and significantly increase the cost of care. There is increasing appreciation that controlled mechanical ventilation (a mode in which each breath is triggered by the ventilator), especially when used for longer time periods, can induce significant diaphragmatic dysfunction. This VIDD, or ventilator induced diaphragmatic dysfunction, may hinder or delay efforts to free the patient from the

A Practical Guide to Mechanical Ventilation, First Edition.
Edited by Jonathon D. Truwit and Scott K. Epstein.
© 2011 John Wiley & Sons, Ltd. Published 2011 by John Wiley & Sons, Ltd.

mechanical ventilator. Given the risks of prolonged mechanical ventilation the clinician must identify when the patient has improved to a degree that efforts can shift to rapidly removing the patient from the ventilator. Indeed, one of he most important question an intensive care unit physician can ask each day at the bedside is "Can this patient breathe spontaneously today?"

3.1.2   Weaning vs. liberation and discontinuation

The process of freeing the patient from the ventilator has been referred to as *weaning*, *liberation*, or *discontinuation* (Table 3.1.1). Historically, the term weaning was used because the process of removing the patient from the mechanical ventilator and taking out the artificial airway occurred by a gradual and deliberate process. Specifically, it was believed that the work of breathing had to be gradually transferred from machine to patient in a controlled and stepwise fashion. Only when the patient could breathe completely unassisted (or nearly so), and for a considerable period, would clinicians consider removing the endotracheal tube. With this understanding, debate occurred as to the best approach for gradually transferring work of breathing and new mechanical ventilator modes were developed or older ones adapted for the purpose. For example, IMV (intermittent mandatory ventilation) was thought to specifically foster this process; reducing the respiratory rate by 40% would transfer 40% of the work; reduction of 75% would transfer 75% of the work, and so on, or so it was once believed.

This effort eventually culminated in two large randomized controlled trials designed to identify the optimal weaning strategy [2, 3]. These investigations compared T-piece, pressure support ventilation (PSV) and IMV (using study designs

Table 3.1.1   Definitions.

Term	Definition
Constant positive airway pressure (CPAP)	A mode of spontaneous breathing trial. Constant positive airway pressure is delivered throughout the respiratory cycle. CPAP can be delivered through the ventilator or with an external device.
Decannulation	Removal of a tracheostomy tube
Discontinuation or liberation	The process of freeing the patient from mechanical ventilation. A determination of whether a patient still requires ventilatory support. It encompasses readiness testing, trials of spontaneous breathing, and, if needed, gradual or progressive withdrawal of ventilatory support. It is exclusive of the process of extubation.
Extubation – planned	Removal of the endotracheal tube by the clinician. This usually follows a successful SBT or process of gradual withdrawal from ventilatory support.

Table 3.1.1 (*Continued*)

Term	Definition
Extubation – unplanned	Deliberate (by the patient) or accidental removal of the endotracheal tube.
Intermittent mandatory ventilation (IMV)	Mode of mechanical ventilation in which the clinician sets the tidal volume and respiratory rate. Weaning typically occurs by a stepwise reduction in the number of breaths delivered by the ventilator. By adding pressure support, the patient's spontaneous breaths can be supported with inspiratory pressure.
Pressure support level (PSV), low level	A mode of ventilatory support that can also be used for a trial of spontaneous breathing. Each breath is triggered by the patient and supported by a clinician-determined level of inspiratory pressure support. As a mode for the SBT, low levels of PSV can help overcome the work of breathing imposed by the endotracheal tube and the ventilatory apparatus.
Prolonged mechanical ventilation	Requirement for >21 days of mechanical ventilation.
Protocol	An organized approach to discontinuing mechanical ventilation. The goal is to regularize or standardize care. One attractive feature is that a protocol can be effectively implement by non-physicians. Protocols can focus on readiness testing, spontaneous breathing trials or strategies for progressive withdrawal.
Readiness testing	A set of objective and subjective criteria used to determine whether a patient is ready to undertake a trial of spontaneous breathing (SBT).
Spontaneous breathing trial (SBT)	A period of breathing without ventilatory assistance or with minimal ventilatory support (on CPAP or low level of pressure support). Successful completion of the SBT usually indicates that a patient no longer requires ventilatory support. SBTs typically last from 30–120 min.
SBT assessment criteria	A set of objective and subjective criteria used to determine whether a patient is tolerating a trial of spontaneous breathing.
T-piece (-tube) trial	A mode of spontaneous breathing trial. The patient is disconnected from the ventilator and breathes exclusively through the endotracheal tube (ETT). The tubing connected perpendicularly to the ETT allows for the patient to breathe humidified oxygen or room air.
Ventilator dependence	Condition where the patient cannot be successfully removed from the ventilator. In general, this is said to occur after 3–6 months of failed weaning attempts.
Weaning – Historic	The process of freeing the patient from mechanical ventilation.
Weaning – Current	The process of gradual or progressive withdrawal of ventilation support. Required in only 20–25% of patients ventilated for more than 24 h.
Weaning predictors	Physiologic tests designed to identify the presence or absence of an imbalance between the load on the respiratory system and the capacity of the respiratory muscles (or respiratory drive) to effectively respond to that load.

with important differences) and found that the latter technique was clearly inferior: patients randomized to IMV took longer to wean from the ventilator than with the other modes. Interestingly, these studies, designed to identify the best mode of weaning, were instrumental in demonstrating that the majority of patients do not require a gradual process for freeing them from the ventilator. Most patients who were judged ready to undergo a T-piece trial tolerated that trial and could be extubated, the vast majority successfully. In contrast, a minority of patients did not tolerate this initial spontaneous breathing trial (SBT). These patients were randomized to more deliberate weaning strategies. This observation has led experts to reconsider application of the term weaning to this process. The terms liberation [4] or discontinuation [5] may better reflect the entire process of freeing the patient from the ventilator; that is, the patient is liberated when they are no longer in need of mechanical ventilatory support. With this scheme the term weaning might best be applied to the minority of patients who do not tolerate the SBT and require a gradual process or *progressive withdrawal*.

With the recognition that most patients tolerate their initial SBT, emphasis has shifted to identifying when a patient is ready to undergo such a trial. The time from intubation until readiness for spontaneous breathing constitutes a pre-discontinuation phase. During this time the patient may manifest profound gas exchange abnormalities (e.g., $FiO_2 > 0.60$ on high levels of PEEP), severely deranged respiratory mechanics (e.g., necessitating full ventilatory support and heavy sedation or neuromuscular blockade), profound respiratory muscle dysfunction, depressed control of breathing, or hemodynamic instability. Attempts to significantly reduce the level of ventilatory support or to allow such a patient to breath spontaneously (with minimal assistance) are ill advised and dangerous. Therefore, the challenge to the clinician is to recognize when this phase ends. In patients intubated for rapidly reversible processes (e.g., cardiogenic pulmonary edema) this phase may last just a few hours. In contrast, in patients with acute lung injury and multi-organ failure this phase may take weeks to resolve, if at all. Detecting the end of this phase requires the use of *readiness testing*, recognizing that respiratory failure has partially or totally resolved, respiratory muscle function has improved, and the patient is ready to breathe spontaneously. To this end, a series of objective criteria has been developed to assist the clinician in identifying the earliest time the patient can safely undergo a trial of spontaneous breathing [5]. Absolute requirements for readiness include adequate oxygenation, hemodynamic stability, and sufficient respiratory drive and respiratory muscle capacity to trigger the ventilator and take a spontaneous breath. Additional objective criteria include *weaning predictors or parameters*, a battery of physiologic measurements (negative inspiratory force, frequency to tidal volume ratio) designed to recognize an imbalance between respiratory load and respiratory muscle capacity. Respiratory therapists and critical care nurses can successfully implement readiness testing by using written guidelines or a *protocol*.

Once readiness criteria are satisfied the patient undergoes a spontaneous breathing trial (without ventilator assistance or on low levels of support) to assess whether mechanical ventilatory support is still required [6]. The spontaneous breathing trial must be carefully assessed by bedside clinicians. This is optimally achieved by using SBT assessment criteria, a set of objective and subjective measurements, to assess tolerance for the trial [5]. Criteria include vital signs (respiratory rate, heart rate, blood pressure), oxygenation and gas exchange, and signs indicating increased work of breathing. Patients tolerating the SBT are considered for removal of the endotracheal tube while those intolerant are placed back on full ventilatory support. The latter group may benefit from a more gradual process or progressive withdrawal of ventilator support. Successful discontinuation from mechanical ventilation depends on identifying and correcting treatable causes for weaning failure. This is best achieved by a systematic evaluation for reversible processes that contribute to increased work of breathing, decreased respiratory muscle strength, or the presence of significant cardiac or psychological dysfunction. Progressive withdrawal can occur by stepwise reduction in the level of pressure support, or in the respiratory rate during IMV, or by employing T-piece or CPAP trials of increasing duration. Once some minimal level of support or duration of unsupported breathing is tolerated the patient is considered to no longer require ventilatory support. Once the patient tolerates spontaneous breathing the clinician must address whether the endotracheal tube is still required; can the patient be extubated (Figure 3.1.1)?

3.1.3 Extubation

Over the last decade it has been appreciated that determining whether a patient still requires mechanical ventilatory support and whether the endotracheal tube is still required are distinct and separate questions (Table 3.1.2). *Extubation failure* has been defined as the need for reintubation within the first 48 to 72 hours after removal of the endotracheal tube and occurs in approximately 15% of patients undergoing planned extubation [7]. Others have used a more liberal definition of post-extubation respiratory failure with the recognition that not all patients need to be reintubated. In fact, some patients with post-extubation respiratory failure (manifested by tachypnea, hypercapnia, and signs of increased work of breathing) can be successfully managed with noninvasive ventilation and do not require reintubation. The determinants of success and the pathophysiologic cause for failure of discontinuation of ventilatory support and extubation are distinct.

Discontinuation (or *weaning*) *failure* typically occurs secondary to an imbalance between the load on the respiratory system and respiratory muscle capacity. Although extubation failure can occur secondary to load–capacity imbalance, it often results from an inability to protect the airway and thus is an integrated function of cough strength, volume of respiratory secretions, patency of the upper airway, and mental status. Moreover, the physiologic and clinical predictors used

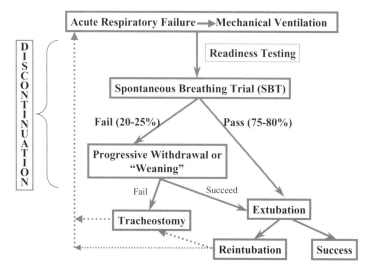

Figure 3.1.1 Overview. After mechanical ventilation is initiated for acute respiratory failure clinicians should focus on determining the earliest time for a trial of spontaneous breathing. Readiness testing applies objective criteria to determine when a SBT can be safely undertaken. The majority of patients will pass their first SBT indicating that mechanical ventilatory support is no longer required. Those not tolerating the SBT are systematically assessed for reversible causes of failure. Once treated further attempts to remove the patient from mechanical ventilation are indicated. This usually takes the form or progressive withdrawal or weaning, a more deliberate stepwise approach. This entire process can be referred to discontinuation or liberation from ventilatory support. Once a patient no longer needs mechanical ventilation the clinician addresses the separate question of whether the patient still requires the endotracheal tube. When the answer is no, the patient undergoes extubation. Patients intolerant of weaning trials or those requiring reintubation may require placement of a tracheostomy tube if it appears that discontinuation of mechanical ventilation will take an additional week or more at a minimum.

to determine likelihood of success and risk for failure are different for discontinuation and extubation. Lastly, the outcomes associated with discontinuation failure and extubation failure appears to be different. Although failed trials of spontaneous breathing are associated with increased duration of mechanical ventilation and length of stay, survival has not been shown to be adversely affected. In contrast, extubation failure substantially prolongs duration of ventilation and length of stay and, in many studies, is associated with increased mortality [7].

3.1.4   Prolonged mechanical ventilation, ventilator-dependence

Up to 10% of patients ventilated for at least 24–48 h prove difficult to liberate from the ventilator (some of these patients may have undergone extubation but required

Table 3.1.2 Comparison of discontinuation of mechanical ventilation and extubation.

	Discontinuation	Extubation
Definition	• Determination of whether patient still requires ventilatory support. Discontinuation of ventilatory support.	• Determination of whether patient still needs an endotracheal tube. Removal of the endotracheal tube.
Reasons for failure	• Imbalance between respiratory load and the capacity of the respiratory muscles • Cardiac dysfunction • Psychological dysfunction	• Inadequate cough • Excessive respiratory secretions • Upper airway obstruction • Abnormal mental status • Factors responsible for discontinuation failure can also cause extubation failure
Measurements used to predict success/failure	• Oxygenation • Respiratory mechanics (compliance, resistance) • Minute ventilation • Respiratory muscle strength • Breathing pattern • Work of breathing	• Cough strength • Volume of respiratory secretions • Patency of upper airway (cuff leak test) • Assessment of mental status
Outcome for failure	• Increased duration of mechanical ventilation, ICU stay, hospital stay • No definite increase in hospital mortality • Increased need for tracheostomy	• Increased duration of mechanical ventilation, ICU stay, hospital stay • Increased hospital mortality • Increased need for tracheostomy

reintubation) and are said to require *prolonged mechanical ventilation,* generally defined as the need for 21 or more days of ventilation [8]. Many of these patients have the endotracheal tube removed and a tracheostomy tube placed, though the optimal timing of this remains hotly debated. The tracheostomy tube provides a secure airway that, assuming the patient is otherwise medically stable, allows for transfer to a non-acute care setting. If further attempts at discontinuation from mechanical ventilation prove successful, efforts are made to remove the tracheostomy tube, a process called *decannulation.* Some patients prove intolerant of weaning efforts for many months (greater than 3–6) and are considered *ventilator dependent.* A portion of this group may require mechanical ventilation for only a part of each day or may be managed with non-invasive ventilation. Patients reaching this stage often require chronic hospitalization though a proportion, depending on human and financial resources, can be managed at home.

3.1.5 A new classification of weaning

A new classification of weaning was recently proposed at an international conference of experts [9]. With this approach *simple weaning* is said to occur when a patient tolerates the first SBT and is successfully extubated. This group may constitute 70% of patients who recover sufficiently to undergo a trial of spontaneous breathing. *Difficult weaning* is defined as a failure to tolerate the initial SBT, with successful weaning requiring up to three SBTs or up to seven days from the first SBT. Prolonged weaning is present when the patient fails three or more SBTs or it takes more than seven days after the first SBT for weaning to be successful. Approximately one in three patients undergoing SBTs will be classified as either difficult or prolonged weaning. It has been suggested that mortality is higher with difficult and prolonged weaning. Specific pathophysiologic factors associated with and predictors for these weaning subtypes remain to be defined.

References

1. Epstein, S. (2006) Complications in ventilator supported patients, in *Principles and Practice of Mechanical Ventilation* (ed. M. Tobin), McGraw Hill, New York, pp. 877–902.
2. Brochard, L., Rauss, A., Benito, S. *et al.* (1994) Comparison of three methods of gradual withdrawal from ventilatory support during weaning from mechanical ventilation. *Am. J. Respir. Crit. Care Med.*, **150** (4), 896–903.
3. Esteban, A., Frutos, F., Tobin, M.J. *et al.* (1995) A comparison of four methods of weaning patients from mechanical ventilation. Spanish Lung Failure Collaborative Group. *N. Engl. J. Med.*, **332** (6), 345–350.
4. Hall, J.B. and Wood, L.D. (1987) Liberation of the patient from mechanical ventilation. *JAMA*, **257** (12), 1621–1628.
5. MacIntyre, N.R., Cook, D.J., Ely, E.W., Jr *et al.* (2001) Evidence-based guidelines for weaning and discontinuing ventilatory support: a collective task force facilitated by the American College of Chest Physicians; the American Association for Respiratory Care; and the American College of Critical Care Medicine. *Chest*, **120** (6 Suppl.), 375S–395S.
6. Ely, E.W., Baker, A.M., Dunagan, D.P. *et al.* (1996) Effect on the duration of mechanical ventilation of identifying patients capable of breathing spontaneously. *N. Engl. J. Med.*, **335** (25), 1864–1869.
7. Epstein, S.K. (2002) Decision to extubate. *Intensive Care Med.*, **28** (5), 535–546.
8. MacIntyre, N.R., Epstein, S.K., Carson, S. *et al.* (2005) Management of patients requiring prolonged mechanical ventilation: report of a NAMDRC consensus conference. *Chest*, **128** (6), 3937–3954.
9. Boles, J.M., Bion, J., Connors, A. *et al.* (2007) Weaning from mechanical ventilation. *Eur. Respir. J.*, **29** (5), 1033–1056.

3.2 Readiness testing and weaning predictors

Scott K. Epstein

Office of Educational Affairs, Tufts University School of Medicine, Boston, MA, USA

3.2.1 Illustrative case

A 72-year-old woman with severe community-acquired pneumonia has been intubated for six days. She steadily improved over the last 48 hours on broad spectrum antibiotics. On Day 6, at 7 a.m., she is awake and alert. The patient is 152 cm tall and weighs 47 kg. A No. 7 endotracheal tube is in place (internal diameter = 7 mm). On physical examination, she is afebrile, with a pulse of 70 beats per minute, blood pressure of 110/60, and respiratory rate of 22 breaths per minute. Ventilator settings are volume assist-control ventilation, FiO_2 0.35, positive end-expiratory pressure (PEEP) 5 cm H_2O, rate 18 breaths per minute, and tidal volume 350 ml. The respiratory therapist has determined the negative inspiratory force (NIF) to be −35 cm H_2O. The frequency tidal volume ratio (f/V_T), recorded during one minute of disconnection from ventilatory support, was 133 (respiratory rate 32 breaths per minute, tidal volume 240 ml). Should this patient undergo a spontaneous breathing trial (SBT)? If a SBT is to be conducted, what mode should be used?

3.2.2 Introduction

Given the numerous complications associated with invasive mechanical ventilation the clinician must work to discontinue mechanical ventilation as soon as it is safe

A Practical Guide to Mechanical Ventilation, First Edition.
Edited by Jonathon D. Truwit and Scott K. Epstein.
© 2011 John Wiley & Sons, Ltd. Published 2011 by John Wiley & Sons, Ltd.

to do so. Rapid discontinuation from mechanical ventilation must be balanced against the risks of premature trials of spontaneous breathing, allowing a patient to breathe without assistance before they are ready. Those risks include precipitating cardiac dysfunction, psychological discouragement, and respiratory muscle fatigue or structural injury to the muscles (e.g., diaphragm). Each of these risks may hinder further efforts to liberate the patient from the ventilator.

3.2.3 Assessment of readiness for spontaneous breathing

Assessment of readiness can commence within hours of the initiation of mechanical ventilation in patients intubated for rapidly reversible processes. For example, patients intubated for cardiogenic pulmonary edema will improve rapidly with afterload reduction, diuretics and nitrates. Patients ventilated for some drug over-doses will have restitution of adequate central respiratory drive as the ingested drug is metabolized, excreted or when an antidote is administered. Other causes of acute respiratory failure are characterized by excessive work of breathing and/or respiratory muscle dysfunction. The latter may include an element of respiratory muscle fatigue, a process that will reverse with muscle rest. Under these conditions full ventilatory support should be maintained for 24–48 hours before evaluating the patient for a trial of spontaneous breathing.

Subjective assessment alone appears to be insufficient in identifying patients ready for spontaneous breathing trials. Therefore, subjective criteria to assess patient readiness for spontaneous breathing can be supplemented, or replaced, by objective assessments that serve as surrogate markers of recovery (Table 3.2.1) [1]. Adequate oxygenation and hemodynamic stability are absolute prerequisites for considering the patient ready to safely undertake a trial of spontaneous breathing.

Table 3.2.1 Criteria used to determine readiness for trials of spontaneous breathing.

Required criteria
1. $PaO_2/FiO_2 \geq 150$[a] or $SaO_2 \geq 90\%$ on $FiO_2 \leq 40\%$ and positive end-expiratory pressure (PEEP) ≤ 5 cm H_2O
2. Hemodynamic stability (no or low dose vasopressor medications, e.g., dopamine at a dose ≤ 5 mcg/kg/min)

Additional criteria[b]
1. Weaning parameters: respiratory rate ≤ 35 breaths/min, spontaneous tidal volume >5 ml/kg, negative inspiratory force (NIF) <-20 to -25 cm H_2O, $f/V_T < 105$ breaths/min/l
2. Hemoglobin $\geq 8–10$ mg/dl
3. Core temperature $\leq 38–38.5$ degrees Celsius
4. Mental status awake and alert or easily arousable

---

[a]A threshold of $PaO_2/FiO_2 \geq 120$ can be used for patients with chronic hypoxemia. Some patients require higher levels of PEEP to avoid atelectasis during mechanical ventilation.
[b]Some authorities consider these criteria to be optional (see text).

Additional criteria, such as adequate hemoglobin, mental status and absence of fever, have been used but little data exist to confirm their utility. For example, patients with depressed neurological status, as assessed by the Glasgow Coma Scale, can still successfully wean and tolerate extubation [2]. Similarly, patients managed with a restrictive blood transfusion strategy (goal hemoglobin of 7–9 mg/dl) had the same duration of mechanical ventilation and probability of successful weaning as patients transfused liberally to achieve a hemoglobin >10 mg/dl [3]. Therefore, one should be cautious in denying a trial of weaning in a patient solely because of depressed mental status or low hemoglobin. Nevertheless, under certain circumstances (e.g., presence of severe anemia in a patient with significant ischemia or cardiac dysfunction) an argument can be made for correcting a reduced hemoglobin prior to SBTs. In summary, these additional objective assessments should serve as guidelines rather than rigid criteria because up to 30% of patients *never* satisfying objective readiness criteria can still ultimately be liberated from mechanical ventilation [4].

3.2.4 Weaning predictors

The logic for using physiologic measurements ("*weaning predictors*") to predict readiness for spontaneous breathing is strong, especially for predictors that indicate increased load on the respiratory system (work of breathing), decreased capacity of the respiratory muscles, or a combination of the two. Clinical signs such as excess activity of the sternocleidomastoid muscle, thoracoabdominal paradox or respiratory alternans suggest load–capacity imbalance but these are neither sensitive nor specific and are dependent on the skill of the observer. Numerous weaning tests (predictors) have been investigated over the last three decades and some of these are routinely applied in the care of ventilated patients (Table 3.2.2) [5]. Parameters such as compliance, resistance, minute ventilation, and negative inspiratory force are assessed during full ventilatory support. Other parameters, such as respiratory rate and tidal volume, are best measured during a brief period of disconnection from the ventilator, though measurement through the ventilator, on no or low levels of support, is possible. Complex physiologic measurements, such as work of breathing and esophageal pressure determination, require the placement of a specialized catheter in the esophagus. The invasive nature of the measurement and the cost of the equipment make it unlikely that such techniques will find routine application in the care of ventilated patients. Some ventilators now offer noninvasive measurements of complex physiologic parameter, such as the airway occlusion pressure (P0.1), the negative pressure generated in the first 100 ms of inspiration. The airway occlusion pressure reflects respiratory drive and when elevated may indicate a respiratory system responding to increased load or decreased capacity. Unfortunately, the predictive value of the ventilator determined airway occlusion measurement has not been sufficiently validated.

Table 3.2.2   Tests used to predict weaning outcome ("weaning predictors").

Measurements of oxygenation and gas exchange
   PaO_2/FiO_2, PaO_2/PAO_2
   Alveolar–arterial O_2 gradient
   Dead space, V_D/V_T
Simple measurements of respiratory load and muscular capacity
   Negative inspiratory force, maximal inspiratory pressure
   Respiratory system compliance (static or dynamic)
   Respiratory system resistance
   Minute ventilation
   Respiratory frequency
   Tidal volume
   Maximal voluntary ventilation
   Vital capacity
Measurements integrating multiple factors
   Frequency–tidal volume ratio, f/V_T
   CROP index (compliance, respiratory rate, oxygenation, pressure)
Complex integrative measurements requiring special equipment
   Airway occlusion pressure
   P0.1/MIP
   Work of breathing
   Oxygen cost of breathing
   Gastric intramucosal pH

Table 3.2.3   Calculating sensitivity, specificity, positive and negative predictive values, and accuracy for a weaning predictor (f/V_T).

Outcome of discontinuation or weaning	$f/V_T \leq 105$ breaths/l/min (positive test)	$f/V_T > 105$ breaths/l/min (negative test)
Success	True positive (TP)	False negative (FN)
Failure	False positive (FP)	True negative (TN)

Sensitivity = TP/(TP + FN), Specificity = TN/(TN + FP).
Positive Predictive Value, PPV = TP/(TP + FP).
Negative Predictive Value, NPV = TN/(TN + FN).
Accuracy = (TP + TN)/(TP + FP + TN + FN).

The best approach to analyzing predictors is to use a 2×2 table to compare test results (using a threshold value) to discontinuation or weaning outcome (Table 3.2.3). This table provides sensitivity, specificity, positive and negative predictive values, and accuracy. The term *sensitivity* addresses the question, "Of patients successfully discontinued or weaned from mechanical ventilation, what proportion will have a positive test?" The term *specificity* addresses the question, "Of patients who fail, what proportion have a negative test?" Positive and negative predictive values address the following questions respectively: "What is probability of success when

Table 3.2.4 Likelihood ratios for a test.

Likelihood ratio	Definition	Change in probability of success or failure
LR positive	Sensitivity/(1-specificity)	LR = 1–2, none/minimal LR = 2–5, small LR = 5–10, moderate LR > 10, large
LR negative	(1-sensitivity)/specificity	LR = 0.5–1, none/minimal LR = 0.3–0.5, small LR = 0.1–0.3, moderate LR < 0.1, large

From: Epstein, S.K. Weaning from mechanical ventilation: the rapid shallow breathing index.
Reproduced with permission: UpToDate, Basow, D.S. (Ed.), Reproduced with permission: UpToDate,
Waltham, MA, 2010.

my patient has a positive test? "What is the probability of failure when my patient has a negative test?" It is crucial to realize that sensitivity and specificity are properties of the test itself, independent of the particular patient sample in whom the test is used. The positive predictive value (PPV) and negative predictive value (NPV) depend on the prevalence of the condition being measured.

Another method of analysis is the determination of the likelihood ratios (LRs) for a test (Table 3.2.4). The LR for a positive test (LR+) is the odds that a patient with success will have a positive test (e.g., frequency–tidal volume ratio, f/$V_T \leq 105$ breaths/min/l) compared with the odds that a patient who fails would have a positive test. The LR for a negative test (LR−) is the odds that a patient with success will have a negative test (e.g., f/$V_T > 105$ breaths/min/l) compared with the odds that a patient who fails would have a negative test. The LRs can be simply computed using sensitivity and specificity. A LR = 1 indicates that the probability of success or failure is the same after the test (post-test probability) as it was before the test (pre-test probability) (e.g., the test is not helpful). When the LR > 1 the probability of success increases, and when the LR < 1 the probability of success decreases. The greater the deviation from one the more powerful the test is as a predictor (Table 3.2.4). By using the pre-test probability, the LR, and a simple nomogram, the post-test probability can be determined quickly using a ruler [6].

3.2.4.1 Specific predictors

3.2.4.1.1 Oxygenation and gas exchange

Indices of oxygenation perform poorly as predictors. One explanation is that trials of spontaneous breathing are only considered in patients satisfying minimum oxygenation requirements, such as a $SaO_2 \geq 90\%$ or $PaO_2 \geq 60\,mm\,Hg$ on $FiO_2 \leq 0.40$–0.50. Given that resolution of severe hypoxemia is a prerequisite for initiating spontaneous breathing trials, the outcome of the latter is determined more by the balance between load and capacity than by oxygenation. Not surprisingly an increase in dead space indicates increased risk for failure, though relatively few studies have examined this parameter. To determine dead space an arterial blood gas or end-tidal CO_2 from capnometry is required, along with a method for measuring mixed expired CO_2 concentration.

3.2.4.1.2 Passive and dynamic mechanics

The presence of abnormal mechanics, reduced compliance and increased airways resistance, indicate the presence of increased work of breathing and thus might suggest higher risk for spontaneous breathing trial failure. While on the ventilator, with the patient relaxed, it is relatively easy to measure compliance and resistance. Dynamic compliance is the tidal volume divided by the difference between peak airway pressure and PEEP. Static compliance is the tidal volume divided by the difference between plateau pressure and PEEP. Compliance measurements are underestimated in the presence of intrinsic PEEP. Resistance is measured as the difference between peak airway and plateau pressure divided by flow (using constant inspiratory flow setting). Nevertheless, mechanics determined during passive inflation with the ventilator do not differ substantially or reliably between those who fail and those who succeed. Even when differences are present, the considerable overlap of values seen with success and failure precludes useful and accurate application of these measurements to predict outcome.

3.2.4.1.3 Assessing respiratory muscle function (negative inspiratory force and maximal inspiratory pressure)

The pressure that can be generated against an occluded airway during a one second maximal inspiratory effort, initiated near residual volume (RV), is a measure of global inspiratory muscle strength. By attaching an aneroid manometer to the opening of the endotracheal tube and asking the patient to maximally inspire against an occluded airway, the negative inspiratory force (NIF) or maximal inspiratory pressure (MIP) can be measured. The MIP also depends upon coordination, the state of the chest wall compliance, lung volume, respiratory drive, patient effort/cooperation and investigator technique and, therefore, may not be reliable in patients undergoing mechanical ventilation. Effort can be improved by using a one-way valve that allows the patient to expire but not inspire. By keeping the valve occluded for up to 20–25 seconds the patient is pushed below FRC toward RV and a reliable maximal effort is produced. In general, studies of NIF have shown low PPVs (NIF < −20 but patient fails), an observation for which there are several explanations [6]. A single maneuver may not reflect respiratory muscle strength or does not ensure adequate endurance. In addition, even if muscle strength is good it does not take into account the load against which the muscles must contract.

3.2.4.1.4 Minute ventilation

In healthy, resting subjects, minute ventilation is approximately 5–6 l/min. In general, total minute ventilation is increased in mechanically ventilated patients and gives an estimate of the demands placed on the respiratory system. Numerous factors increase minute ventilation including conditions of increased carbon dioxide production (fever, hypermetabolic states), metabolic acidosis, hypoxemia, increased dead space, and increased central drive. At higher levels of minute ventilation, work of breathing per minute rises. In general, higher values for minute ventilation are associated with weaning failure. The negative predictive value for elevated minute ventilation is typically <0.50, indicating that half or more of patients with minute ventilation greater than 10–15 l/min are still successfully weaned.

3.2.4.1.5 Vital capacity

The vital capacity (VC) is the maximum volume of gas exhaled after a full inspiration. Typically the patient is instructed to inhale to total lung capacity (TLC) and then exhale to residual volume. In essence, the VC maneuver integrates respiratory muscle function with the impedance against which the muscles must contract. Values in healthy patients range from 65 to 75 ml/kg. As with the MIP, the VC is highly dependent on patient cooperation and effort. Indeed, it has been noted that fewer than half of patients can comply with the maneuver and test precision is poor (repeated measures in the same patient vary widely). These technical difficulties may help explain why the predictive accuracy of the vital capacity measurement has been poor.

3.2.4.1.6 Respiratory frequency, tidal volume, and the frequency to tidal volume ratio

Respiratory frequency typically increases in patients with high workload or with respiratory muscle weakness and, therefore, should be a good indicator of an imbalance between these components and increased risk for weaning failure. Although it may seem that frequency can easily be determined, this may not be the case. For example, relying on the digital read out on the ventilator may underestimate respiratory rate because efforts that fail to trigger the ventilator are not registered. Careful inspection of the pressure–time or flow–time curves can be used to detect these untriggered breaths. Respiratory frequency can be influenced by many other factors, including anxiety or pain. *Tidal volume* is expected to be low in patients with respiratory muscle dysfunction or elevated work of breathing. It must be remembered that tidal volume is a derived variable when determined using a spirometer. Errors in either minute ventilation or in the measurement of respiratory rate will lead to an error in tidal volume estimate.

Patients with either elevated respiratory load or reduced respiratory muscle function tend to breath rapidly and shallowly, thus the ratio of respiratory frequency to tidal volume has been extensively studied [7]. The maneuver is safe and easy to perform: the patient is disconnected from the ventilator, the endotracheal tube is connected to a spirometer (while the patient breathes humidified room air or oxygen), the minute ventilation (V_E) is measured over 60 s, the tidal volume (V_T) is calculated using the V_E and the measured respiratory rate ($V_T = V_E/f$), and the ratio is calculated (f/V_T, breaths/min/l). Values greater than 100–105 breaths/min/l, during unsupported breathing, are indicative of rapid shallow breathing and are associated with weaning failure. The f/V_T also can be measured on partial support modes using the digital readout from the ventilator to determine respiratory frequency and tidal volume. The f/V_T is lower on partial support modes compared to unsupported ventilation through the endotracheal tube and the predictive threshold has not been robustly defined [8]. One must be cautious using the digital readout when the patient displays trigger asynchrony. These ineffective inspiratory efforts fail to trigger the ventilator and are ignored by the respiratory frequency sensing mechanism of the ventilator. This can result in a falsely low report of the respiratory frequency and an underestimation of the f/V_T. Conversely, a number of factors may lead to a higher f/V_T, including: anxiety, female gender, narrow endotracheal tube size, sepsis or pneumonia, older age, supine positioning, fever, and preceding lung disease.

Ideally, clinical decision making guided by these weaning predictors would accelerate liberation from mechanical ventilation while avoiding the adverse consequences of failed weaning trials. Recently, the use of these objective physiologic criteria and their role in assessing readiness has been reassessed [1, 5]. Important problems in observational studies of weaning predictors have been identified: weaning predictors are frequently used *a priori* to determine which patients undergo weaning; the method and timing of measurement differs between studies and are subject to large coefficients of variation; insufficient blinding of clinicians determining weaning tolerance; and there is often an absence of objective criteria to determine weaning tolerance. These factors will inflate the purported accuracy of weaning predictors.

A comprehensive evidence-based medicine review concluded that relatively few predictors led to clinically significant changes in the probability of weaning success or failure [5]. Only five predictors measured during ventilatory support (negative inspiratory force, maximal inspiratory pressure, minute ventilation, P0.1/MIP, CROP [Compliance, Respiratory rate, Oxygenation, and Pressure]) had possible value in predicting weaning outcome. Of these, only the latter two had likelihood ratios suggesting clinical utility, but the small number of patients studied precludes recommending their application. Three other parameters (respiratory frequency, tidal volume, f/V_T), measured during 1–3 minutes of unassisted breathing, were more accurate, but even these tests were associated with only small to moderate changes in the probability of success or failure, respectively (LR positive <5, LR negative >0.1).

In a recent randomized controlled trial, all ventilated patients underwent a five component daily screen to assess readiness for spontaneous breathing [9]. To pass the screen *all* of the following had to be present $PaO_2/FiO_2 \geq 150$ (on PEEP < 5 cm H_2O), hemodynamic stability, acceptable mental status, adequate cough, and $f/V_T < 105$ breaths/min/l. Based on randomization, in one group the f/V_T was not used for weaning decision making while in the other only patients with $f/V_T < 105$ breaths/min/l underwent a SBT. Those passing the screen automatically underwent a two-hour spontaneous breathing trial and were then considered for extubation if the SBT was tolerated. The group randomized to use of the f/V_T took longer to wean from the ventilator. This result may derive either from the limited predicted value of weaning predictors or from the inherent safety of a closely monitored spontaneous breathing trial. In other words, a failed SBT may not cause harm if the patient is carefully observed and rapidly returned to full ventilatory support at the earliest signs of trouble. This concept is supported by a study that used phrenic nerve stimulation which found that diaphragmatic muscle fatigue did not occur in patients failing a spontaneous breathing trial on a T-piece [10]. It must be appreciated that in this study patients were returned to ventilatory support as soon as signs of weaning intolerance occurred. It is likely that fatigue, and possibly structural respiratory muscle injury, would ensue if the failed weaning trial was unduly extended. Therefore, it appears that weaning predictors are not routinely helpful in deciding whether or not to initiate a SBT (Table 3.2.5). In other words, the best diagnostic test for whether or not a patient needs ventilatory support is the SBT itself [11]. Indeed, a recent trial found that greater than 50% of patients passed a SBT when readiness was assessed without using weaning predictors [12]. Nevertheless, these tests may still prove valuable. They may help the reluctant clinician realize a patient is ready for spontaneous breathing. They may aid decision making in patients in whom the risks associated with weaning failure are prohibitively high. In a patient in whom a failed discontinuation

Table 3.2.5 Summary recommendations for using clinical factors and weaning predictors in deciding if a patient is ready to undergo a spontaneous breathing trial.

Recommendation	Level of supporting evidence
Readiness testing should be based principally on adequate oxygenation and hemodynamic stability (Table 3.2.1).	High quality (multiple, large randomized and observational studies)
Approximately 75% of patients satisfying readiness criteria tolerate an initial trial of spontaneous breathing (they do not require slower progressive withdrawal from ventilatory support).	High quality (multiple, large randomized and observational studies)
Weaning predictors are usually of minimal help in deciding whether to initiate spontaneous breathing trials. Among available weaning predictors, the frequency–tidal volume ratio is the most accurate.	High quality (single randomized controlled trial, systematic evidence-based literature review and meta-analysis)

trial could prove especially dangerous (e.g., a patient with significant coronary disease) tests that yield even small or moderate changes in probability of success/ failure may be clinically relevant. These physiologically-based tests may prove useful in guiding the evaluation of patients with weaning failure in an effort to identify reversible causes of weaning intolerance. For example, in a patient failing weaning trials, an elevated f/V_T would indicate probable imbalance between respiratory load and respiratory muscle capacity. A reduced negative inspiratory force would confirm the latter. Conversely, if a patient failing weaning trials has normal weaning predictors, the clinician should focus or cardiac or psychogenic causes.

3.2.5 Readiness testing

After objective criteria are satisfied, the patient undergoes formal readiness testing by breathing spontaneously on low levels of pressure support ventilation (PSV), continuous positive airway pressure (CPAP, 5 cm H_2O), or unassisted through a T-piece. Some form of spontaneous breathing trial is generally mandatory because nearly 40% of patients directly extubated after satisfying readiness criteria alone require reintubation.

The best approach to carrying out the spontaneous breathing trial has been debated. Proponents of T-piece argue that it best approximates the work of breathing the patient will experience after extubation. In contrast, other experts prefer low levels of pressure support to counterbalance the resistive workload that may be imposed by a narrow endotracheal tube. The pressure support level required to offset this imposed load varies widely, from 3 to 14 cm H_2O, and is difficult to determine noninvasively. Therefore, in any individual patient, a given level of pressure support may either over- or under-compensate for the imposed work. In general, 5–8 cm H_2O of pressure support appears to be the best compromise for these considerations.

Randomized trials comparing pressure support to T-piece and CPAP to T-piece have shown the techniques to be roughly equivalent in terms of successful weaning and extubation [13, 14]. When the patient must breathe through a small endotracheal tube (e.g., ≤7 mm) or tube with a lumen narrowed by inspissated secretions the tube-related imposed work of breathing may be substantial. Under those circumstances, using pressure support to overcome the additional work may be superior to T-piece. This may explain why some patients who fail a T-piece succeed when immediately switched to low level PSV and can then be successfully extubated [15]. There are also practical advantages to performing a spontaneous breathing trial through the ventilator (CPAP or PSV mode): no additional equipment is required; ventilator alarm and monitoring systems can be utilized to promptly identify the patient who is intolerant of weaning; and, if needed, ventilatory support can be simply and rapidly reestablished. Another form of mechanical ventilation, automatic tube compensation (ATC) has been suggested as a more accurate solution to overcoming the work of breathing imposed by a narrow endotracheal tube. With this approach the level of pressure support is adjusted during the respiratory cycle, based on the characteristics of the endotracheal tube (e.g., internal diameter), to overcome the imposed work of breathing without over-compensating. To date, spontaneous breathing trials conducted on ATC have not proved to be more accurate predictors of weaning or extubation success than those carried out with T-piece, CPAP or PSV.

In general, tolerance for a 120-minute trial of spontaneous breathing signals that a patient no longer requires ventilatory support. Yet, one study found no difference in success rate when comparing patients randomized to either 30- or 120-minute T-piece breathing. Of note, these investigators examined only the first attempt at spontaneous breathing. A similar, but much smaller and significantly underpowered trial, found no difference between 30- and 120-minutes of PSV of 7 cm H_2O during an initial SBT. The ideal duration for subsequent spontaneous breathing trials or for trials performed with partial support modes remains unknown, but it may be longer than 120 minutes. As an example, a study of 75 COPD patients, ventilated for at least 15 days, found a *median* time to trial failure of 120 minutes. Thus it would be expected that extubating all such patients after 120 minutes would result in a dangerously high reintubation rate. All these considerations aside, most experts continue to recommend a trial of approximately 120 minutes as an adequate test to assess whether the patient still needs ventilatory support (Table 3.2.6). A T-piece trial of 30 minutes is reasonable for the first SBT [11].

Careful assessment during a spontaneous breathing trial is based on both objective and subjective criteria (Table 3.2.7). Although these criteria are collectively widely applied, the individual components have not been subjected to rigorous validation to identify the optimal thresholds. Some criteria are non-specific and may reflect processes other than physiologic weaning intolerance. For example, tachypnea and tachycardia may result from patient anxiety rather than true physiologic impairment. Conversely, these criteria may not always identify patients with true physiologic imbalance. More sophisticated breathing pattern analysis (during or

Table 3.2.6 Summary recommendations for the use of spontaneous breathing trials to assess whether a patients still requires ventilatory support.

Recommendation	Level of evidence
Readiness testing is best performed with a 120-min spontaneous breathing trial conducted on T-piece or on low levels of CPAP or pressure support. (In many circumstances, a 30-min T-piece trial is adequate for the initial SBT.) Tolerance for the trial signals readiness for liberation from mechanical ventilation.	High quality; based on multiple randomized trials.
Tolerance for the spontaneous breathing trial is assessed by monitoring vital signs, oximetry, gas exchange and absence of clinical signs indicative of increased work of breathing.	High quality; based on multiple, large prospective trials.

Table 3.2.7   Criteria indicating that a patient is not tolerating a trial of spontaneous breathing.

Objective criteria
1. $SaO_2 < 0.90$ or $PaO_2 < 60\,mm\,Hg$ on $FiO_2 > 0.40$–0.50 or $PaO_2/FiO_2 < 120$–150
2. Increase in $PaCO_2 > 10\,mm\,Hg$ or decrease in pH > 0.10
3. Respiratory rate >35 breaths/min
4. Heart rate >140 bpm or an increase >20% of baseline
5. Systolic blood pressure <90 mm Hg or >160 mm Hg or change of >20% from baseline
Subjective criteria
1. Presence of signs of increased work of breathing including thoracoabdominal paradox or excessive use of accessory respiratory muscles
2. Presence of other signs of distress such as diaphoresis or agitation

just after the SBT) may identify patients who still require ventilatory support despite satisfying conventional SBT assessment criteria, but these complex measurements require further study.

If a patient fails the spontaneous breathing trial the clinician must embark on an investigation to identify the cause for failure with a goal of elucidating reversible factors. In addition, the clinician must decide how long to rest the patient before further attempts are made at discontinuation. Whether to continue with daily SBTs, change to a more gradual mode of discontinuation (e.g., weaning) or a combination of the two must be decided. For patients who pass the SBT, the clinician then turns their attention to the separate issue of whether the endotracheal tube is still required; can the patient be extubated?

3.2.6   Illustrative case continued

The intensive care unit team decided to proceed with the SBT based on the patient's normal hemodynamics and adequate oxygenation ($PaO_2/FiO_2 \geq 150$ on PEEP $\leq 5\,cm$ H_2O). The increased f/V_T was attributed to several factors including older age, female gender, and the narrow endotracheal tube. The team also reasoned that a well-monitored SBT has proven to be a safe test for the need for mechanical ventilatory support. The SBT was conducted on PSV $5\,cm\,H_2O$ to account for possible increased imposed work of breathing resulting from the narrow endotracheal tube. The patient tolerated the two-hour SBT and was successfully extubated.

References

1. MacIntyre, N.R., Cook, D.J., Ely, E.W., Jr. *et al.* (2001) Evidence-based guidelines for weaning and discontinuing ventilatory support: a collective task force facilitated by the American College of Chest Physicians; the American Association for Respiratory Care; and the American College of Critical Care Medicine. *Chest*, **120** (6 Suppl.), 375S–395S.

2. Coplin, W.M., Pierson, D.J., Cooley, K.D. *et al.* (2000) Implications of extubation delay in brain-injured patients meeting standard weaning criteria. *Am. J. Respir. Crit. Care Med.*, **161** (5), 1530–1536.

3. Hebert, P.C., Blajchman, M.A., Cook, D.J. *et al.* (2001) Do blood transfusions improve outcomes related to mechanical ventilation? *Chest*, **119** (6), 1850–1857.

4. Ely, E.W., Baker, A.M., Evans, G.W. *et al.* (1999) The prognostic significance of passing a daily screen of weaning parameters. *Intensive Care Med.*, **25** (6), 581–587.

5. Meade, M., Guyatt, G., Cook, D. *et al.* (2001) Predicting success in weaning from mechanical ventilation. *Chest*, **120** (6 Suppl.), 400S–424S.

6. Epstein, S.K. (2000) Weaning parameters. *Respir. Care Clin. N. Am.*, **6** (2), 253–301, v–vi.

7. Yang, K.L. and Tobin, M.J. (1991) A prospective study of indexes predicting the outcome of trials of weaning from mechanical ventilation. *N. Engl. J. Med.*, **324** (21), 1445–1450.

8. El-Khatib, M.F., Zeineldine, S.M. and Jamaleddine, G.W. (2008) Effect of pressure support ventilation and positive end expiratory pressure on the rapid shallow breathing index in intensive care unit patients. *Intensive Care Med.*, **34** (3), 505–510.

9. Tanios, M.A., Nevins, M.L., Hendra, K.P. *et al.* (2006) A randomized, controlled trial of the role of weaning predictors in clinical decision making. *Crit. Care Med.*, **34** (10), 2530–2535.

10. Laghi, F., Cattapan, S.E., Jubran, A. *et al.* (2003) Is weaning failure caused by low-frequency fatigue of the diaphragm? *Am. J. Respir. Crit. Care Med.*, **167** (2), 120–127.

11. Boles, J.M., Bion, J., Connors, A. *et al.* (2007) Weaning from mechanical ventilation. *Eur. Respir. J.*, **29** (5), 1033–1056.

12. Girard, T.D., Kress, J.P., Fuchs, B.D. *et al.* (2008) Efficacy and safety of a paired sedation and ventilator weaning protocol for mechanically ventilated patients in intensive care (Awakening and Breathing Controlled trial): a randomised controlled trial. *Lancet*, **371** (9607), 126–134.

13. Esteban, A., Alia, I., Gordo, F. *et al.* (1997) Extubation outcome after spontaneous breathing trials with T-tube or pressure support ventilation. The Spanish Lung Failure Collaborative Group. *Am. J. Respir. Crit. Care Med.*, **156** (2 Pt 1), 459–465.

14. Jones, D.P., Byrne, P., Morgan, C. *et al.* (1991) Positive end-expiratory pressure vs T-piece. Extubation after mechanical ventilation. *Chest*, **100** (6), 1655–1659.

15. Ezingeard, E., Diconne, E., Guyomarc'h, S. *et al.* (2006) Weaning from mechanical ventilation with pressure support in patients failing a T-tube trial of spontaneous breathing. *Intensive Care Med.*, **32** (1), 165–169.

3.3 Physiological barriers

Scott K. Epstein

Office of Educational Affairs, Tufts University School of Medicine, Boston, MA, USA

3.3.1 Illustrative case

An 82-year-old man has been intubated for 10 days after complicated surgery for a ruptured abdominal aortic aneurysm. His course has been complicated by hospital-acquired pneumonia and acute renal failure. He has a history of Type II diabetes mellitus and hypertension. By Day 5 the ventilator settings were volume assist control ventilation with FiO_2 0.30, positive end-expiratory pressure (PEEP) 5 cm H_2O, respiratory rate 16 breaths/min, and tidal volume 500 ml. An arterial blood gas revealed pH 7.44, $PaCO_2$ 35 mm Hg, and PaO_2 79 mm Hg. Renal function has normalized with a creatinine of 0.8 mg/dl. On physical examination he is awake and alert, temperature 37 °C, pulse 90 beats per minute, and respiratory rate 18 breaths per minute. The endotracheal tube is a No. 8.5 (internal diameter 8.5 mm). Spontaneous breathing trials (SBTs) on Days 7–9 were terminated after 15 minutes or less because the patient developed diaphoresis, tachypnea (35 breaths/min), tachycardia (115 beats/min) and hypertension (180/100). Weaning predictors have demonstrated favorable results with a negative inspiratory force (NIF) of −60 cm H_2O, total minute ventilation <10 l/min, and frequency–tidal volume ratio (f/V_T) of 80 breaths/min/l. How should the patient be evaluated and treated?

3.3.2 Introduction

As many as one third of patients cannot tolerate the initial trial of spontaneous breathing and require a more prolonged process for discontinuation of mechanical

A Practical Guide to Mechanical Ventilation, First Edition.
Edited by Jonathon D. Truwit and Scott K. Epstein.
© 2011 John Wiley & Sons, Ltd. Published 2011 by John Wiley & Sons, Ltd.

ventilation. A large body of research has identified many of the mechanisms underlying discontinuation failure. Therefore, intolerance for spontaneous breathing and
weaning trials should prompt a thorough investigation for the underlying cause with
the goal of identifying, and ultimately treating, reversible factors (Figure 3.3.1)
(Tables 3.3.1 and 3.3.2) [1, 2].

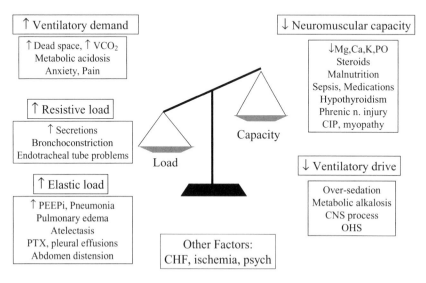

Figure 3.3.1 Overview of barriers that limit discontinuation and weaning from mechanical
ventilation. Most patients fail because of an imbalance between the load on the respiratory system
(increases in ventilatory demand, resistive work of breathing, elastic work of breathing) and
neuromuscular capacity. (Reproduced with permission [1].)

Table 3.3.1   Barriers to weaning: increased load.

Barrier to weaning	Examples	Therapeutic consideration
↑ Ventilatory demand		
Hypoxemia	1. Atelectasis	1. ↑ PEEP
	2. Morbid obesity, abdominal distension	2. Keep patient in upright position, >45°
	3. Underlying lung disease	3. ↑ FiO$_2$
	4. ↑ peripheral O$_2$ utilization (anxiety, fever, sepsis)	4. Sedation, antipyretics, antibiotics
↑ Dead space	1. Hyperinflation	1. Bronchodilators, steroids, ↓ minute ventilation
	2. Intravascular volume depletion	2. Intravenous fluids
	3. Pulmonary embolism	3. Anticoagulation

Table 3.3.1 (*Continued*)

Barrier to weaning	Examples	Therapeutic consideration
↑CO_2 production (VCO_2)	1. Fever 2. Overfeeding 3. Increased metabolic rate	1. Antipyretics 2. ↓ calories administered 3. Treat underlying cause (sepsis, hyperthyroidism)
Metabolic acidosis	1. Renal Failure	1. Dialysis, Bicarbonate
Neuropsychiatric	1. Delirium 2. Anxiety 3. Pain	1. Antipsychotics (e.g., haldol, olanzepine) 2. Sedative hypnotic agents (e.g., lorazepam) 3. Opiates (e.g., morphine, fentanyl)
↑ Resistive load		
Bronchoconstriction	1. COPD and asthma	1. Bronchodilators, steroids
Airway edema	1. COPD and asthma 2. Lower respiratory tract infection	1. Steroids 2. Antibiotics
↑ Secretions	1. Tracheobronchitis 2. Pneumonia	1. Antibiotics, airway suctioning 2. Antibiotics, airway suctioning
Respiratory equipment	1. Endotracheal or tracheal tube luminal narrowing 2. Heat and moisture exchangers (HME)	1. Replace tube or consider extubation 2. Remove HME during SBT or change to heated humidifier
↑ Elastic load		
Dynamic hyperinflation	1. COPD and asthma 2. States associated with ↑ minute ventilation (fever, hypoxemia, anxiety)	1. Bronchodilators, steroids, ↓ minute ventilation, add extrinsic PEEP to help patient trigger the ventilator 2. Antipyretics, ↑ FiO_2, sedation
Pulmonary edema	1. Congestive heart failure 2. Acute lung injury	1. Diuretics, inotropic agents 2. Lung protective strategy with ↓ tidal volume (e.g., 6 ml/kg IBW), titrate PEEP
Other alveolar filling	Pneumonia	Antibiotics
Atelectasis	1. After low spontaneous tidal volumes 2. Excess respiratory secretions 3. Process obstructing airway	1. ↑ tidal volume, ↑ PEEP 2. Chest physiotherapy and airway suctioning 3. Bronchoscopy
Pleural disease	1. Pleural effusion 2. Pneumothorax (PTX)	1. Thoracentesis, pigtail catheter drainage 2. Chest tube
Chest wall disease Abdominal distension	1. Morbid obesity 2. Ileus 3. Ascites	1. Wean with patient sitting at ≥45° 2. Decompress abdomen with NGT suction, treat causes of ileus (d/c opiates, correct hypokalemia) 3. Paracentesis

Table 3.3.2 Barriers to weaning: decreased respiratory muscle capacity.

Barrier to weaning	Examples	Therapeutic consideration
↓ Neuromuscular capacity		
Electrolyte abnormality	1. ↓ Magnesium (Mg) 2. ↓ Calcium (Ca) 3. ↓ Potassium (K) 4. ↓ Phosphorus (PO)	1–4. Assess electrolyte concentrations and replete if deficiencies detected
Medications	1. Corticosteroids 2. Neuromuscular blocking agents (NMBs)	1., 2. Minimize use of these agents and, if possible, avoid simultaneous use 2. Use of train of four monitoring to avoid excess use of NMBs, dose NMBs cautiously in setting of hepatic or renal disease
Metabolic conditions	1. Malnutrition 2. Hypothyroidism 3. Adrenal insufficiency	1. Enteral or parenteral feeding (avoid overfeeding) 2. Thyroid hormone replacement 3. Hydrocortisone
Inflammatory states	1. Severe sepsis	1. Antibiotics, consider activated protein C, consider corticosteroids
Neuropathy	1. Phrenic nerve injury (post-CABG, trauma) 2. Guillain–Barre syndrome 3. Critical illness polyneuropathy (CIP)	1. Prevention is key, recovery takes months to a year 2. Plasmapharesis or gamma globulin 3. Supportive care, tight glucose control, spontaneous recovery in weeks to months
Myopathy	1. Critical illness myopathy 2. VIDD	1. Minimize duration and dose of corticosteroids, supportive care, recovery in weeks to months 2. Avoid prolonged controlled mechanical ventilation
↓ Ventilatory Drive		
Excess Sedation	1. Use of intravenous sedation 2. Failure to use a sedation algorithm or sedation scoring system	1. Use sedation algorithm driven by a sedation scoring system (e.g., SAS, RASS) 2. Use strategy of daily cessation of sedation
Metabolic Alkalosis	1. NG suctioning 2. Alkali administration 3. Post-hypercapnic 4. Volume depletion, overdiuresis 5. Chloride depletion 6. Corticosteroids	1. Maintain intravascular volume, use PPI or H_2 blocker 2. Be cautious in administering sodium bicarbonate 3. Target baseline $PaCO_2$ when setting ventilator. 4. Maintain euvolemia 5. Replete chloride and potassium 6. Acetazolamide (Diamox)

Table 3.3.2 *(Continued)*

Barrier to weaning	Examples	Therapeutic consideration
CNS Process	1. Stroke 2. Meningoencephalitis 3. Toxic metabolic encephalopathy	1. Avoid sedative hypnotics, avoid ↓ cerebral perfusion 2. Antibiotics 3. Correct metabolic abnormalities, use antidotes for toxic ingestions
Sleep apnea	1. Central sleep apnea 2. Obesity hypoventilation syndrome (OHS)	1., 2. Avoid sedative hypnotic medications. Avoid overventilation (hypocapnia), consider respiratory stimulants (progesterone, theophylline, doxapram)

3.3.3 Hypoxemia

Hypoxemia is an unusual cause of discontinuation or weaning failure because adequate oxygenation is a prerequisite for initiating spontaneous breathing trials. For patients without chronic lung disease and chronic hypoxemia a $PaO_2/FiO_2 \geq 150$ (e.g., $PaO_2 \geq 60\,mm\,Hg$ on an FiO_2 of 0.40) indicates adequate oxygenation [3]. For patients with chronic hypoxemia (e.g., oxygen dependent COPD) a lower PaO_2/FiO_2 is acceptable (e.g., ≥ 120). Hypoxemia, from whatever cause, leads to increased minute ventilation, increased work of breathing and, therefore, can further hinder efforts to successfully discontinue mechanical ventilation.

A number of mechanisms can lead to worsening oxygenation during spontaneous breathing. Low tidal volume breathing promotes atelectasis, resulting in shunt (zone of lung with perfusion without ventilation) and decreased oxygenation. This scenario is common in morbidly obese patients or those with significant abdominal distension (e.g., ascites). Keeping such patients in the upright position (elevating the head of the bed to >45°) or using PEEP to prevent expiratory alveolar collapse may help.

During spontaneous breathing when the work of breathing is significantly elevated, the respiratory muscles dramatically increase oxygen extraction resulting in consumption of up to 50–60% of total oxygen consumption. If oxygen delivery (a function of cardiac output and oxygen carrying capacity) fails to increase in response, the oxygen content of blood returning to the heart (measured by mixed venous oxygen saturation) is significantly reduced [4]. This reduction in mixed venous oxygen content magnifies the effect of ventilation–perfusion inequality or shunts and causes worsening hypoxemia. When the PaO_2 falls this may further compromise oxygen delivery to respiratory muscles and the heart. Therefore, strategies designed to maximize cardiac performance (to improve oxygen delivery) and minimize peripheral oxygen consumption may help improve the PaO_2.

3.3.4 Respiratory drive

Depressed central respiratory drive occasionally contributes to weaning intolerance, though more commonly it leads to a delay in the initiation of weaning. Recent studies indicate that strategies for minimizing sedation by using either a sedation algorithm (driven by a sedation scoring system) [5] or daily interruption of sedation [6] may result in shorter duration of mechanical ventilation. Decreased drive can also result from a direct central nervous system insult (e.g., stroke, encephalitis), underlying abnormal control of breathing (e.g., central sleep apnea) or metabolic alkalosis.

Typically, patients with weaning intolerance display evidence of increased respiratory drive, a response to an imbalance between disordered respiratory mechanics (increased load on the system) and respiratory muscle dysfunction. Increased respiratory drive may also result from hypoxemia, increased dead space ventilation, increased carbon dioxide production, metabolic acidosis, or a primary increase in central drive because of neuropsychiatric disease (e.g., anxiety). Studies examining different parameters for estimating respiratory drive (mean inspiratory flow or the airway occlusion pressure, P0.1) indicate that these are abnormally elevated in patients who fail to tolerate a trial of spontaneous breathing. Indeed, respiratory drive during discontinuation and weaning failure is comparable to that seen in patients with acute respiratory failure [7]. The airway occlusion pressure is measured during the first 100 ms of inspiration as the patient breathes against a closed valve. By taking advantage of the time delay required to open the demand valve in the inspiratory circuit some newer ventilators allow P0.1 to be measured automatically without special equipment.

Increased respiratory drive itself can result in weaning failure by increasing the amount of respiratory work per minute. In the presence of expiratory airflow limitation (COPD, asthma) increased respiratory drive can worsen dynamic hyperinflation resulting in increased inspiratory work of breathing and gas exchange abnormalities. Treatment should be directed at the underlying cause(s), such as correction of hypoxemia, acidosis, and reducing work of breathing (Table 3.3.1). On occasion judicious use of sedation may be useful to reduce a non-physiologic elevation in respiratory drive. Cautious use may be indicated in patients with COPD in whom high levels of minute ventilation significantly worsen dynamic hyperinflation and the associated inspiratory work of breathing.

3.3.5 Increased load, increased work of breathing

An increased load on the respiratory system most often arises because of increased airways resistance or increased elastance (decreased respiratory system compliance). Studies demonstrate that resistance is higher and compliance lower in patients who fail to tolerate weaning compared to those who succeed. Moreover, patients who fail show steady deterioration in these measurements over the course of a trial of spontaneous breathing [8].

3.3.5.1 Increased resistive work

Increased resistive work can occur because of intrinsic airway narrowing related to bronchoconstriction and inflammation, as seen in patients with COPD or asthma. Alternatively, the airway lumen can be narrowed by the presence of increased respiratory secretions from pneumonia or tracheobronchitis. Increased resistive work can also result from extrinsic factors such as the ventilator apparatus. For example, heat and moisture exchange (HME) devices and the ventilator tubing and valves can impose an excessive resistive load. Heat and moisture exchange devices also increase dead space and the requirement for minute ventilation. Narrow endotracheal tubes (e.g., inner diameter ≤ 7 mm) impose a substantial increase in resistive work of breathing. The inner diameter of larger endotracheal tubes decreases over time, usually due to accumulation of secretions on the inner walls of the tube.

Several methods can be used to detect the presence of increased airways resistance. Although the presence of wheezing indicates increased resistance it does not quantify the magnitude. Airways resistance can be estimated by comparing the difference between peak inspiratory pressure and the plateau pressure; the larger the difference the greater the resistance. Airways resistance greater than 20 cm $H_2O/l/s$ is associated with weaning failure. Most ventilators automatically compute resistance by using the equation (assuming a relaxed patient and constant flow):

$$R = (\text{Peak pressure} - \text{plateau pressure})/\text{Flow}$$

Increased airways resistance may also contribute to weaning intolerance by worsening expiratory airflow and increasing dynamic hyperinflation (see below) and by making it more difficult to trigger the ventilator. Physiologic and clinical studies show that inhaled bronchodilators (e.g., albuterol) effectively decrease airways resistance. Under idealized, experimental conditions, four puffs delivered from a metered dose inhaler (MDI) using a spacer device appear optimal [9]. Higher albuterol doses result in tachycardia (and increase the risk for transient hypokalemia) without further reducing airways resistance. In the real world intensive care unit setting, airways resistance measurements can be used to optimize bronchodilator delivery. For example, in the absence of side effects, bronchodilator dose may be increased until no further reduction in airways resistance can be detected.

3.3.5.2 Increased elastic work

As with resistive work, patients destined to fail weaning confront higher elastic load than those who ultimately succeed. Increased elastic work (decreased compliance) results from any process that increases the amount of pressure required to generate a given tidal volume (excluding work needed to overcome resistance). Common factors include those causing alveolar filling (cardiogenic pulmonary edema, acute lung injury, pneumonia, alveolar hemorrhage) or alveolar collapse (atelectasis). Factors external to the lung, such as pleural (effusions, pneumothorax) and chest/abdominal wall (ascites, ileus), increase the elastic work of the entire respiratory system. Expiratory flow limitation results in dynamic hyperinflation (called intrinsic or auto-PEEP) shifting tidal breathing to the flat, non-compliant curve of the pressure–volume curve. In other words, generating a 500 ml tidal breath entails much greater inspiratory work in the hyperinflated patient than it does in the patient breathing at normal lung volumes.

Increased elastic work is signaled by an elevation in both the peak inspiratory pressure and the plateau pressure. Static compliance (Cstat = Tidal Volume / (Plateau pressure − PEEPi) can be measure automatically by the ventilator with values less than 70 ml/cm H_2O considered abnormal. The presence of dynamic hyperinflation also increases work of breathing by imposing an inspiratory threshold load on the system. In this setting, excess work must be performed to halt the inward recoil of the respiratory system (chest wall and lung) before a negative intrathoracic pressure can be generated to allow for inspiration to occur. In this case application of extrinsic PEEP (typically set at approximately 80% of the measured intrinsic PEEP) can decreased the inspiratory work by making it easier for the patient to trigger the ventilator [10]. Caution is recommended as use of extrinsic PEEP at levels exceeding the intrinsic PEEP can impede exhalation and actually worsen dynamic hyperinflation.

3.3.6 Decreased respiratory muscle capacity

Decreased respiratory muscle strength is frequently observed in patients intolerant of weaning, with a number of clinically relevant mechanisms identified (Table 3.3.3). Critical illness myopathy can occur secondary to the use of high dose corticosteroids (with or without concomitant neuromuscular blocking agents). Such patients may demonstrate flaccid quadriparesis (greatest in proximal muscles), an elevated creatine phosphokinase, and electromyography studies consistent with a myopathic process. Critical illness neuromyopathy is an axonal motor and sensory neuropathy occurring in the setting of severe sepsis and multiple organ failure. These patients demonstrate limb muscle weakness and depressed deep tendon reflexes [11].

Evidence from animal models demonstrates that controlled mechanical ventilation (CMV) can damage respiratory muscles, a process now referred to as ventilator induced diaphragmatic dysfunction (VIDD) [12]. In this entity diaphragmatic pressure generating capacity and endurance are diminished in a time-dependent manner (increasing weakness with more prolonged mechanical ventilation). Potential

Table 3.3.3 Causes of neuromuscular weakness.

- Decreased diaphragmatic pressure generation secondary to dynamic hyperinflation
- Phrenic nerve injury after cardiac surgery (cold induced injury or ischemia)
- Critical illness neuromyopathy (usually in setting of sepsis and multiple organ failure)
- Ventilator induced diaphragmatic dysfunction (VIDD) – muscle atrophy, muscle fiber remodeling, oxidant stress, structural injury
- Acute myopathy (from high dose corticosteroids with or without concomitant neuromuscular blockade)
- Effects of neuromuscular blocking agents (especially in setting of hepatic or renal failure)
- Effects of endocrinopathy (e.g., hypothyroidism, adrenal insufficiency) or malnutrition
- Electrolyte imbalance
- Underlying neuromuscular disease (e.g., Guillain–Barre syndrome, Myasthenia gravis, Amyotrophic lateral sclerosis, etc.)
- Sepsis induced myopathy

mechanisms include muscle atrophy, remodeling of muscle fibers, oxidant-induced stress, and structural injury. This entity differs fundamentally from critical illness neuromyopathy because neuromuscular transmission is preserved. Triggered modes of ventilation such as assist control can attenuate VIDD. It remains to be definitively proven in critically ill patients, primarily because of the numerous confounding factors present in the majority of such patients.

Older studies suggested that respiratory muscle fatigue was an important finding in weaning failure, and manifested as increased respiratory frequency and thoracoabdominal paradox (abnormal inward motion of the abdomen during inspiration). In contrast, others noted that rapid shallow breathing and thoracoabdominal paradox appeared immediately during a spontaneous breathing trial and did not progress during failed weaning. This timing indicates these clinical events are more likely to be a response to increased loading rather than fatigue. This hypothesis was confirmed when it was demonstrated that normal volunteers subjected to high inspiratory loads developed thoracoabdominal paradox in the absence of fatigue [13]. Magnetic stimulation of the phrenic nerve in the cervical region allows for the study of diaphragmatic function during weaning. Using this well validated technique it was demonstrated that patients intolerant of a well-monitored SBT failed to develop evidence for low frequency respiratory muscle fatigue [14]. It must be remembered that patients were carefully observed in this study and returned to full ventilatory support as soon as any signs of weaning intolerance were noted. Although not proven in patients, loaded breathing in animals can injure the respiratory muscles without the development of fatigue.

One approach to determining whether the respiratory system is confronting a potentially fatiguing load is to compute the tension time index (TTI). This index is the product of the respiratory duty cycle (inspiratory time, T_i, divided by the time between each breath, T_{tot}) and the ratio of mean inspiratory pressure required on each breath divided by maximal inspiratory pressure ($TTI = T_i/T_{tot} * P_i/P_{imax}$).

It is known that weaning intolerance is characterized by a tension time index above a threshold value of 0.15, at which respiratory muscle fatigue will invariably ensue in normal patients. Indeed, the time to task failure is equal to $0.1 \ (TTI)^{-3.6}$ [12]. Therefore, if patients confronting such a load are not returned to ventilatory support expeditiously respiratory muscle fatigue will likely develop. The consequences are significant because the respiratory muscles may require more than 24 hours to recover from fatigue [15]. Subsequent weaning trials, undertaken before fatigue reversal, will fail and may subject the respiratory muscles to irreversible structural injury. Fortunately, clinical signs of discontinuation or weaning intolerance appear to precede the development of fatigue, thus serving as an early warning sign to return the patient to full ventilatory support.

3.3.7 Cardiac limitation to weaning

Cardiac disease can cause weaning intolerance via a number of mechanisms. Firstly, increased work of breathing, or the associated release in catecholamines, can cause myocardial ischemia (detected by nuclear technique or continuous EKG [ECG] monitoring). Secondly, the transition from positive pressure ventilation to spontaneous (negative pressure) breathing can increase left ventricular preload and afterload, elevating transmural pulmonary artery occlusion pressure and causing pulmonary edema [16]. Thirdly, patients intolerant of SBTs often fail to appropriately increase cardiac output and stroke volume during the trial [4]. Patients at risk for the latter may demonstrate an elevated BNP (brain natriuretic peptide) [17] or N-terminal pro-BNP [18] prior to the weaning trial or an elevated N-terminal pro-BNP at the end of the trial. In one study, a pre-SBT BNP >275 pg/dl correlated with a longer duration of weaning [18]. A decrease in left ventricular ejection fraction has been observed in COPD patients undergoing T-piece trials, an effect that can be partially offset by the use of pressure support [19]. The stress of weaning is considerabl, as it results in increased levels of plasma insulin, cortisol, and glucose [20]. Lastly, positive fluid balance has been associated with weaning failure [21].

Clinicians should maintain a high index suspicion for cardiac causes limiting weaning, especially in patients with known heart disease, those with risk factors for coronary artery disease, or those in whom other barriers to weaning cannot be identified. Transthoracic or transesophageal echocardiography can be safely performed in intubated patients and can be used to define the presence of systolic dysfunction, diastolic dysfunction, or significant valvular heart disease. Continuous multilead electrocardiography can be performed during weaning trials to identify weaning-related myocardial ischemia. Treatment of volume overload should be with diuretics. Indeed, positive fluid balance has been noted in patients with weaning failure [21]. When ischemia is suspected, beta blockers and nitrates are used to reduce myocardial work and optimize coronary blood flow. Beta-1 selective agents are generally well tolerated in patients with COPD, though the lowest effective dose should be sought. Inhaled anticholinergic agents can be used in instances where increased wheezing results. If necessary, the short acting agent esmolol can be used to assess whether bronchospasm will occur in a patient at risk.

3.3.8   Psychological factors limiting weaning

Psychological factors can limit weaning but the frequency and magnitude of the problem is unknown. Criteria used to indicate weaning intolerance (e.g., agitation, diaphoresis, tachycardia and tachypnea), can also be manifestations of anxiety or psychological distress. Small uncontrolled reports note that biofeedback, relaxation techniques, hypnosis, or therapy for depression (using methylphenidate) can contribute to successful weaning. In one small randomized, controlled trial, relaxation biofeedback using frontalis and respiratory muscle electromyography reduced the duration of mechanical ventilation [22]. Delirium is present in the majority of ventilated patients and its presence is correlated with prolonged duration of intubation. When compared to benzodiazepines, dexmedetomidine (an alpha agonist) was associated with less delirium and shorter time to extubation [23]. Additional randomized controlled trials with agents aimed at preventing or reversing delirium should be available in the near future.

Psychological factors should be considered in patients with underlying psychiatric disease, those with abnormal mental status or when delirium is present. In addition, psychological factors should be considered in patients failing SBTs or weaning when no plausible physiological cause can be identified (e.g., not detectable abnormalities in respiratory mechanics, respiratory muscle function or cardiac function).

3.3.9   Once limiting factors are identified and treated

Once reversible etiologies of weaning intolerance are identified and treated, further efforts to liberate the patient from the ventilator are indicated. The clinician must now decide on which approach to take. How long should the patient rest before undertaking another trial? Because respiratory muscle fatigue does not usually occur during a well-monitored SBT, there is little logic for completely resting the patient on controlled mechanical ventilation with the intent of reversing fatigue. Should the patient undergo daily spontaneous breathing trials? Should the patient undergo a slow reduction in ventilator support until minimal or no support is required? Should these approaches be combined?

3.3.10   Illustrative case continued

The intensive care unit team suspected weaning intolerance was secondary to cardiac causes. In reviewing his records it was noted that the patient had gained 11 liters of fluid since admission. A chest radiograph showed cardiomegaly and small bilateral effusions. During the patient's next SBT (conducted on a T-tube) a continuous electrocardiogram revealed 2 mm ST segment depressions in leads V2 through V4. The changes rapidly resolved with return to full ventilatory support. A brain natruiretic peptide (BNP) level was increased at 500 pg/dl. A subsequent transthoracic echocardiogram revealed a reduced left ventricular ejection fraction of 35%. The patient was started on asprin, metoprolol, lisinopril and topical nitrates. Furosemide was given, resulting in a negative fluid balance over the next 48 hours. A repeat BNP level was recorded at 130 pg/dl. A subsequent two-hour SBT was tolerated and the patient was successfully extubated.

References

1. Epstein, S. (2003) Weaning from ventilatory support, in *Textbook of Pulmonary Diseases* (eds J. Crapo, J. Glassroth, J. Karlinsky *et al.*), Lippincott, Williams & Wilkins, Philidelphia, pp. 1089–1101.
2. Epstein, S.K. (2002) Weaning from mechanical ventilation. *Respir. Care*, **47** (4), 454–466; discussion 466–458.
3. MacIntyre, N.R., Cook, D.J., Ely, E.W., Jr *et al.* (2001) Evidence-based guidelines for weaning and discontinuing ventilatory support: a collective task force facilitated by the American College of Chest Physicians; the American Association for Respiratory Care; and the American College of Critical Care Medicine. *Chest*, **120** (6 Suppl.), 375S–395S.
4. Jubran, A., Mathru, M., Dries, D. *et al.* (1998) Continuous recordings of mixed venous oxygen saturation during weaning from mechanical ventilation and the ramifications thereof. *Am. J. Respir. Crit. Care Med.*, **158** (6), 1763–1769.
5. Brook, A.D., Ahrens, T.S., Schaiff, R. *et al.* (1999) Effect of a nursing-implemented sedation protocol on the duration of mechanical ventilation. *Crit. Care Med.*, **27** (12), 2609–2615.
6. Kress, J.P., Pohlman, A.S., O'Connor, M.F. *et al.* (2000) Daily interruption of sedative infusions in critically ill patients undergoing mechanical ventilation. *N. Engl. J. Med.*, **342** (20), 1471–1477.
7. Del Rosario, N., Sassoon, C.S., Chetty, K.G. *et al.* (1997) Breathing pattern during acute respiratory failure and recovery. *Eur. Respir. J.*, **10** (11), 2560–2565.
8. Jubran, A. and Tobin, M.J. (1997) Pathophysiologic basis of acute respiratory distress in patients who fail a trial of weaning from mechanical ventilation. *Am. J. Respir. Crit. Care Med.*, **155** (3), 906–915.
9. Dhand, R., Duarte, A.G., Jubran, A. *et al.* (1996) Dose-response to bronchodilator delivered by metered-dose inhaler in ventilator-supported patients. *Am. J. Respir. Crit. Care Med.*, **154** (2 Pt 1), 388–393.
10. Ranieri, V.M., Giuliani, R., Cinnella, G. *et al.* (1993) Physiologic effects of positive end-expiratory pressure in patients with chronic obstructive pulmonary disease during acute ventilatory failure and controlled mechanical ventilation. *Am. Rev. Respir. Dis.*, **147** (1), 5–13.
11. De Jonghe, B., Bastuji-Garin, S., Durand, M.C. *et al.* (2007) Respiratory weakness is associated with limb weakness and delayed weaning in critical illness. *Crit. Care Med.*, **35** (9), 2007–2015.
12. Vassilakopoulos, T., Zakynthinos, S. and Roussos, C. (2006) Bench-to-bedside review: weaning failure – should we rest the respiratory muscles with controlled mechanical ventilation? *Crit. Care*, **10** (1), 204.

13. Tobin, M.J., Perez, W., Guenther, S.M. *et al.* (1987) Does rib cage-abdominal paradox signify respiratory muscle fatigue? *J. Appl. Physiol.*, **63** (2), 851–860.
14. Laghi, F., Cattapan, S.E., Jubran, A. *et al.* (2003) Is weaning failure caused by low-frequency fatigue of the diaphragm? *Am. J. Respir. Crit. Care Med.*, **167** (2), 120–127.
15. Laghi, F., D'Alfonso, N. and Tobin, M.J. (1995) Pattern of recovery from diaphragmatic fatigue over 24 hours. *J. Appl. Physiol.*, **79** (2), 539–546.
16. Lemaire, F., Teboul, J.L., Cinotti, L. *et al.* (1988) Acute left ventricular dysfunction during unsuccessful weaning from mechanical ventilation. *Anesthesiology*, **69** (2), 171–179.
17. Mekontso-Dessap, A., de Prost, N., Girou, E. *et al.* (2006) B-type natriuretic peptide and weaning from mechanical ventilation. *Intensive Care Med.*, **32** (10), 1529–1536.
18. Grasso, S., Leone, A., De Michele, M. *et al.* (2007) Use of N-terminal pro-brain natriuretic peptide to detect acute cardiac dysfunction during weaning failure in difficult-to-wean patients with chronic obstructive pulmonary disease. *Crit. Care Med.*, **35** (1), 96–105.
19. Richard, C., Teboul, J.L., Archambaud, F. *et al.* (1994) Left ventricular function during weaning of patients with chronic obstructive pulmonary disease. *Intensive Care Med.*, **20** (3), 181–186.
20. Koksal, G.M., Sayilgan, C., Sen, O. *et al.* (2004) The effects of different weaning modes on the endocrine stress response. *Crit. Care*, **8** (1), R31–R34.
21. Upadya, A., Tilluckdharry, L., Muralidharan, V. *et al.* (2005) Fluid balance and weaning outcomes. *Intensive Care Med.*, **31** (12), 1643–1647.
22. Holliday, J.E. and Hyers, T.M. (1990) The reduction of weaning time from mechanical ventilation using tidal volume and relaxation biofeedback. *Am. Rev. Respir. Dis.*, **141** (5 Pt 1), 1214–1220.
23. Riker, R.R., Shehabi, Y., Bokesch, P.M. *et al.* (2009) Dexmedetomidine vs midazolam for sedation of critically ill patients: a randomized trial. *JAMA*, **301** (5), 489–499.

3.4 Modes used during discontinuation

Scott K. Epstein

Office of Educational Affairs, Tufts University School of Medicine, Boston, MA, USA

3.4.1 Illustrative case

A 48-year-old woman has been intubated for 10 days for severe sepsis manifested as shock, renal failure, and respiratory failure secondary to acute lung injury. After improving and satisfying readiness criteria she has failed spontaneous breathing trials (pressure support 5 cm H_2O) on three consecutive days. Tachypnea and signs of increased work of breathing have characterized each episode. A No. 8 endotracheal tube (8 mm internal diameter) is in place. Ventilator settings have been volume assist control ventilation with FiO_2 0.40, positive end-expiratory pressure (PEEP) 5 cm H_2O, respiratory rate 16 breaths/min and tidal volume 400 ml. A negative inspiratory force (NIF) is only −15 cm H_2O and the frequency tidal volume ratio (f/V_T) is markedly elevated at 175 breaths/min/l. The patient has undergone a thorough evaluation for reversible causes of weaning failure and none have been identified. What approach should be used to try to liberate the patient from mechanical ventilation?

3.4.2 Introduction

Once the reversible factors causing weaning intolerance have been identified and corrected, further efforts to discontinue mechanical ventilation are indicated. One

A Practical Guide to Mechanical Ventilation, First Edition.
Edited by Jonathon D. Truwit and Scott K. Epstein.
© 2011 John Wiley & Sons, Ltd. Published 2011 by John Wiley & Sons, Ltd.

issue is how long to rest a patient after a failed weaning effort. The answer depends on whether respiratory muscle fatigue has occurred. As noted in the previous chapter, respiratory muscle fatigue does not usually occur if there is timely return of the patient to full ventilatory support at the earliest signs of intolerance for a spontaneous breathing trial [1]. Under these circumstances, only a brief period of rest is required before the next attempt at discontinuation. As an example, a large randomized controlled trial found no difference in outcome for patients given multiple daily spontaneous breathing trials and those given a single daily trial [2]. In contrast, if the clinician suspects that respiratory muscle fatigue has complicated a failed spontaneous breathing trial then 24 hours of rest on full support should precede the next weaning effort. This may be the case when there was a delay in returning the patient to ventilatory support or profound signs of respiratory failure or distress occurred during the trial. Suggestive findings may include thoracoabdominal paradox or hypercapnia. An equally relevant consideration is whether or not reversible barriers to weaning remain active. Subjecting a patient with inadequately treated airways disease or active cardiac disease to multiple daily weaning attempts makes little sense and poses substantial risk to the patient. Rather further attempts should await resolution of the barrier to weaning.

3.4.3   Weaning modes (modes of progressive withdrawal)

The clinician must next decide whether to perform another spontaneous breathing trial (SBT) or to more gradually reduce ventilatory support (progressive withdrawal) (Table 3.4.1). The latter approach theoretically slowly shifts work from

Table 3.4.1 Modes of progressive withdrawal.

Mode	Method of decreasing level of ventilator support	Duration of tolerance indicating readiness for liberation
T-piece	Increase as tolerated or increase incrementally	2 h
CPAP, 5 cm H_2O	Increase as tolerated or increase incrementally	2 h
PSV	Decrease PSV level by 2–4 cm H_2O two or more times each day	2–24 h at 5–8 cm H_2O
SIMV	Decrease by 2–4 breaths/min two or more times each day	2–24 h at IMV ≤ 5 breaths/min
SIMV + PSV	Decrease by 2–4 breaths/min two or more times each day followed by decrease PSV level by 2–4 cm H_2O two or more times each day	2–24 h at 5–8 cm H_2O (IMV = 0)

CPAP = constant positive airway pressure; PSV = pressure support ventilation; SIMV = synchronized intermittent mandatory ventilation.

ventilator to patient. It remains unproven whether this process reconditions (or trains) the respiratory muscles. Alternatively, a slower process may provide time needed for recovery as further clinical improvement results in a reduction in respiratory load or an increase in respiratory muscle strength and endurance.

3.4.4 T-piece

In this approach the patient is removed from ventilatory support and allowed to breathe through the endotracheal tube connected to a source of humidified gas. Discrete T-piece trials are undertaken for increasing periods [3]. Each discrete trial is for a predetermined duration of time (e.g., 5, 15, 30, 60 and 120 min), as long as the patient is tolerating the trial based on objective and subjective criteria (Table 3.2.7, Chapter 3.2). The initial trial duration can be selected based on the duration of the original SBT. For example, if the patient failed at 60 minutes, the initial trial will be 60 minutes. Each discrete trial is separated by a variable period of rest on ventilatory support. Progression through the process depends on the successful completion of each step. For example, if the patient tolerates the five-minute trial, the next trial will be for 15 minutes. If the 15-minute trial is tolerated it will be followed by a 30-minute trial. If the 15-minute trial is not tolerated, the subsequent trial will again be for 15 minutes. Once there is tolerance for a trial of sufficient duration (e.g., 120 min) the patient is considered successfully weaned from the ventilator and consideration can shift to decisions about extubation.

Proponents of this approach argue the technique is ideal for reconditioning or training the respiratory muscles, because periods of increasing work are interspersed with respiratory muscle rest. Critics contend that by forcing the patient to pass through each step, weaning is unnecessarily delayed. Therefore, some patients tolerating a five-minute trial, if given the opportunity, will tolerate 120 minutes of spontaneous breathing, thus declaring themselves liberated from the ventilator several days earlier than anticipated. In support of this concept, one study noted that 30% of difficult to wean chronic obstructive pulmonary disease (COPD) patients ventilated for at least two weeks immediately tolerated a prolonged period of unsupported breathing [4]. Therefore, an alternative to the incremental approach is to allow each SBT to be limited by tolerance for the trial (e.g., daily spontaneous breathing trials) rather than using fixed time duration [2]. Once 120 minutes of spontaneous breathing is successfully completed, the patient is effectively discontinued from mechanical ventilation.

3.4.5 Continuous positive airway pressure (CPAP)

Progressive withdrawal can be conducted with continuous positive airway pressure (CPAP) (from zero to 5 cm H_2O) using the same approaches outlined above for T-piece. Progressive withdrawal with CPAP has two potential advantages. It allows the weaning process to occur with the patient connected to the ventilator, and therefore monitoring of the patient is facilitated (e.g., ventilator alarms can alert the clinician to the presence of inadequate or excessive minute ventilation, low tidal volume, or significant tachypnea). In patients with expiratory airflow obstruction, using 5 cm H_2O of CPAP decreases inspiratory work by counterbalancing dynamic hyperinflation and intrinsic PEEP. One disadvantage is that inspiratory work may be required to open demand valves and trigger the ventilator. Using flow triggering (flow-by) helps lessen the work associated with triggering.

3.4.6 Pressure support ventilation (PSV)

With pressure support ventilation (PSV), all breaths are patient triggered and each breath is limited by the clinician-determined pressure level. With PSV the delivered tidal volume depends on the pressure level, patient effort (respiratory drive and respiratory muscle strength), mechanics of the respiratory system and the duration of the breath. The latter is determined by patient effort with cycling from inspiration to expiration dependent on flow – expiration occurs when inspiratory flows falls to a low level (e.g., 5 l/min) or a certain percentage of the peak inspiratory flow (e.g., 25%). With very high levels of pressure support patient effort is minimal. As the pressure support level is decreased patient effort increases incrementally. When using pressure support to wean, the pressure level is initially set at a value that results in an acceptable respiratory rate, often less than 30–35 breaths per minute. Thereafter, one or more times each day the clinician attempts to reduce the pressure support level by 2–4 cm H_2O [2, 3]. If the reduction in pressure support is not accompanied by a significant increase in respiratory rate (e.g., >30–35 breaths/min), or other signs of intolerance, that level is maintained for some period (often 6–24 h). If the patient continues to tolerate the lower level of pressure support, a further reduction of 2–4 cm H_2O is undertaken. If a reduction in pressure support level leads to an unacceptable increase in respiratory rate, or other signs of intolerance, pressure support is increased until the respiratory rate is again less than 30–35 breaths/min. In general, that higher level of pressure support will be maintained for at least 6–24 hours before another attempt at reduction is undertaken. Once the patient tolerates a minimal level of pressure support (e.g., 5–8 cm H_2O) for a given period (e.g., 2–24 h), weaning can be considered successful. Some clinicians will add an additional trial of CPAP or T-piece after the minimal level of pressure support is achieved. At least one investigation suggests that this additional SBT is unnecessary [5].

Proponents of pressure support argue that this mode allows for a more gradual transfer of respiratory load from ventilator to patient. Pressure support assists in overcoming the imposed work of breathing related to the endotracheal tube. By conducting weaning on the ventilator the sophisticated ventilator monitoring system can be used to ensure patient tolerance for the reduction in ventilatory support. Critics of pressure support argue that the degree of unloading offered at any given pressure level is difficult to predict. They further argue that this mode may not provide adequate rest because patients perform some work on every breath.

3.4.7   Intermittent mandatory ventilation (IMV)

In this approach, the mandatory or IMV rate is initially set at a value that results in an acceptable overall respiratory rate, often less than 30–35 breaths/min. Some will start at an IMV rate that is one half of the total respiratory rate observed during assist control ventilation (e.g., prior to weaning) [3]. In fact, IMV is now delivered as synchronized IMV (SIMV) where the ventilator monitors patient effort and assists a set number of breaths per minute. With each assisted breath the patient receives a tidal volume set by the clinician. Any additional breaths are patient triggered and unsupported. This differs substantially from pressure support where every breath is patient initiated and each is supported. One or more times each day the clinician attempts to reduce the IMV rate by 2–4 breaths/min. If the reduction in IMV rate is not accompanied by a significant increase in respiratory rate (e.g., >35 breaths/min), or other signs of intolerance, that machine rate is maintained for some period (often 6–24 h). If the patient continues to tolerate the lower IMV rate, a further reduction of 2–4 breaths/min is undertaken. If a reduction in IMV rate leads to an unacceptable increase in respiratory rate, or other signs of intolerance, the machine rate is increased until the total respiratory rate is again less than 30–35 breaths/min. In general, that higher IMV rate will be maintained for at least 6–24 hours before another attempt at reduction is undertaken. Once the patient is able to tolerate some minimal IMV rate (e.g., 0–4 breaths/min) for a given period (e.g., 2–24 h) weaning is considered to be successful.

Proponents of IMV argue that the stepwise reduction in the number of machine delivered breaths will lead to a proportionate shift in work of breathing from ventilator to patient. The assumption is that patients do all respiratory work on unassisted breaths and little or no work on the assisted, mandatory breaths. In this interpretation, inspiratory muscles contract briefly to trigger the ventilator (assisted breath) but that contraction ceases immediately upon machine delivery of gas. With these assumptions, at an IMV rate of 15 and total respiratory rate of 20 (five unassisted breaths), the patient would do just 25% of total respiratory work. At an IMV rate of 10 and total respiratory rate of 20, the patient would do 50% of total respiratory work. At an IMV rate of five and total respiratory rate of 20, the patient would do 75% of total respiratory work. In fact, elegant physiologic studies clearly demonstrate that this is not the case [6]. As anticipated, at high IMV rates patients do little if any work on assisted breaths, while work of breathing is substantial during the few spontaneous (patient triggered, unassisted) breaths. As the machine rate is decreased, not only is considerable work performed on spontaneous breaths but similar respiratory effort occurs during the assisted ("supported") breaths. Apparently, the neuromuscular apparatus adapts poorly to changing loads because respiratory muscle contraction and electromyographic activity during lower levels of SIMV is similar during both intervening (unsupported) and mandatory (supported) breaths. With this physiologic insight, critics of IMV point out that even at relatively high machine rates patients are forced to do considerable work for long periods.

3.4.8   Combined IMV and pressure support

By adding pressure support to the non-mandatory breaths in IMV it has been demonstrated that work of breathing for both the intervening *and* mandatory breaths decreases when compared to either technique alone [7]. Therefore, this strategy would appear to overcome the limitation of SIMV. In this approach, the mandatory (IMV) rate and pressure support level are initially set at values that result in an acceptable overall respiratory rate, often less than 30–35 breaths/min. One or more times each day the clinician attempts to reduce the IMV rate level by 2–4 breaths/min. If the reduction in IMV rate is not accompanied by a significant increase in respiratory rate (e.g., >35 breaths/min), or other signs of intolerance, that machine rate is maintained for some period (often 6–24 h). If the patient continues to tolerate the lower IMV rate, a further reduction of 2–4 breaths/min is undertaken. If a reduction in IMV rate leads to an unacceptable increase in respiratory rate, the machine rate is increased until the total respiratory rate is again less than 30–35 breaths/min. Alternatively, the IMV rate can be maintained while the pressure support is increased to achieve a respiratory rate less than 30–35 breaths/min. In general, these new ventilator settings will be maintained for at least 6–24 hours before another attempt at reduction is undertaken. Once the patient is able to tolerate an IMV rate of zero, the clinician next reduces PSV level by 2–4 cm H_2O one or more times per day, using the same approach outlined above for pressure support weaning. Once the patient is able to tolerate a minimal level of pressure support (e.g., 5–8 cm H_2O) for a given period (e.g., 2–24 h) they are successfully discontinued from mechanical ventilation.

Proponents of combining SIMV with pressure support argue that the addition of the latter component allows this method to realize the goal of a stepwise, proportional transfer of work of breathing from machine to patient. Critics contend that the need to manipulate two variables (IMV rate and pressure support level) adds needless complexity to the process, with the added steps unnecessarily delaying weaning.

3.4.9   Randomized controlled trials

Relatively few well designed randomized controlled trials (RCTs) comparing different modes of progressive withdrawal (weaning) have been published. Two multicenter RCTs directly compared progressive withdrawal techniques in patients who satisfied readiness criteria but failed to tolerate a two-hour spontaneous breathing trial (Table 3.4.2). Brochard *et al.* found that PSV reduced the duration of weaning, when compared to the combined groups receiving either T-piece or SIMV (5.7 vs. 9.3 days) [3]. In this study, the T-piece method entailed an incremental approach with trials of increasing duration. Esteban and coworkers noted that T-piece shortened the median duration of mechanical ventilation, when compared to PSV or SIMV (three vs. four vs. five days, respectively) [2]. In this study, T-piece was applied in the form of a 120-minute SBT, conducted either once or multiple times daily. These contrasting results are likely related to differences in study design and statistical analysis, rather than a true difference in the effectiveness of the

Table 3.4.2 Comparison of two major randomized controlled trials examining different modes of weaning from mechanical ventilation.

	Study of Brochard *et al.*	Study of Esteban *et al.*
Number of patients screened	456	546
Number of patients randomized	109	130
Duration of mechanical ventilation at randomization	14 days	9 days
Weaning modes tested	Pressure support (PSV) SIMV T-piece (incremental)	Pressure support (PSV) SIMV T-piece (once daily) T-piece (multiple daily)
Protocol for weaning	PSV: ↓ by 2–4 cm H2O, 2×/day SIMV: ↓ by 2–4 breaths/min, 2×/day T-piece: progressively increase to 2 h	PSV: ↓ by 2–4 cm H2O, 2x/day SIMV: ↓ by 2–4 breaths/min, 2×/day T-piece (once): as tolerated up to 2 h T-piece (multiple): T-piece or CPAP 5 cm H2O as tolerated multiple times per day (up to 2 h per trial)
Criteria for successful weaning	PSV: 8 cm H2O for 24 h SIMV: 4 breaths/min for 24 h T-piece: 2 h (1–3 times/24 h)	PSV: 5 cm H2O for 2 h SIMV: 5 breaths/min for 2 h T-piece: 2 h (once)
Primary outcome assessed	Weaning success at 21 days	Weaning success at 14 days
Main results	PSV decreased percentage of patients with weaning failure (23% v. T-piece 43%, SIMV 42%) Shorter mean duration of weaning with PSV (5.7 days) compared to pooled T-piece and SIMV patients (9.3 days)	Weaning failure: Once daily T-piece (29%), Multiple daily T-piece (18%), PSV (38%), SIMV (31%) Shorter median duration of weaning with T-piece, once (3 days) and T-piece, multiple (3 days) compared to PSV (4 days) and SIMV (5 days)

techniques. Although the number of patients subjected to the initial readiness trial was large (approximately 500 patients per study), the number eventually randomized to each "weaning" strategy was small (only 30–40 patients per group). On the other hand, the studies were in agreement in finding that SIMV slows the process of liberation, a finding that is concordant with the aforementioned physiologic investigations. As noted above, this effect can be overcome by adding PSV to the unsupported breaths during SIMV. Indeed, one small RCT of 19 COPD patients noted a trend toward shorter weaning duration with SIMV/PSV compared to SIMV alone [8]. One recent study randomized patients to two-hour daily SBTs with T-piece or PSV and found the latter associated with decreased weaning time, duration of mechanical ventilation, and length of intensive care unit stay [9]. These results must be interpreted cautiously as the study was unblinded, the weaning protocol not explicitly stated and the randomization unequal (150 patients to PSV, 110 patients to T-piece).

In sum, these RCTs indicate that IMV should not be used for progressive withdrawal. Progressive withdrawal using either T-piece (or CPAP) or pressure support is reasonable. Combining IMV and pressure support is likely effective but adds complexity by necessitating the adjustment of two, rather than one, parameters. Based on the Esteban study and the extensive experience with SBTs in determining readiness, an approach incorporating daily 120-minute SBTs may be the optimal method. Although further study is needed, combining daily SBTs with one of the recommended progressive withdrawal strategies is likely to be effective (Table 3.4.3). It must be re-emphasized that whenever a patient fails to tolerate a reduction in ventilatory support, the clinician must reassess for reversible causes of weaning failure.

3.4.10 Computerized weaning

One recent RCT examined the use of a closed loop knowledge-based system compared to usual care [10]. The computer-driven ventilator continuously adjusts the level of pressure support by 2–4 cm H_2O to keep the patient in a "zone of comfort" (defined as a respiratory rate 15–30 bpm; tidal volume above a clinician-set minimal threshold; $PetCO_2$ below a clinician-set maximal threshold). Once a minimal level of PSV is achieved, a SBT is automatically conducted and the physician prompted if the SBT proves successful. Using this design, computer-driven ventilation resulted in decreased duration of weaning and total duration of ventilation without adverse events or increase in the need for reintubation. A subsequent single-center RCT, using the same automated system, found no difference between conventional and computerized weaning [11]. This mode of weaning is currently only available on one ventilator model. Further study is warranted before the approach can be recommended. To date, there is no robust data to indicate that other closed loop modes, such as volume support, volume assured pressure support, and adaptive

Table 3.4.3 Evidence-based recommendation for weaning modes.

Weaning issue	Supporting evidence
Daily SBTs are preferred to slow reductions in ventilatory support. Multiple daily SBTS are reasonable provided there is no clinical evidence of respiratory muscle fatigue. If respiratory muscle fatigue is suspected, 24 h of rest on full ventilatory support should be given before another weaning attempt.	Moderate quality; based on physiologic studies and a large RCT.
Progressive withdrawal of ventilatory support can be carried out with T-piece, pressure support or a combination of pressure support and SIMV. It is unknown if coupling daily SBTs with progressive withdrawal is advantageous.	Moderate quality; based on two large and one small RCT.
Automatic weaning modes deserve further investigation	Moderate quality; based on two RCTs
SIMV alone should not be used for weaning.	High quality; based on two large RCTs and physiologic studies.
NIV can be used to facilitate weaning in select patients with acute on chronic respiratory failure from COPD.	High quality; based on six randomized and several uncontrolled trials.

support ventilation, facilitate the process of weaning compared to the techniques discussed above.

3.4.11 Noninvasive ventilation

Noninvasive ventilation (NIV) effectively treats acute respiratory failure complicating COPD and also benefits select patients with acute hypoxemic failure, including those with acute cardiogenic pulmonary edema. A number of RCTs have explored the use of NIV in patients having trouble weaning from mechanical ventilation. One study examined COPD patients with acute on chronic hypercapnic respiratory failure (mean $PaCO_2 \sim 90$ mm Hg) who failed an initial T-piece trial. Patients were randomized to standard pressure support weaning *or* immediate extubation to NIV (pressure support mode) delivered via a full-face mask and standard intensive care unit ventilator [12]. The NIV group had statistically significant reductions in duration of mechanical ventilation, length of intensive care unit stay, and 60-day mortality. Another investigation of acute on chronic respiratory failure patients found NIV reduced duration of invasive mechanical ventilation, though other outcomes were unchanged [13]. A third investigation randomized patients who had failed three SBTs, 77% of whom had chronic lung disease [14]. NIV was associated with shorter duration of mechanical ventilation, shorter intensive care unit and hospital stay, fewer tracheostomies, higher intensive care unit survival, and a lower incidence of nosocomial pneumonia and septic shock. A meta-analysis that included five of these studies, with 80% of the patients having COPD, found that NIV improved outcome (fewer days on mechanical ventilation, shorter length of stay, less ventilator associated pneumonia and improved survival) [15]. Therefore, NIV can be considered for weaning in a highly select group of patients with acute on chronic lung disease. Important caveats include the following: SBT readiness criteria must be satisfied; extubation criteria must be satisfied (e.g., adequate mental status, effective cough, and manageable volume of respiratory secretions); and the patient must be a good candidate for NIV (able to breath spontaneously for at least 5–10 minutes and not deemed to be a difficult reintubation). The benefits of NIV include a reduction in the acquisition of pneumonia, lower sedation requirements, and better recognition of readiness for extubation, particularly when psychological factors or the imposed work of breathing are contributing to weaning failure. Larger studies, including patients with other forms of respiratory failure and well-defined selection criteria are required before this technique can be generally recommended.

3.4.12 What happens to the patient who cannot be weaned

Approximately 10% of patients undergoing mechanical ventilation for at least 24–48 hours are unable to be successfully weaned during their intensive care unit stay. This may be a result of ongoing critical illness and multi-organ failure, severe pre-existing lung disease, or persistent abnormalities of respiratory function (increased load and decreased respiratory muscle capacity). The vast majority of these patients will undergo a tracheostomy. When stable these patients will typically be transferred to a weaning unit, located either within the acute care hospital, or to a free standing long-term acute care facility. These venues have proven effective at successfully liberating patients from mechanical ventilation. A recent multicenter observational study of >1400 patients found that 50% of such patients were successfully discontinued from the ventilator [16, 17].

3.4.13 Illustrative case continued

The patient was changed to pressure support ventilation with a PSV level of 15 cm H_2O, PEEP 5 cm H_2O and FiO_2 0.40. On these settings her respiratory rate was 22 breaths/min with tidal volume ranging from 420 to 440 ml. Over the next three days the team systematically reduced the PSV level by 2–4 cm H_2O as the patients' respiratory rate remained less than 30 breaths/min. A repeat NIF was improved at –45 cm H_2O and the f/V_T fell to 90 breaths/min/l. The patient then tolerated six hours of PSV 5 cm H_2O and underwent successful extubation.

References

1. Laghi, F., Cattapan, S.E., Jubran, A. *et al.* (2003) Is weaning failure caused by low-frequency fatigue of the diaphragm? *Am. J. Respir. Crit. Care Med.*, **167** (2), 120–127.

2. Esteban, A., Frutos, F., Tobin, M.J. *et al.* (1995) A comparison of four methods of weaning patients from mechanical ventilation. Spanish Lung Failure Collaborative Group. *N. Engl. J. Med.*, **332** (6), 345–350.

3. Brochard, L., Rauss, A., Benito, S. *et al.* (1994) Comparison of three methods of gradual withdrawal from ventilatory support during weaning from mechanical ventilation. *Am. J. Respir. Crit. Care Med.*, **150** (4), 896–903.

4. Vitacca, M., Vianello, A., Colombo, D. *et al.* (2001) Comparison of two methods for weaning patients with chronic obstructive pulmonary disease requiring mechanical ventilation for more than 15 days. *Am. J. Respir. Crit. Care Med.*, **164** (2), 225–230.

5. Koh, Y., Hong, S.B., Lim, C.M. *et al.* (2000) Effect of an additional 1-hour T-piece trial on weaning outcome at minimal pressure support. *J. Crit. Care*, **15** (2), 41–45.

6. Imsand, C., Feihl, F., Perret, C. *et al.* (1994) Regulation of inspiratory neuromuscular output during synchronized intermittent mechanical ventilation. *Anesthesiology*, **80** (1), 13–22.

7. Leung, P., Jubran, A. and Tobin, M.J. (1997) Comparison of assisted ventilator modes on triggering, patient effort, and dyspnea. *Am. J. Respir. Crit. Care Med.*, **155** (6), 1940–1948.

8. Jounieaux, V., Duran, A. and Levi-Valensi, P. (1994) Synchronized intermittent mandatory ventilation with and without pressure support ventilation in weaning patients with COPD from mechanical ventilation. *Chest*, **105** (4), 1204–1210.

9. Matic, I. and Majeric-Kogler, V. (2004) Comparison of pressure support and T-tube weaning from mechanical ventilation: randomized prospective study. *Croat. Med. J.*, **45** (2), 162–166.

10. Lellouche, F., Mancebo, J., Jolliet, P. *et al.* (2006) A multicenter randomized trial of computer-driven protocolized weaning from mechanical ventilation. *Am. J. Respir. Crit. Care Med.*, **174** (8), 894–900.

11. Rose, L., Presneill, J.J., Johnston, L. *et al.* (2008) A randomised, controlled trial of conventional versus automated weaning from mechanical ventilation using SmartCare/PS. *Intensive Care Med.*, **34** (10), 1788–1795.

12. Nava, S., Ambrosino, N., Clini, E. *et al.* (1998) Noninvasive mechanical ventilation in the weaning of patients with respiratory failure due to chronic obstructive pulmonary disease. A randomized, controlled trial. *Ann. Intern. Med.*, **128** (9), 721–728.

13. Girault, C., Daudenthun, I., Chevron, V. *et al.* (1999) Noninvasive ventilation as a systematic extubation and weaning technique in acute-on-chronic respiratory failure: a prospective, randomized controlled study. *Am. J. Respir. Crit. Care Med.*, **160** (1), 86–92.

14. Ferrer, M., Esquinas, A., Arancibia, F. *et al.* (2003) Noninvasive ventilation during persistent weaning failure: a randomized controlled trial. *Am. J. Respir. Crit. Care Med.*, **168** (1), 70–76.

15. Burns, K.E., Adhikari, N.K. and Meade, M.O. (2006) A meta-analysis of noninvasive weaning to facilitate liberation from mechanical ventilation. *Can. J. Anaesth.*, **53** (3), 305–315.

16. Scheinhorn, D.J., Hassenpflug, M.S., Votto, J.J. *et al.* (2007) Post-ICU mechanical ventilation at 23 long-term care hospitals: a multicenter outcomes study. *Chest*, **131** (1), 85–93.

17. Scheinhorn, D.J., Hassenpflug, M.S., Votto, J.J. *et al.* (2007) Ventilator-dependent survivors of catastrophic illness transferred to 23 long-term care hospitals for weaning from prolonged mechanical ventilation. *Chest*, **131** (1), 76–84.

3.5 Extubation

Scott K. Epstein

Office of Educational Affairs, Tufts University School of Medicine, Boston, MA, USA

3.5.1 Illustrative case

E.F. is a 67-year-old woman with chronic obstructive pulmonary disease (COPD) who was intubated eight days ago for severe community-acquired pneumonia. Sputum culture showed mixed flora. She was treated with intravenous methylprednisolone, levofloxacin, and the combination of albuterol and ipratropium delivered via a metered dose inhaler with spacer. She was ventilated using volume assist control ventilation. For the first 72 hours she required continuous intravenous sedation but this was discontinued 48 hours ago and she has become more alert and interactive. At 8 a.m. this morning her physical examination demonstrated the following vital signs: temperature 37, pulse 91, blood pressure 136/67, respiratory rate 24 (machine rate 16), weight 60 kilograms. Lungs revealed fair air entry bilaterally with an inspiratory:expiratory ratio of 1:4 and faint expiratory wheezes. She did not use accessory respiratory muscles to breathe and no thoracoabdominal paradox was noted. Cardiac examination was within normal limits. No cyanosis or edema was noted. Ventilator settings: rate 16 breaths/min, tidal volume 400 ml, PEEP 5 cm H_2O, and FiO_2 0.30. Total minute ventilation on the ventilator was 9.6 l/min. Peak airway pressure was 23 cm H_2O with a plateau pressure of 11 cm H_2O. An arterial

A Practical Guide to Mechanical Ventilation, First Edition.
Edited by Jonathon D. Truwit and Scott K. Epstein.
© 2011 John Wiley & Sons, Ltd. Published 2011 by John Wiley & Sons, Ltd.

blood gas showed a pH of 7.34, $PaCO_2$ 60 mm Hg, and PaO_2 67 mm Hg, consistent with a chronic respiratory acidosis. The chest radiograph showed the No. 7 endotracheal tube to be in good position and mild hyperinflation was noted. A right lower lobe infiltrate was significantly improved from the admission chest X-ray. The patient has just tolerated a 120-minute spontaneous breathing trial on continuous positive airway pressure (CPAP) of 5 cm H_2O. Is the patient ready to undergo extubation? What additional tests should be performed to further determine the risk for extubation failure? How should the endotracheal tube be removed? What is the probability that she will develop respiratory distress after extubation? If she requires reintubation, how may her outcome be affected? What modalities may reduce her risk for developing extubation failure?

3.5.2 Introduction

Once it has been determined that ventilatory support is no longer required, the clinician must then decide whether or not the patient can tolerate removal of the endotracheal tube (e.g., extubation). This decision to extubate is of considerable importance, as both delayed extubation and failed extubation are associated with increased duration of mechanical ventilation and increased mortality. Developing predictive tools and optimizing extubation decisions requires knowledge of the risk factors for, and causes of, extubation failure. The method for removing the tube may be important though this area has been little investigated. Despite applying available predictive tools, approximately 25% of patients develop clinically significant respiratory distress within 48–72 hours of extubation [1]. A proportion of these patients will improve with medical interventions that specifically address the underlying cause of their post-extubation respiratory failure. Another group will improve with the application of noninvasive mechanical ventilation. Approximately 50% of patients do not respond to medical therapy or noninvasive ventilation (NIV) and require reinsertion of an endotracheal tube (reintubation).

3.5.3 Risk factors for extubation failure

The prevalence of extubation failure (usually defined as the need for reintubation), occurring within 24–72 hours of planned extubation, ranges from 2 to 25%, with medical, pediatric, and multidisciplinary intensive care unit (ICU) patients at highest risk [2]. The risk appears to be much lower (e.g., approximately 5%) among cardiothoracic, general surgical, and trauma patients. Certain patient types appear to be at very high risk for extubation failure. For example, some studies indicate that as many as one third of neurological patients fail to tolerate removal of the endotracheal tube [3]. A number of other factors have been identified that appear to be associated with elevated risk for extubation failure (Table 3.5.1) [2]. Although many of these factors are intrinsic to the patient some, such as ICU physician

Table 3.5.1 Risk factors for extubation failure.

- Medical, pediatric, or multidisciplinary ICU patient
- Older age
- Pneumonia as cause for mechanical ventilation
- Higher severity of illness at the time of extubation
- Use of continuous intravenous sedation
- Abnormal mental status, delirium
- Semirecumbent positioning
- Transport out of ICU for procedures
- Decreased physician and nurse staffing in the ICU

staffing and nurse-to-patient ratios, relate more to the process of how care is delivered.

It has already been noted that extubation without testing the patient with a spontaneous breathing trial (SBT) is potentially dangerous, with nearly 40% of such patients failing and requiring reintubation [4]. Previous chapters have discussed the utility of the SBT for determining whether ventilatory support is still required. Because extubation typically follows successful completion of an SBT, the mode and duration of the trial could influence extubation outcome. For example, partial support modes (e.g., CPAP, pressure support) may over-assist the patient, leading to extubation in a patient not yet ready to fully sustain unassisted breathing. In addition, when work imposed by the endotracheal tube or ventilatory circuit is substantial, the pressure support ventilation (PSV) level required to offset the additional load ranges widely and may be difficult to predict. Studies comparing the various SBT modes (T-piece, CPAP, low level pressure support) note little, if any, difference in 48-hour reintubation rates.

The duration of the pre-extubation SBT is potentially important, as too short a trial can result in premature removal of the endotracheal tube and subsequent reintubation. Although two studies suggested extubation after 30 minutes of T-piece or low-level pressure support (7 cm H_2O) is no riskier than after 120 minutes, caution is recommended [5, 6]. These studies looked only at the patient's first SBT and extension of this observation to subsequent SBTs is not warranted.

3.5.4 Causes of extubation failure (Table 3.5.2)

3.5.4.1 Imbalance between respiratory load and capacity

The distinction between discontinuation or weaning failure (inability to tolerate spontaneous breathing free of ventilatory support) and extubation failure (inability to tolerate removal of the translaryngeal tube) has been noted earlier. Nevertheless, the respiratory muscle capacity and load imbalance that frequently characterizes weaning failure may also lead to extubation failure. For example, nearly half of all patients with extubation failure demonstrate hypercapnia, hypoxemia, or signs of

Table 3.5.2 Causes for extubation failure.

- Imbalance between load on the respiratory system (work of breathing) and respiratory muscle capacity
- Cardiac disease
- Upper airway obstruction
- Ineffective cough
- Excess respiratory secretions
- Depressed mental status

---

increased work of breathing. This occurs when the spontaneous breathing trial selected by the clinician proves to be inadequate or inaccurate in assessing whether the patient still requires ventilatory support. This can occur if the SBT duration is too short. For example, a patient extubated after tolerating 60 minutes of a SBT may require reintubation. If the SBT had been extended to 120 minutes, respiratory distress (signs of discontinuation intolerance) would have developed and the patient returned to full ventilatory support without undergoing extubation. In this case, the patient would have been classified as a failure of weaning. Another mechanism is when partial support provides over-assistance, allowing the patient to tolerate the SBT when they would have failed if less support had been provided. Alternatively, the traditional parameters (e.g., respiratory rate, oxygen saturation, blood pressure, heart rate, and blood gases) used to detect tolerance during the SBT may be insensitive in detecting early signs of load–capacity imbalance. Indeed, several recent investigations suggest that more sophisticated analysis of the breathing pattern (measuring the variability from one breath to the next) may be more accurate in detecting load–capacity imbalance [7]. The common theme is that patients are mistakenly identified as no longer requiring ventilatory support and undergo "premature" extubation. Under these conditions, it may be said that weaning failure is manifested as extubation failure.

3.5.4.2 Cardiac disease

The transition from positive to negative intrathoracic pressure occurring when a patient goes from full ventilatory support to spontaneous unsupported breathing may precipitate heart failure. Negative intrathoracic pressure increases both preload and afterload and has been associated with significant elevation of the pulmonary artery occlusion pressure [8]. If the SBT is conducted on partial support, intrathoracic pressure may remain positive during the SBT. When the patient undergoes extubation, there is a rapid shift to the negative intrathoracic pressure associated with spontaneous unassisted breathing, possibly precipitating cardiac failure. Indeed, cardiac-related extubation failure appears more likely to occur when a partial support mode is used to determine readiness for extubation. When a T-piece (or CPAP of 0 cm H_2O) is used during the SBT the unfavorable loading effects of negative intrathoracic pressure occur *prior* to extubation. The patient then manifests signs and symptoms related to cardiac dysfunction during the SBT, leading them to be returned to the ventilator rather than undergoing extubation.

3.5.4.3 *Upper airway obstruction*

Extubation failure can result from upper airway obstruction, an etiology that may be difficult to detect prior to endotracheal tube removal. Injury to the upper airway can occur at the time of extubation, while the endotracheal tube is in place, or at the time of tube removal. Glottic or subglottic narrowing may result from laryngotracheal trauma and can take the form of inflammation, granuloma formation, ulceration, or edema. Such lesions may frequently occur and explain why the work of breathing after extubation may equal or exceed that observed with a T-piece. Subglottic stenosis can result from over-inflation of the endotracheal tube balloon, resulting in ischemic injury to the tracheal mucosa. The risk for such injury increases with the duration of intubation, overly large or excessively mobile endotracheal tubes, excess cuff pressure, tracheal infection, and female gender.

3.5.4.4 *Clearance of respiratory secretions*

Efficient clearance of respiratory secretions depends on a number of factors, including adequate laryngeal function, expiratory muscle function, and effective cough. Laryngeal dysfunction can result from the presence of the nasogastric tube, depressed mental status, or the adverse effects of sedative/hypnotic and narcotic agents. These medications can further negatively impact upper airway protective mechanisms by leading to a depressed mental status. Increased airway secretions can occur secondary to endotracheal tube irritation, non-infectious airway inflammation, lower or upper respiratory tract infection, or aspirated secretions originating from the naso- or oropharynx. Secretions from these latter sources can accumulate between the glottis and the balloon of the endotracheal tube and be difficult to adequately suction.

3.5.4.5 *Cough*

To generate an effective cough the spontaneously breathing patient must take in a large tidal volume and then effectively close the glottis. The expiratory muscles (most prominently the abdominals; rectus abdominus, transverse abdominus, and the obliques) contract against the closed glottis leading to a large increase in intrathoracic pressure. The glottis then opens allowing rapid and turbulent gas flow to escape from the airway. The turbulent nature of the expiratory flow helps in the removal of mucus and secretions from the airway. Therefore, ineffective cough can result from glottic incompetence, expiratory muscle dysfunction, inspiratory muscle weakness, and narcotic administration. Weakening of the tracheal wall (tracheomalacia) resulting from injury related to prolonged intubation also impedes cough as the trachea collapses during the forced expiratory maneuver.

3.5.4.6 Abnormal mental status

A severely depressed mental status typically precludes discontinuation of mechanical ventilation because of significant hypercapnia and respiratory acidosis. Less severe depression of mental status can lead to extubation failure because of an inability to protect the airway. This is especially important when cough is ineffective or when respiratory secretions are abundant. In fact, if cough is adequate and respiratory secretions are not abundant, altered mental status alone only slightly increases the risk for extubation failure [9].

3.5.5 Outcome of extubation

Patients with unnecessarily delayed extubation are at increased risk for pneumonia, experience longer ICU stays, and have higher hospital mortality compared to patients with timely extubation. Therefore, the clinician works to extubate the patient as soon as feasible. The outcome for patients who tolerate extubation for a minimum of 24–72 hours is favorable, with hospital mortality rates generally below 10%. In contrast, ICU and hospital mortality is markedly higher among patients who fail and require reintubation within 24–72 hours after extubation. Extubation failure also prolongs the duration of mechanical ventilation, length of ICU and hospital stay, need for post-acute care hospitalization, the need for tracheostomy, and increases hospital costs. In one study of medical ICU patients, reintubation resulted in 12 additional days on mechanical ventilation, 21 additional days in the ICU, and 30 additional days in hospital [10].

The explanation for the increased mortality with extubation failure may be related to clinical deterioration between the time the endotracheal tube is removed and the eventual re-establishment of ventilatory support. In fact, delayed time to reintubation is associated with increased mortality [11]. The concept is important because it implies that early re-establishment of mechanical support could prevent deterioration and lead to improved outcome. The latter is supported by a prospective follow-up study where the authors found that reducing median time to reintubation (from 21 h in historic controls to 6 h) resulted in lower hospital mortality (from 43% in historic controls to 20%) [12]. In addition, recent studies demonstrated that early use of noninvasive ventilation in patients at increased risk for extubation failure resulted in lower reintubation rates and lower ICU mortality (see below).

3.5.6 Prediction of extubation outcome (Table 3.5.3)

With both delayed extubation and extubation failure associated with poor outcome, the rationale for using tests to better predict extubation outcome is strong. Patients deemed to have *low risk* for extubation failure require only routine post-extubation care and possibly a shorter period of post-extubation ICU observation. Patients at *moderate risk* may be candidates for strategies designed to prevent post-extubation

Table 3.5.3 Parameters used to predict extubation outcome.

1. Weaning parameters applied during, near the end, or after the completion of a spontaneous breathing trial
   - Respiratory frequency, tidal volume, frequency–tidal volume ratio
   - Minute ventilation recovery time
   - Breathing pattern (coefficient of variation, entropy)
2. Parameters that assess airway patency and protection
   - Maximal expiratory pressure
   - Peak expiratory flow rate
   - Cough strength
   - Secretion volume
   - Suctioning frequency
   - Cuff leak test (qualitative, quantitative)
   - Neurologic function (Glasgow Coma Scale, CAM-ICU, following four commands)
3. Other factors
   - Positive fluid balance

respiratory failure (e.g., early noninvasive ventilation). Such patients also merit a longer post-extubation period of surveillance in the ICU with the intent of rapidly detecting respiratory failure, allowing for prompt re-establishment of ventilatory support. Patients at *highest risk* should generally not be extubated. Such patients should be considered for a tracheostomy tube.

The decision to extubate cannot be based solely on routine screening criteria for weaning (e.g., adequate oxygenation, hemodynamic stability), as nearly 40% of these patients require reintubation. As note above, important information is gained by successful completion of an adequate spontaneous breathing trial as 80–95% passing the trial will also tolerate extubation. Unfortunately, routine observation during a successful SBT, including standard assessments of oxygen saturation, blood pressure, heart rate, and respiratory frequency, does not identify patients at increased risk for extubation failure [13].

3.5.6.1 Discontinuation or weaning parameters

In seeking to improve prediction of extubation outcome, and taking into consideration the pathophysiologic basis for weaning failure, investigators have studied the large group of weaning parameters reviewed in Chapter 3.2. Not surprisingly, because of the distinct pathophysiologic basis for extubation failure, these parameters (when measured prior to a SBT) perform poorly in predicting extubation outcome. Higher f/V_T is associated with increased risk for extubation failure but the likelihood ratios indicate that overall probability of success or failure changes only minimally [14]. Measuring parameters (e.g., frequency–tidal volume ratio) at the *end* of a successful SBT (and analyzing the change occurring during the SBT)

Table 3.5.4   Extubation predictors based on etiologies for extubation failure.

Cause of extubation failure	Specific extubation predictors
Upper airway obstruction	• Qualitative cuff leak test • Quantitative cuff leak test
Inadequate cough	• Qualitative assessment of spontaneous or suction catheter induced cough • Inability to cough secretions onto a white card placed a few centimeters from the opening of the endotracheal tube • Peak expiratory flow rate
Excess respiratory secretions	• Quantitative or qualitative assessment of the volume of secretions • Frequency of suctioning required to manage secretions
Abnormal mental status	• Glasgow coma scale score • CAM-ICU to detect delirium • Ability to follow four simple commands (open eyes, follow with eyes, grasp hand, stick out tongue)

may prove more useful in predicting extubation outcome but further study is needed.

Another newly developed test is the minute ventilation recovery time [15]. In this test, the minute ventilation is recorded after the patient is returned to the ventilator at the end of the SBT and compared to the minute ventilation present prior to the start of the SBT (the former is typically greater than the latter). Specifically, it has been noted that patients who take longer to recover to the their pre-SBT minute ventilation are more likely to require reintubation.

Many clinicians routinely obtain an arterial blood gas (ABG) at the end of the SBT. Recent studies indicate that this ABG infrequently informs extubation decision making [16]. This author obtains an ABG when a patient is at risk for hypoventilation (e.g., ongoing sedation, presence of central nervous system pathology, history of central hypoventilation syndrome) to ensure adequate ventilation. On occasion an ABG may clarify that tachypnea at the end of the SBT is not related to true weaning intolerance but rather a result of anxiety. Under these circumstances the ABG may disclose a significant acute respiratory alkalosis. Tests aimed specifically at those factors are likely to prove most useful in predicting extubation outcome (Table 3.5.4).

3.5.6.2   Parameters that assess upper airway patency and the capacity for airway protection

Unlike the decision to allow a patient to breathe spontaneously through an artificial airway, the decision to extubate is influenced by assessment of upper airway

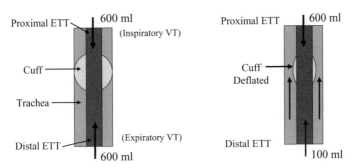

Figure 3.5.1 Schematic of the quantitative cuff leak test. In the left panel, with the cuff inflated, there is no difference between the inspired and expired tidal volume; the cuff leak is zero. In the right panel, with the cuff deflated, the expired tidal volume is much less that the inspiratory tidal volume. In this case, the cuff leak volume is 500 ml (83% of the inspired volume).

patency and the capacity to protect that airway. Upper airway obstruction increases the resistive work of breathing after endotracheal tube removal, often resulting in extubation failure. Assessment of airway patency prior to tube removal is challenging. Mechanical ventilators can measure both inspired and expired tidal volume. The latter value is calculated by analyzing the gas expired *through* the endotracheal tube. With the endotracheal tube cuff fully inflated, the volume of expired tidal gas should equal the amount of inspired tidal volume, because little or no gas leaks around the tube (Figure 3.5.1). If the cuff is fully deflated, and assuming a normally patent upper airway, then the measurable volume of expired tidal gas should be much lower than the inspired tidal volume. In other words, much of the volume leaks or is expired around, rather than through, the endotracheal tube. If the upper airway is abnormally narrow then despite cuff deflation, most of the expired gas returns to the ventilator through the endotracheal tube: there is very little leak. The clinician at the bedside can hear this cuff leak. Absence of an audible air leak after deflation of the endotracheal tube cuff (*qualitative cuff leak test*) has been associated with increased risk for post-extubation stridor, but the subjective nature of the test is a limiting factor.

Another approach is indirect measurement of the volume of gas escaping around the tube during cuff deflation. This *quantitative cuff leak* is calculated by averaging the difference (during six consecutive breaths) between inspiratory and expiratory volume (after balloon deflation) while the patient breathes on volume assist control ventilation. When cuff leak volume is less than 110–130 ml or less than 10–25% of the inspired tidal volume (positive cuff leak test), the risk for post-extubation stridor and reintubation is significantly elevated. Yet, some patients with little leak (positive test) can still be successfully extubated. These false positive test results can result from secretions adhering to the outside of the tube that block gas from escaping around the tube during cuff deflation. This apparent "upper airway obstruction" resolves with removal of the endotracheal tube. A positive test can also occur when exhaled tidal volume is spuriously elevated because of a higher than expected inspiratory tidal volume. The latter may occur when the patient augments machine delivered tidal volume with spontaneous gas inspired around the tube when the cuff is deflated. Delivering inspired tidal volume and then deflating the cuff to allow for expiration to occur can eliminate this confounder.

When performing the cuff leak test the clinician must be careful not to allow accidental unplanned extubation to occur. With cuff deflation the endotracheal tube has increased freedom to move and may induce significant cough as the tip touches the airway wall. Firmly holding on to the tube during the cuff leak test decreases the cough and the risk for unplanned extubation.

The ability to generate an effective cough is crucial for protecting the airway after removal of the endotracheal tube. Expiratory muscle function is essential for effective cough but objective measurements of cough strength are challenging. By attaching either a flow- (pneumotach) or pressure-measuring device to the endotracheal tube, peak cough flow rates and maximal expiratory pressure can be measured, respectively. More commonly clinicians use a subjective measure of cough strength. For example, presence of a strong catheter stimulated or spontaneous cough (e.g., compared to one considered to be absent or weak) is predictive of extubation success.

Several strategies have been employed to assess the burden of respiratory secretions. A qualitative assessment is possible by viewing the flow–volume curve available on many ventilators. A "sawtooth" pattern on the flow–volume curve may indicate the presence of airway secretions, though the volume of secretions cannot be determined with this method. In addition, fluid sloshing around the ventilator tubing can produce the same appearance. Estimates of secretion volume have been used, with the presence of moderate or abundant secretions increasing the relative risk for reintubation compared to patients with no or small amounts of secretions. The reproducibility of this measurement is suspect. Some investigators have assiduously collected all suctioned secretions to generate a quantitative measurement but this technique is cumbersome. One strategy for assessing secretion volume is to determine the frequency of airway suctioning: the relative risk for extubation failure increases for patients requiring endotracheal suctioning more frequently than every two hours. The combination of weak cough *and* moderate to abundant secretion volume appears to be a better predictor of extubation failure than either parameter alone.

3.5.6.3 Assessment of mental status

Brain dysfunction can contribute to extubation failure by causing hypoventilation or by decreasing the patient's capacity to protect the airway. A commonly used method for assessing mental status is the Glasgow Coma Scale (GCS) score (range

3–15). When applied to predicting extubation failure, studies of the GCS have come to conflicting results about the association of a low score with increased risk for reintubation. The reason is that abnormal mental status alone is insufficient to determine extubation risk. For example, in a study of brain injured patients 80% of patients with GCS $\leq$ 8 (including 10/11 with a GCS $\leq$ 4) tolerated extubation [9]. Patients with delirium are at increased risk for extubation failure. Delirium can be assessed using a Confusion Assessment Method adapted for use in the ICU (CAM-ICU) [17]. Others assess mental status based on the patient's capacity to follow four simple commands: open eyes, follow with eyes, grasp hand, stick out tongue. For example, in one study patients unable to complete all four simple tasks were more than four times as likely to require reintubation as those capable of completing all four commands [18].

The greatest risk for extubation failure occurs when abnormal mental status coexists with other risk factors, such as inadequate cough or excessive respiratory secretions. In other words, the capacity of the patient to protect their airway is an integrated function of cough strength, pharyngeal muscle competency, secretion volume, and mental status. Extubation failure is likely to occur when cough is ineffective, a propensity for aspiration is present, secretions are abundant, and encephalopathy is present [18].

3.5.7 Technique of extubation

Although much thought and effort has been devoted to the best approach to wean patients from mechanical ventilation little attention has been given to the method for removing the endotracheal tube. Most authorities agree that the procedure should be carefully explained to the patient prior to removing the tube. All necessary equipment should be at the bedside for immediate use. This includes an apparatus for suctioning both the pharyngeal and tracheal airway, a bag–valve–mask, a mask or nasal cannula to deliver oxygen, apparatus for delivering noninvasive ventilation, equipment for establishing an emergency surgical airway, and an intubation kit.

Airway suctioning is mandatory to remove any residual secretions. Secretions can accumulate on top of the balloon of the endotracheal tube. These subglottic secretions are not accessible to suction catheters placed through the endotracheal tube or into the mouth. Therefore, some clinicians will keep the suction catheter in the endotracheal tube as the cuff is deflated and the tube is removed. This allows subglottic secretions to be removed along with the endotracheal tube. One concern with this technique is that prolonged application of negative pressure (from the suction catheter) will predispose to atelectasis.

The approach used by the author is to initially suction the airway, first with the cuff deflated and then with it reinflated. At this point, using either the bag–valve–mask or the ventilator, a single large tidal volume breath is delivered with the intent of reversing atelectasis. The cuff is then deflated again and the tube removed. A source of oxygen is immediately applied using a mask or nasal cannula. The patient is encouraged to take deep breaths and to cough.

3.5.8 Prevention of extubation failure

Patients deemed to be anything other than low risk for extubation failure should be considered for preventive measures. Patients with excess respiratory secretions can be given antibiotic therapy (if the sputum is purulent) and ipratropium bromide delivered via a metered dose inhaler with spacer. If secretions originate in the nose or sinuses then adding an antihistamine, topical decongestant, and topical anti-inflammatory agent (e.g., nasal corticosteroid) may be useful.

Previous work suggested that corticosteroids, given just prior to extubation, were ineffective in preventing post-extubation upper airway obstruction in adults. More recently, it was found that an injection of methylprednisolone (given 24 h prior to extubation) reduced the risk for post-extubation stridor in patients with a cuff leak volume <25% of inspired tidal volume [19]. Another study of >750 patients ventilated for at least 36 hours found that 80 mg of methylprednisolone given 12 hours prior to extubation virtually eliminated the need for reintubation secondary to laryngeal edema [20].

Swallowing dysfunction and increased risk for aspiration is common in extubated patients. Approximately one third of patients ventilated for 18 or more hours manifest defective airway protective mechanisms. The incidence of swallowing dysfunction increases with more prolonged duration of ventilation and may take a week or more to resolve. The elderly, those with abnormal mental status and patients undergoing prolonged mechanical ventilation are at highest risk for aspiration. Based on these observations it is prudent to keep patients NPO for 12–24 hours after extubation. Patients with one or more of the risk factors noted above should undergo a formal swallowing assessment before being permitted to eat and drink.

Two recently published randomized controlled trials found that immediate post-extubation application of noninvasive ventilation in patients at *highest risk* for extubation failure is effective in preventing reintubation and may reduce mortality. In one study patients were deemed at high risk if one or more the following were present: more than one consecutive failed weaning trial, chronic heart failure, $PaCO_2 > 45$ mm Hg (blood gas drawn immediately after extubation), weak cough, or the presence of other comorbid conditions (COPD, active malignancy, cirrhosis, chronic renal failure, etc.) [21]. A second study used NIV if age >65 years or cardiac failure present or APACHE >12 at the time of extubation [22]. As with the case of using NIV to facilitate weaning, SBT readiness criteria must be satisfied, extubation criteria must be satisfied (e.g., adequate mental status, effective cough, and manageable volume of respiratory secretions), and the patient must be a good candidate for NIV (able to breath spontaneously for at least 5–10 minutes and not deemed to be a difficult reintubation).

3.5.9 Treatment of post-extubation respiratory distress

A major factor in the decision to extubate is consideration of the effectiveness of treatment for extubation failure. When effective therapy for extubation failure does not exist, direct extubation may not be feasible. For example, in a patient unable to protect the airway, and not expected to improve in the near future, the best approach is tracheostomy. If effective post-extubation therapy exists, clinicians may be more aggressive in proceeding with extubation.

Treatment for extubation failure can be divided into specific therapy (aimed at the proximate cause for failure – for example, nebulized racemic epinephrine, intravenous corticosteroids, and heliox for laryngospasm or laryngeal edema; diuretics and nitroglycerin for cardiac ischemia and heart failure; bronchodilators and steroids for obstructive lung disease) and non-specific therapy (e.g., re-establishment of ventilatory support). The invasive nature of reintubation may lead clinicians to overly rely upon medical strategies when treating extubation failure. Yet, data showing higher mortality with longer time to reintubation suggest that clinicians should rapidly assess the response to specific therapy and not hesitate in reintubating patients failing to improve.

With the above considerations in mind and the experience using NIV to facilitate weaning and its prophylactic use in patients at high risk for extubation failure, a strategy of using NIV (usually delivered via a full-face mask) in patients failing extubation has been investigated. As noted in the section on prevention, an advantage of this technique is the potential for early application at the first sign of respiratory distress or deterioration. A number of uncontrolled series suggested that NIV could prevent the need for reintubation in approximately two thirds of patients experiencing extubation failure. In contrast, a single-center study found that NIV did not prevent the need for reintubation when used in a cohort of patients with established post-extubation respiratory failure (overall rate of reintubation 70%) [23]. A multicenter study randomized 221 patients to either standard care or NIV (delivered using a full-face mask and standard ICU ventilator) if they had two or more of the following criteria (within 48 h of extubation): hypercapnia ($PaCO_2 > 45$ mm Hg or a $\geq 20\%$ increase from pre-extubation); clinical signs of increased work of breathing or respiratory muscle fatigue; respiratory rate >25 breaths/min for two consecutive hours; respiratory acidosis (pH < 7.33 with $PaCO_2 > 45$ mm Hg); and hypoxemia ($SaO_2 < 90\%$ or $PaO_2 < 80$ mm Hg on $FiO_2 \geq 0.5$) [1]. No differences were found in need for reintubation, length of ICU or hospital stay. Patients randomized to NIV experienced a higher ICU mortality, perhaps related to the longer time between extubation and reintubation than that experienced by patients randomized to standard post-extubation care. Unfortunately, only 10% of patients had COPD, a group very likely to benefit from NIV. Indeed, a case-control investigation of 30 COPD patients with post-extubation hypercapnic failure, found that noninvasive pressure support reduced the need for reintubation when compared to carefully matched historic controls [24].

In summary, use of NIV should be considered in patients with COPD who experience post-extubation respiratory failure, assuming the patient is a good candidate for noninvasive ventilation. Caution should be applied when using NIV in other patient populations after extubation. If NIV is used it is essential that the patient demonstrates unequivocal evidence of improvement within 1–4 hours of initiation. Factors to be assessed include dyspnea, respiratory rate, use of accessory respiratory muscles, and the $PaCO_2$. In the absence of improvement within four hours, the patient should be considered for reintubation.

3.5.10   Unplanned extubation

Unintended removal of the endotracheal tube (unplanned extubation) can be life threatening, especially when it occurs in a hemodynamically unstable patient or one with persistent severe hypoxemia. Unplanned extubation may occur in up to 3–16% of patients or 1–2 events per every 100 ventilator days. Unplanned extubation can either be accidental or deliberate. In the latter instance, an often agitated, confused, patient grabs the endotracheal tube and intentionally removes it. Patients at highest risk for deliberate unplanned extubation are those requiring sedation or physical restraint. The vast majority of patients with accidental unplanned extubation require immediate reintubation. In contrast, patients with deliberate unplanned extubation, especially if weaning trials have already been initiated, typically do not require reintubation [25].

3.5.11   Illustrative case continued

E.F. underwent a cuff leak test and this was negative: inspired volume 400 ml, expired volume 35 ml, or a cuff leak volume of 365 ml. She required airway suctioning infrequently, every four hours, and demonstrated a strong cough. She was mildly lethargic on examination but easy to arouse. She correctly followed all commands and had a GCS of 15. Based on these criteria the patient underwent planned extubation. She did well for the first 24 hours but gradually developed an increased respiratory rate of 32, use of accessory respiratory muscles and an elevated $PaCO_2$. Noninvasive ventilation was initiated using a full-face mask and bilevel ventilation (IPAP 12 cm H_2O, EPAP 5 cm H_2O). Within 30 minutes she was no longer using accessory respiratory muscles and the respiratory rate decreased to 24. Over the next two days she spent about 70% of the time on NIV. Subsequently, she was weaned to nocturnal NIV and then off completely at the time of transfer to the ward.

References

1. Esteban, A., Frutos-Vivar, F., Ferguson, N.D. *et al.* (2004) Noninvasive positive-pressure ventilation for respiratory failure after extubation. *N. Engl. J. Med.*, **350** (24), 2452–2460.

2. Epstein, S.K. (2002) Decision to extubate. *Intensive Care Med.*, **28** (5), 535–546.
3. Vallverdu, I., Calaf, N., Subirana, M. *et al.* (1998) Clinical characteristics, respiratory functional parameters, and outcome of a two-hour T-piece trial in patients weaning from mechanical ventilation. *Am. J. Respir. Crit. Care Med.*, **158** (6), 1855–1862.
4. Zeggwagh, A.A., Abouqal, R., Madani, N. *et al.* (1999) Weaning from mechanical ventilation: a model for extubation. *Intensive Care Med.*, **25** (10), 1077–1083.
5. Esteban, A., Alia, I., Tobin, M.J. *et al.* (1999) Effect of spontaneous breathing trial duration on outcome of attempts to discontinue mechanical ventilation. Spanish Lung Failure Collaborative Group. *Am. J. Respir. Crit. Care Med.*, **159** (2), 512–518.
6. Perren, A., Domenighetti, G., Mauri, S. *et al.* (2002) Protocol-directed weaning from mechanical ventilation: clinical outcome in patients randomized for a 30-min or 120-min trial with pressure support ventilation. *Intensive Care Med.*, **28** (8), 1058–1063.
7. Wysocki, M., Cracco, C., Teixeira, A. *et al.* (2006) Reduced breathing variability as a predictor of unsuccessful patient separation from mechanical ventilation. *Crit. Care Med.*, **34** (8), 2076–2083.
8. Lemaire, F., Teboul, J.L., Cinotti, L. *et al.* (1988) Acute left ventricular dysfunction during unsuccessful weaning from mechanical ventilation. *Anesthesiology*, **69** (2), 171–179.
9. Coplin, W.M., Pierson, D.J., Cooley, K.D. *et al.* (2000) Implications of extubation delay in brain-injured patients meeting standard weaning criteria. *Am. J. Respir. Crit. Care Med.*, **161** (5), 1530–1536.
10. Epstein, S.K., Ciubotaru, R.L. and Wong, J.B. (1997) Effect of failed extubation on the outcome of mechanical ventilation. *Chest*, **112** (1), 186–192.
11. Epstein, S.K. and Ciubotaru, R.L. (1998) Independent effects of etiology of failure and time to reintubation on outcome for patients failing extubation. *Am. J. Respir. Crit. Care Med.*, **158** (2), 489–493.
12. Epstein, S.K. (2002) Extubation. *Respir. Care*, **47** (4), 483–492; discussion 493–485.
13. Esteban, A., Alia, I., Gordo, F. *et al.* (1997) Extubation outcome after spontaneous breathing trials with T-tube or pressure support ventilation. The Spanish Lung Failure Collaborative Group. *Am. J. Respir. Crit. Care Med.*, **156** (2 Pt 1), 459–465.
14. Frutos-Vivar, F., Ferguson, N.D., Esteban, A. *et al.* (2006) Risk factors for extubation failure in patients following a successful spontaneous breathing trial. *Chest*, **130** (6), 1664–1671.
15. Martinez, A., Seymour, C. and Nam, M. (2003) Minute ventilation recovery time: a predictor of extubation outcome. *Chest*, **123** (4), 1214–1221.
16. Salam, A., Smina, M., Gada, P. *et al.* (2003) The effect of arterial blood gas values on extubation decisions. *Respir. Care*, **48** (11), 1033–1037.
17. Ely, E.W., Shintani, A., Truman, B. *et al.* (2004) Delirium as a predictor of mortality in mechanically ventilated patients in the intensive care unit. *JAMA*, **291** (14), 1753–1762.
18. Salam, A., Tilluckdharry, L., Amoateng-Adjepong, Y. *et al.* (2004) Neurologic status, cough, secretions and extubation outcomes. *Intensive Care Med.*, **30**, 1334–1339.
19. Cheng, K.C., Hou, C.C., Huang, H.C. *et al.* (2006) Intravenous injection of methylprednisolone reduces the incidence of postextubation stridor in intensive care unit patients. *Crit. Care Med.*, **34** (5), 1345–1350.
20. Francois, B., Bellissant, E., Gissot, V. *et al.* (2007) 12-h pretreatment with methylprednisolone versus placebo for prevention of postextubation laryngeal oedema: a randomised double-blind trial. *Lancet*, **369** (9567), 1083–1089.
21. Nava, S., Gregoretti, C., Fanfulla, F. *et al.* (2005) Noninvasive ventilation to prevent respiratory failure after extubation in high-risk patients. *Crit. Care Med.*, **33**, 2465–2470.
22. Ferrer, M., Valencia, M., Nicolas, J.M. *et al.* (2006) Early non-invasive ventilation averts extubation failure in patients at risk. A randomized trial. *Am. J. Respir. Crit. Care Med.*, **173** (2), 164–170.

23. Keenan, S.P., Powers, C., McCormack, D.G. *et al.* (2002) Noninvasive positive-pressure ventilation for postextubation respiratory distress: a randomized controlled trial. *JAMA*, **287** (24), 3238–3244.

24. Hilbert, G., Gruson, D., Portel, L. *et al.* (1998) Noninvasive pressure support ventilation in COPD patients with postextubation hypercapnic respiratory insufficiency. *Eur. Respir. J.*, **11** (6), 1349–1353.

25. Epstein, S.K., Nevins, M.L. and Chung, J. (2000) Effect of unplanned extubation on outcome of mechanical ventilation. *Am. J. Respir. Crit. Care Med.*, **161** (6), 1912–1916.

3.6 Adjuncts to facilitate weaning

Scott K. Epstein[1] and Marjolein de Wit[2]

[1] Office of Educational Affairs, Tufts University School of Medicine, Boston, MA, USA
[2] Division of Pulmonary and Critical Care Medicine, Virginia Commonwealth University, Richmond, VA, USA

3.6.1 Illustrative case

The intensive care unit (ICU) team was consulted on a 59-year-old woman intubated for three days with an exacerbation of chronic obstructive pulmonary disease (COPD). The patient had failed a trial on noninvasive ventilation prior to intubation. To date her ICU course had been uncomplicated. She had been managed on inhaled bronchodilators, intravenous corticosteroids, antibiotics, ranitidine, subcutaneous heparin, and continuous intravenous sedation (propofol and lorazepam). Physical examination revealed a thin female with a generalized decrease in muscle mass (height 170 cm, weight 45 kg) who was intubated and lying in the supine position. The patient was stable with a temperature of 37 °C, blood pressure 125/65, pulse 70 beats/min, and respiratory rate 14 breaths/min, She did not respond to verbal command though moved all four extremities in response to physical stimulus (RASS, Richmond Agitation Sedation Score, −4). The remainder of the neurologic examination was non-focal. Chest examination revealed poor air entry bilaterally, clear lung fields but a markedly prolonged expiratory time. The rest of the examination was unremarkable. Ventilator settings were volume assist control ventilation: FiO_2 0.30, PEEP 5 cm H_2O, rate 14 breaths/min, tidal volume 500. The peak inspiratory pressure was 24 cm H_2O with a plateau pressure of 18 cm H_2O. An arterial

A Practical Guide to Mechanical Ventilation, First Edition.
Edited by Jonathon D. Truwit and Scott K. Epstein.
© 2011 John Wiley & Sons, Ltd. Published 2011 by John Wiley & Sons, Ltd.

blood gas revealed: pH 7.34, $PaCO_2$ 65 mm Hg, PaO_2 69 mm Hg. A chest radiograph showed hyperinflation without infiltrates. The No. 8 endotracheal tube was positioned 3 cm above the carina.

3.6.2   Introduction

The previous chapters have delineated the physiologic barriers to successful liberation from mechanical ventilation. It has been emphasized that identification followed by effective treatment of these barriers is essential to discontinue mechanical ventilation. This chapter focuses on additional strategies used to avoid or reverse barriers to weaning (Table 3.6.1).

3.6.3   Minimizing sedation

The vast majority of patients requiring intubation and mechanical ventilation need some form of sedation, beginning with the intubation itself. When establishing airway access patients typically receive a short acting sedative hypnotic, often followed by a single dose of a neuromuscular blocking agent (e.g., succinylcholine, pancuronium). Rapidly acting agents such as propofol or etomidate are often used, though the latter should not be used because it is associated with adrenal insufficiency. Once intubation is complete ongoing treatment is often necessary to counteract the pain of the endotracheal tube and the frequent discomfort associated with poor patient ventilator interaction. Pain may also result from invasive catheters, endotracheal suction, underlying musculoskeletal disease or prolonged bed rest. Therefore, most patients will require pharmacologic analgesia, with opiates the most commonly used medications (morphine, fentanyl, remifentanil). These agents cause respiratory depression and have the potential to delay weaning from mechanical ventilation.

Table 3.6.1   Potential adjuncts to facilitate weaning from mechanical ventilation.

- Minimizing sedation using a sedation algorithm or daily interruption of sedation[a]
- Glycemic control (glucose <180 mg/dl)[a]
- Pharmacologic treatment for anxiety, depression, and delirium
- Use of Biofeedback strategies
- Nutritional support
- Growth hormone and anabolic steroids
- Increasing hemoglobin (e.g., transfusion, erythropoietin)
- Positioning (elevating the head of the bed to 45°)[b]
- Respiratory muscle training
- Whole body rehabilitation including early mobilization[b]

[a]Supported by well conducted randomized controlled trials.
[b]Randomized controlled trials show a reduction in ventilator associated pneumonia.

Intravenous sedation may be administered as intermittent boluses, continuous infusions, or a combination of the two. The most commonly administered medications are benzodiazepines (lorazepam, midazolam) and propofol. As with opiates, these medications cause respiratory depression. Dexmedetomidine, a selective alpha-2 agonist, appears to not cause significant respiratory depression.

3.6.3.1 Sedation protocols

Studies demonstrate that continuous intravenous sedation is associated with increased duration of mechanical ventilation and length of ICU and hospital stay [1]. Randomized trials show that protocols directed at minimizing the use of continuous sedative infusions shorten the duration of mechanical ventilation [2, 3]. One approach is to have sedation administration driven by a sedation scoring system, such as the Sedation Agitation Score (SAS) [4] or the Richmond Agitation Sedation Score (RASS) [5] (Table 3.6.2). Using this tool, sedation is either increased or decreased to achieve a predetermined level of sedation. The level of sedation sought changes depending on the patient's condition. For example, with ongoing severe respiratory failure and difficulty with oxygenation or ventilation the goal is for the patient to do no respiratory work. In a patient intubated 24 hours ago for severe ARDS, requiring FiO_2 100% and PEEP 15 cm H_2O, the goal might be a RASS of -3 to -5 to ensure that all breaths are machine triggered. The goal is complete cessation of spontaneous respiration, absence of respiratory muscle oxygen consumption, and suppression of expiratory muscle action that may counterbalance the beneficial effects of PEEP. In contrast, when the same patient has improved (e.g., FiO_2 40–50%, PEEP 5–8 cm H_2O) and the emphasis shifts to liberation from the ventilator, the goal might be a RASS of 0 to -2.

Sedation driven by a scoring system can be pursued "informally", that is, the bedside caregiver adjusts medications as they see fit (e.g., every hour, every 2–4 h, etc.) to achieve the desired level of sedation. In contrast, sedation can be given by a protocol where the caregiver targets a level of sedation, at fixed time intervals, using an algorithm that provides drug dosages and frequency of administration. In a study of 321 medical ICU patients ventilated for acute respiratory failure protocol-directed sedation reduced duration of mechanical ventilation, length of intensive care unit and hospital stay, and the need for tracheostomy [2]. Figure 3.6.1 shows the algorithm used in the Medical Respiratory ICU at the Virginia Commonwealth University Medical Center.

Another approach for reducing the amount of intravenous sedation administered is a strategy of daily cessation of sedative infusions. In a randomized controlled trial (RCT) of 128 medical ICU patients, daily cessation of sedation was associated with decreased duration of mechanical ventilation, decreased length of ICU stay, and less need for neurodiagnostic procedures [3]. Subsequent analyses from the same group show that this strategy is safe in patients with coronary artery disease and reduces the number of ICU complications [6, 7]. With this approach sedation

Table 3.6.2 Two commonly used sedation scoring systems.

Sedation Agitation Score (SAS) [4]		Richmond Agitation Sedation Score (RASS) [5]	
Score	Description	Score	Description
7	Dangerous agitation: Pulling at endotracheal tube and catheters, climbing out of bed, striking at staff, thrashing about	+4	Combative: Overtly combatizzve or violent; immediate danger to staff
6	Very agitated: Does not calm despite verbal reassurance, requires physical restraints, biting endotracheal tube	+3	Very agitated: Pulls on/removes tube(s) or catheter(s) or aggressive behavior toward staff
5	Agitated: Anxious or mildly agitated, attempting to sit up, calms down to verbal instruction	+2	Agitated: Frequent non-purposeful movement or patient–ventilator dyssynchrony
4	Calm and cooperative: Calm, awakens easily, follows commands	+1	Restless: Anxious or apprehensive but movements not aggressive or vigorous
3	Sedated: Difficult to arouse, awakens to verbal stimuli or gentle shaking but drifts off again, follows simple commands	0	Alert and Calm
2	Very sedated: Arouses to physical stimuli but does not communicate or follow commands, may have spontaneous movements	−1	Drowsy: Not fully alert, but has sustained (>10s) awakening with eye contact to voice
1	Unarousable: Minimal or no response to noxious stimuli, does not communicate or follow commands	−2	Light sedation: Briefly (<10s) awakens with eye contact to voice
		−3	Moderate sedation: Any movement (but no eye contact) to voice
		−4	Deep sedation: No response to voice, but any movement to physical stimulation
		−5	Unarousable: No response to voice or physical stimulation

is stopped completely and the patient assessed. A patient is deemed "awake" if able to perform three of the following four actions: opens eyes to voice, uses eyes to follow upon command, squeezes hand on request, and sticks out tongue on request. If sedation must be reinstituted it is done so at one half the previous dose [3].

Based on the above studies, mechanically ventilated patients should be managed by either a sedation algorithm or daily interruption of sedation. A randomized controlled trial directly comparing a sedation algorithm to daily interruption found the

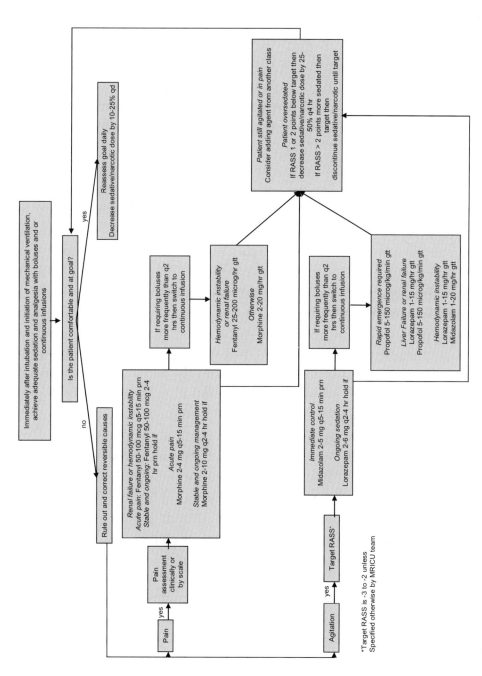

Figure 3.6.1 Sedation algorithm developed for use in the Medical Respiratory Intensive Care Unit at Virginia Commonwealth University Medical Center. (Reproduced with permission from Marjolein de Wit, MD).

latter was associated with greater time on mechanical ventilation and increased length of stay. This study contained many patients with alcohol or substance abuse, suggesting that this population is better managed by protocol titration of sedation [8]. When daily interruption of sedation is used, continuous infusion of propofol appears to be superior to intermittent bolus dosing with lorazepam. The former strategy is associated with decreased days on the ventilator [9]. Further studies are required to determine if one of these strategies is superior in different patient populations. A recent RCT comparing midazolam to dexmedetomidine (an alpha 2 agonist) found the latter was associated with less time on mechanical ventilation [10]. Another study used a "wake up and breathe" strategy by randomizing patients to a daily spontaneous awakening trial (SAT) followed by a spontaneous breathing trial (SBT) compared to a group receiving only the SBT. Those receiving the combined SAT and SBT experienced increased time off of mechanical ventilation, decreased time in coma, decreased length of hospital and ICU stay and improved one year survival. The improved outcome most likely resulted from the patients receiving the SAT being awake and ready for extubation once the SBT was tolerated [11].

3.6.4   Treatment of psychological barriers to weaning including use of biofeedback

Psychological barriers to weaning undoubtedly occur, but the prevalence is unknown. These may result directly from critical illness, underlying psychiatric disease, medications, the ICU environment, or sleep deprivation [12]. Recent work by Ely *et al.* demonstrates a high prevalence of delirium in critically ill mechanically ventilated patients [13]. Delirium is an independent predictor for increased mortality and is associated with more prolonged mechanical ventilation [14]. Delirium may be either hyperactive (agitated) or hypoactive, with the latter more common and difficult to diagnose [15]. Non-pharmacologic therapeutic approaches should be considered, including establishing a normal sleep–wake cycle, ensuring comfortable positioning, and enhancing supportive communication. When pharmacologic intervention proves necessary, butyrophenones (e.g., haloperidol) are most often used to treat agitated delirium. The optimal pharmacologic approach to hypoactive delirium, and the impact on outcome, remains under investigation. Two studies suggest that dexmedetomidine is associated with less delirium than benzodiazepines [10, 16].

Anxiety may manifest as agitation, diaphoresis, and tachypnea, findings that are often thought to indicate physiological weaning intolerance. Pharmacologic treatment for anxiety and agitation, and the associated risks, has been discussed above. Several brief reports suggest that hypnosis, relaxation techniques, or biofeedback may promote successful liberation from the ventilator. Biofeedback may facilitate weaning by decreasing respiratory rate and increasing tidal volume. This is achieved by increasing the patient's voluntary control of breathing, enhancing patient confidence, and decreasing anxiety. In an unblinded randomized controlled trial (patients initiating weaning after a minimum of seven days), the investigators studied relaxation biofeedback in an effort to avoid muscle fatigue and induce anxiolysis [17]. The biofeedback group received several interventions, including feedback on tidal volume (using a computer screen to compare actual tidal volume to a threshold value), computerized visual feedback on frontalis muscle tension (using an electromyogram) and communication (e.g., encouragement). The biofeedback group required 12 fewer days of mechanical ventilation but the study's numerous methodologic issues raise questions about external validity of the results.

Depression is also common in ICU patients and may hinder efforts to wean from mechanical ventilation. Traditional antidepressants have a slow onset of action, but uncontrolled reports suggest that the rapid-onset psychostimulant, methylphenidate, may facilitate liberation from the ventilator.

3.6.5 Nutritional support

Malnutrition is common in advanced cardiac and respiratory disease, malignancy, and immunosuppressed states and is exacerbated by the catabolic effects of critical illness [18]. Malnourished patients may demonstrate abnormal control of breathing, reduced respiratory muscle strength and endurance, and increased risk for infection. Indeed, malnutrition has been associated with decreased weaning success.

Nutritional support improves nutritional status but it is unclear whether nutritional support improves outcome for critically ill mechanically ventilated patients [18]. Much of this debate revolves around the issue of whether certain nutritional preparations have specific therapeutic benefits in critical illness (e.g., omega-3 fatty acids, supplementation with glutamine or arginine). The logic of treating patients with pre-existing malnutrition or those who experience more prolonged critical illness is compelling though strong supporting evidence is lacking. Similarly, clear evidence is lacking that earlier institution of nutritional support is superior to later intervention. In general, it is reasonable to start nutrition early in patients with pre-existing malnutrition who will be unable to have adequate oral intake for at least 5–7 days. For those without malnutrition some recommend early nutrition if inadequate oral intake is expected to last for more than one week [19]. Enteral nutrition appears to be as effective as parenteral strategies and is associated with fewer side effects [18]. That said, interruptions in feeding are common in ventilated patients receiving enteral nutrition. These interruptions, often resulting from mechanical problems related to small bore tubes and high residual volumes, may substantially limit caloric intake [20]. A strategy of frequent measurement of gastric residual volumes and use of prokinetic agents can improve the tolerance of early nutrition [21].

Does nutritional support improve weaning success? High fat, low carbohydrate diets (20–40% of calories supplied as fat) have the potential to reduce the respiratory quotient (VCO_2/VO_2) and therefore the amount of minute ventilation required to achieve a given $PaCO_2$. The resulting decrease in respiratory load could prove beneficial in patients with limited ventilatory reserve. Two small, randomized controlled trials, totaling just 52 ICU patients, compared the response to isocaloric enteral formulae. In one study the high fat, low calorie formula was associated with a significant decrease in $PaCO_2$ and shorter time to successful weaning. In the other, a reduction in respiratory quotient did not translate into an improvement in weaning success [22]. A meta-analysis showed no improvement in weaning when comparing parenteral nutrition to no nutrition [23].

Over-feeding is a risk of nutritional support. When excess calories are supplied the respiratory quotient and the amount of carbon dioxide produced rise significantly and the patient must confront an increased ventilatory load. Ideally, caloric intake should be matched closely to energy expenditure but exact measurements are difficult to make. A common approach is to administer approximately 25 kcal/kg per day.

3.6.6   Growth hormone and anabolic steroids

Critical illness is characterized by a catabolic state. The associated structural neuromuscular abnormalities (including respiratory muscles) have led investigators to study whether growth hormone or anabolic steroids can improve weaning outcome. One randomized controlled trial found no difference in duration of weaning or likelihood of weaning success when comparing growth hormone to placebo [24]. Of great concern is two large randomized controlled trials that reported an increase in mortality in critically ill patients receiving growth hormone [25]. A recent randomized, double-blind, placebo-controlled trial compared oxandrolone, an anabolic steroid, to placebo in surgical or trauma patients requiring >7 days of ventilation. Oxandrolone was associated with *increased* duration of mechanical ventilation [26]. Based on the above studies, neither growth hormone nor anabolic steroids can be recommended as adjuncts to weaning.

3.6.7   Strategies for increasing hemoglobin

Many randomized controlled studies require the absence of anemia (usually defined as a hemoglobin >10 mg/dl) as one criterion for spontaneous breathing trial readiness. During weaning from mechanical ventilation the respiratory muscles consume a considerable amount of oxygen. Weaning failure is associated with an inability to adequately increase oxygen delivery [27]. Hemoglobin is a major determinant of oxygen content so increasing this parameter has the potential to increase oxygen delivery to the respiratory muscles and may increase weaning success. Small observational studies of COPD patients suggest potential benefit from transfusion in terms of weaning success. A large multicenter trial randomized critically ill patients to liberal (goal hemoglobin 10–12) or restrictive transfusion (goal hemoglobin 7–9) strategies [28]. In a post-hoc analysis the investigators found no different in weaning success despite markedly different hemoglobin levels in the groups [29]. A subsequent study found no difference in weaning outcomes when comparing erythropoetin to placebo in critically ill patients [30]. So at present there is no evidence that increasing hemoglobin above a level of 7–9 mg/dl improves weaning outcomes.

3.6.8 Glycemic control

Hyperglycemia is a common complication of critical illness and has been associated with adverse outcomes, including critical illness neuromyopathy, a condition associated with delayed weaning and prolonged mechanical ventilation. Therefore, investigators have examined whether strict glycemic control can improve outcome. Two large randomized controlled trials demonstrated that keeping glucose between 80 and 110 mg/dl using insulin infusions was associated with accelerated weaning from mechanical ventilation compared to keeping the glucose between 180 and 210 mg/dl [31, 32]. The same investigators have demonstrated that strict glycemic control reduces the incidence of critical illness neuromyopathy, which may explain the reduction in prolonged mechanical ventilation [33]. The potential impact is important as nearly 50% of patients with sepsis, multi-organ failure or prolonged mechanical ventilation have evidence for critical illness neuromyopathy [34]. Strict glycemic control does increase the risk for hypoglycemia, though the impact on patient outcome has not been well defined. The most recent large randomized trial, including over 6000 patients, found that tight glycemic control (81–108 mg/dl) was associated with more severe hypoglycemia and higher mortality than conventional glycemic control (less than 180 mg/dl) [35]. A meta-analysis suggested possible benefit of tight glycemic control, but only in surgical ICU patients [36].

3.6.9 Positioning

Changing body position can benefit the mechanically ventilated patient. The majority of patients with acute lung injury demonstrate an improvement in PaO_2 when turned from the supine to the prone position. Patients with unilateral lung disease will have an increase PaO_2 when the non-affected lung is placed in the dependent position. Though oxygenation improves in these situations an impact on weaning has not been demonstrated.

Ventilator-associated pneumonia contributes to increased mortality and to increased duration of mechanical ventilation. One mechanism is gastric bacterial colonization followed by aspiration of organisms into the lung. Elevating the head of the bed to 45° reduces this movement of organisms and reduces the incidence of ventilator-associated pneumonia [37]. Although not directly studied this simple and safe maneuver (assuming hemodynamic and neurologic stability) has the potential to shorten the duration of mechanical ventilation.

3.6.10 Respiratory muscle training

Patients who fail weaning from mechanical ventilation often have respiratory muscle weakness when assessed using a negative inspiratory force (NIF) maneuver [38]. Inspiratory muscle endurance is also decreased and worsens with duration of mechanical ventilation [39]. Therefore, clinicians must avoid or correct factors that contribute to respiratory muscle weakness. For example, electrolyte abnormalities (hypokalemia, hypomagnesemia, hypophosphatemia) must be corrected, adequate nutrition delivered (see above), and medications scrutinized (minimizing use of neuromuscular blocking agents and corticosteroids). In addition, strategies for improving respiratory muscle strength and endurance have the potential to improve weaning success. Studies demonstrate improvement in muscle strength, as assessed by NIF, when comparing values measured at the time of weaning failure to those determined when weaning is successful [38]. Whether this reflects a training effect or improvement related to resolution of inflammation and the catabolic state, or improved nutritional status, is uncertain.

Investigators have used inspiratory muscle training techniques to facilitate weaning [40, 41]. One approach uses an adjustable resistive inspiratory training device attached to the endotracheal tube. In observational studies, this approach is associated with improved maximal inspiratory pressure and vital capacity. When applied to patients who have failed weaning, weaning success has been observed. Unfortunately, the only randomized controlled trial showed no effect on weaning outcome when inspiratory muscle training was performed using an insensitive inspiratory trigger threshold to induce inspiratory overload [42]. Therefore, at the present time routine use of respiratory muscle training for difficult to wean patients cannot be recommended.

3.6.11 Whole body rehabilitation

Whole body rehabilitation is extensively employed in difficult to wean mechanically ventilated tracheostomized patients transferred to long-term acute care facilities. Such programs typically focus on both upper and lower extremity training to address the profound weakness present in this cohort. Inspiratory muscle training, using a threshold resistor device, is used to increase respiratory muscle strength and endurance. Rehabilitation is often facilitated by using a portable ventilator until a patient can sustain prolonged periods of spontaneous breathing. Observational studies suggest that this approach shortens the time to weaning success in the long-term setting [43].

There is a nascent literature on early mobilization of mechanically ventilated ICU patients [44, 45]. Interventions include passive and active range of motion, maintaining upright trunk posture and ambulation. Goals of mobilization include improving neuromuscular function, decreasing complications (including pulmonary), and increasing psychological well-being. Such benefits could facilitate weaning and shorten the duration of mechanical ventilation. A recent RCT found that whole body rehabilitation (physical and occupational therapy plus daily interruption of sedation) was well tolerated and safe. This strategy resulted in improved functional outcomes and increased ventilator free days [46].

3.6.12   Illustrative case continued

The ICU team recommended that the head of the bed be elevated to 45°. The patient was changed to the unit's sedation algorithm designed to minimize sedation and targeted a RASS of 0 to −2. Enteral nutrition was initiated (high fat, low carbohydrate formula) with a goal of 25 kcal/kg/day. A glycemic control protocol was instituted and insulin was required to keep the serum glucose level less than 180 mg/dl. By Day 8 the patient was more awake and alert and began daily spontaneous breathing trials on CPAP 5 cm H_2O. On Day 10 a two-hour SBT was tolerated and the patient was successfully extubated.

References

1. Kollef, M.H., Levy, N.T., Ahrens, T.S. *et al.* (1998) The use of continuous i.v. sedation is associated with prolongation of mechanical ventilation. *Chest*, **114** (2), 541–548.
2. Brook, A.D., Ahrens, T.S., Schaiff, R. *et al.* (1999) Effect of a nursing-implemented sedation protocol on the duration of mechanical ventilation. *Crit. Care Med.*, **27** (12), 2609–2615.
3. Kress, J.P., Pohlman, A.S., O'Connor, M.F. *et al.* (2000) Daily interruption of sedative infusions in critically ill patients undergoing mechanical ventilation. *N. Engl. J. Med.*, **342** (20), 1471–1477.
4. Riker, R.R., Picard, J.T. and Fraser, G.L. (1999) Prospective evaluation of the Sedation-Agitation Scale for adult critically ill patients. *Crit. Care Med.*, **27** (7), 1325–1329.
5. Sessler, C.N., Gosnell, M.S., Grap, M.J. *et al.* (2002) The Richmond Agitation-Sedation Scale: validity and reliability in adult intensive care unit patients. *Am. J. Respir. Crit. Care Med.*, **166** (10), 1338–1344.
6. Schweickert, W.D., Gehlbach, B.K., Pohlman, A.S. *et al.* (2004) Daily interruption of sedative infusions and complications of critical illness in mechanically ventilated patients. *Crit. Care Med.*, **32** (6), 1272–1276.
7. Kress, J.P., Vinayak, A.G., Levitt, J. *et al.* (2007) Daily sedative interruption in mechanically ventilated patients at risk for coronary artery disease. *Crit. Care Med.*, **35** (2), 365–371.
8. de Wit, M., Gennings, C., Jenvey, W.I. *et al.* (2008) Randomized trial comparing daily interruption of sedation and nursing-implemented sedation algorithm in medical intensive care unit patients. *Crit. Care*, **12** (3), R70.
9. Carson, S.S., Kress, J.P., Rodgers, J.E. *et al.* (2006) A randomized trial of intermittent lorazepam versus propofol with daily interruption in mechanically ventilated patients. *Crit. Care Med.*, **34** (5), 1326–1332.
10. Riker, R.R., Shehabi, Y., Bokesch, P.M. *et al.* (2009) Dexmedetomidine vs midazolam for sedation of critically ill patients: a randomized trial. *JAMA*, **301** (5), 489–499.
11. Girard, T.D., Kress, J.P., Fuchs, B.D. *et al.* (2008) Efficacy and safety of a paired sedation and ventilator weaning protocol for mechanically ventilated patients in intensive care

(Awakening and Breathing Controlled trial): a randomised controlled trial. *Lancet*, **371** (9607), 126–134.

12. MacIntyre, N.R. (1995) Psychological factors in weaning from mechanical ventilatory support. *Respir. Care*, **40** (3), 277–281.

13. Ely, E.W., Gautam, S., Margolin, R. *et al.* (2001) The impact of delirium in the intensive care unit on hospital length of stay. *Intensive Care Med.*, **27** (12), 1892–1900.

14. Ely, E.W., Shintani, A., Truman, B. *et al.* (2004) Delirium as a predictor of mortality in mechanically ventilated patients in the intensive care unit. *JAMA*, **291** (14), 1753–1762.

15. Pandharipande, P., Cotton, B.A., Shintani, A. *et al.* (2007) Motoric subtypes of delirium in mechanically ventilated surgical and trauma intensive care unit patients. *Intensive Care Med.*, **33** (10), 1726–1731.

16. Pandharipande, P.P., Pun, B.T., Herr, D.L. *et al.* (2007) Effect of sedation with dexmedetomidine vs lorazepam on acute brain dysfunction in mechanically ventilated patients: the MENDS randomized controlled trial. *JAMA*, **298** (22), 2644–2653.

17. Holliday, J.E. and Hyers, T.M. (1990) The reduction of weaning time from mechanical ventilation using tidal volume and relaxation biofeedback. *Am. Rev. Respir. Dis.*, **141** (5 Pt 1), 1214–1220.

18. Heyland, D.K., Dhaliwal, R., Drover, J.W. *et al.* (2003) Canadian clinical practice guidelines for nutrition support in mechanically ventilated, critically ill adult patients. *J. Parenter. Enteral. Nutr.*, **27** (5), 355–373.

19. Roberts, S.R., Kennerly, D.A., Keane, D. *et al.* (2003) Nutrition support in the intensive care unit. Adequacy, timeliness, and outcomes. *Crit. Care Nurse*, **23** (6), 49–57.

20. O'Meara, D., Mireles-Cabodevila, E., Frame, F. *et al.* (2008) Evaluation of delivery of enteral nutrition in critically ill patients receiving mechanical ventilation. *Am. J. Crit. Care*, **17** (1), 53–61.

21. Desachy, A., Clavel, M., Vuagnat, A. *et al.* (2008) Initial efficacy and tolerability of early enteral nutrition with immediate or gradual introduction in intubated patients. *Intensive Care Med.*, **34** (6), 1054–1059.

22. Cook, D., Meade, M., Guyatt, G. *et al.* (2001) Trials of miscellaneous interventions to wean from mechanical ventilation. *Chest*, **120** (6 Suppl.), 438S–444S.

23. Koretz, R.L., Lipman, T.O. and Klein, S. (2001) AGA technical review on parenteral nutrition. *Gastroenterology*, **121** (4), 970–1001.

24. Pichard, C., Kyle, U., Chevrolet, J.C. *et al.* (1996) Lack of effects of recombinant growth hormone on muscle function in patients requiring prolonged mechanical ventilation: a prospective, randomized, controlled study. *Crit. Care Med.*, **24** (3), 403–413.

25. Takala, J., Ruokonen, E., Webster, N.R. *et al.* (1999) Increased mortality associated with growth hormone treatment in critically ill adults. *N. Engl. J. Med.*, **341** (11), 785–792.

26. Bulger, E.M., Jurkovich, G.J., Farver, C.L. *et al.* (2004) Oxandrolone does not improve outcome of ventilator dependent surgical patients. *Ann. Surg.*, **240** (3), 472–478; discussion 478–480.

27. Jubran, A., Mathru, M., Dries, D. *et al.* (1998) Continuous recordings of mixed venous oxygen saturation during weaning from mechanical ventilation and the ramifications thereof. *Am. J. Respir. Crit. Care Med.*, **158** (6), 1763–1769.

28. Hebert, P.C., Wells, G., Blajchman, M.A. *et al.* (1999) A multicenter, randomized, controlled clinical trial of transfusion requirements in critical care. Transfusion Requirements in Critical Care Investigators, Canadian Critical Care Trials Group. *N. Engl. J. Med.*, **340** (6), 409–417.

29. Hebert, P.C., Blajchman, M.A., Cook, D.J. *et al.* (2001) Do blood transfusions improve outcomes related to mechanical ventilation? *Chest*, **119** (6), 1850–1857.

30. Corwin, H.L., Gettinger, A., Pearl, R.G. *et al.* (2002) Efficacy of recombinant human eryth-ropoietin in critically ill patients: a randomized controlled trial. *JAMA*, **288** (22), 2827–2835.
31. Van den Berghe, G., Wouters, P., Weekers, F. *et al.* (2001) Intensive insulin therapy in the critically ill patients. *N. Engl. J. Med.*, **345** (19), 1359–1367.
32. Van den Berghe, G., Wilmer, A., Hermans, G. *et al.* (2006) Intensive insulin therapy in the medical ICU. *N. Engl. J. Med.*, **354** (5), 449–461.
33. Hermans, G., Wilmer, A., Meersseman, W. *et al.* (2007) Impact of intensive insulin therapy on neuromuscular complications and ventilator dependency in the medical intensive care unit. *Am. J. Respir. Crit. Care Med.*, **175** (5), 480–489.
34. Stevens, R.D., Dowdy, D.W., Michaels, R.K. *et al.* (2007) Neuromuscular dysfunction acquired in critical illness: a systematic review. *Intensive Care Med.*, **33** (11), 1876–1891.
35. Finfer, S., Chittock, D.R., Su, S.Y. *et al.* (2009) Intensive versus conventional glucose control in critically ill patients. *N. Engl. J. Med.*, **360** (13), 1283–1297.
36. Griesdale, D.E., de Souza, R.J., van Dam, R.M. *et al.* (2009) Intensive insulin therapy and mortality among critically ill patients: a meta-analysis including NICE-SUGAR study data. *CMAJ*, **180** (8), 821–827.
37. Drakulovic, M.B., Torres, A., Bauer, T.T. *et al.* (1999) Supine body position as a risk factor for nosocomial pneumonia in mechanically ventilated patients: a randomised trial. *Lancet*, **354** (9193), 1851–1858.
38. Vassilakopoulos, T., Zakynthinos, S. and Roussos, C. (1998) The tension-time index and the frequency/tidal volume ratio are the major pathophysiologic determinants of weaning failure and success. *Am. J. Respir. Crit. Care Med.*, **158** (2), 378–385.
39. Chang, A.T., Boots, R.J., Brown, M.G. *et al.* (2005) Reduced inspiratory muscle endurance following successful weaning from prolonged mechanical ventilation. *Chest*, **128** (2), 553–559.
40. Aldrich, T.K., Karpel, J.P., Uhrlass, R.M. *et al.* (1989) Weaning from mechanical ventilation: adjunctive use of inspiratory muscle resistive training. *Crit. Care Med.*, **17** (2), 143–147.
41. Martin, A.D., Davenport, P.D., Franceschi, A.C. *et al.* (2002) Use of inspiratory muscle strength training to facilitate ventilator weaning: a series of 10 consecutive patients. *Chest*, **122** (1), 192–196.
42. Caruso, P., Denari, S.D., Ruiz, S.A. *et al.* (2005) Inspiratory muscle training is ineffective in mechanically ventilated critically ill patients. *Clinics*, **60** (6), 479–484.
43. Martin, U.J., Hincapie, L., Nimchuk, M. *et al.* (2005) Impact of whole-body rehabilitation in patients receiving chronic mechanical ventilation. *Crit. Care Med.*, **33** (10), 2259–2265.
44. Morris, P.E. and Herridge, M.S. (2007) Early intensive care unit mobility: future directions. *Crit. Care Clin*, **23** (1), 97–110.
45. Bailey, P., Thomsen, G.E., Spuhler, V.J. *et al.* (2007) Early activity is feasible and safe in respiratory failure patients. *Crit. Care Med.*, **35** (1), 139–145.
46. Schweickert, W.D., Pohlman, M.C., Pohlman, A.S. *et al.* (2009) Early physical and occupational therapy in mechanically ventilated, critically ill patients: a randomized controlled trial. *Lancet*, **373** (9678), 1874–1882.

3.7 Tracheostomy

Scott K. Epstein

Office of Educational Affairs, Tufts University School of Medicine, Boston, MA, USA

3.7.1 Illustrative case

A 45-year-old woman with acute respiratory failure and multisystem organ dysfunction had been intubated for 10 days. At the time of admission she required vasopressors for shock, had a creatinine of 3 mg/dl, and an APACHE II score of 30. For the first 36 hours she required neuromuscular blockade and heavy sedation. By Day 7 she no longer required vasopressors, the creatinine had improved to 0.9 mg/dl and she was awake and alert needing only occasional sedation. Ventilator settings were volume assist control ventilation with respiratory rate of 16, tidal volume of 400 ml, FiO_2 of 0.4 and PEEP 5 cm H_2O. Some spontaneous respiratory efforts were present but these inconsistently triggered a ventilator-assisted breath. For the last four days she has failed spontaneous breathing trials (PSV 7 cm H_2O), not lasting longer than five minutes, with a respiratory rate >40 and notable use of accessory respiratory muscles to breathe. A negative inspiratory force was −15 cm H_2O. Careful neurologic examination was consistent with critical illness neuromyopathy. On rounds the intensive care unit (ICU) nurse asked if the team should consider placing a tracheostomy tube.

A Practical Guide to Mechanical Ventilation, First Edition.
Edited by Jonathon D. Truwit and Scott K. Epstein.
© 2011 John Wiley & Sons, Ltd. Published 2011 by John Wiley & Sons, Ltd.

3.7.2 Introduction

Tracheostomy refers to the placement of a tube through the anterior neck directly into the trachea. Because the trachea is easily accessible at the bedside it provides ready access for emergency airway cannulation (e.g., in the setting of acute upper airway obstruction) and for chronic airway access after laryngeal surgery. More commonly, in the ICU setting, tracheostomy tubes are placed to allow removal of a translaryngeal endotracheal tube. Indeed, tracheostomy is a frequently performed procedure in critically ill patients. In general, in ICU patients with acute respiratory failure, 10% of patients may require tracheostomy. This number rises when examining patients in a trauma or neurologic ICU or those who require reintubation. The procedure can be performed surgically (in an operating room or at the bedside) or percutaneously at the bedside. Improvements in technique have resulted in a relatively low complication rate. Analysis of observational (retrospective and prospective) studies and randomized trials comparing either tracheostomy and translaryngeal intubation or those comparing early versus late tracheostomy does not yield a definitive answer on whether tracheostomy improves survival [1].

There are a number of possible indications for tracheostomy tube placement in intubated patients with acute respiratory failure (Table 3.7.1). The decision is typically individualized based on specific patient characteristics and wishes. In acute respiratory failure patients the indication is usually failure to wean, failed extubation or prolonged mechanical ventilation. Absolute contra-indications are few, though the risk of the procedure must always be carefully balanced against purported benefits.

Table 3.7.1 Indications and contra-indications for tracheostomy tube placement.

Indications
- Failure to wean from mechanical ventilation
- Repeated extubation failure
- Inability to protect airway or manage secretions in a patient no longer requiring ventilatory support
- Prolonged mechanical ventilation (e.g., >10–21 days)
- Need for stable airway to allow patient transfer to a non-acute ICU setting
- Trauma (severe maxillofacial, laryngeal, tracheal)
- Upper airway obstruction that is not easily or rapidly reversible or is immediately life threatening (large tumors of the aerodigestive tract, edema of tongue, pharynx, and larynx)

Contra-indications
- Soft tissue infection of the neck
- Abnormal anatomy that precludes performing the procedure
- Unstable respiratory failure (refractory hypoxemia or hypercapnia)
- Refractory coagulopathy

3.7.3 Physiologic and non-physiologic benefits of tracheostomy

Tracheostomy tubes have an important effect on respiratory physiology [2]. When analyzing the physiology of tracheostomy tubes comparisons are most appropriately made with the translaryngeal endotracheal tube that will be removed. As with an endotracheal tube, tracheostomy disturbs the normal humidification and warming of inspired air, necessitating the use of heated humidifiers or heat and moisture exchangers. Squamous metaplasia, chronic inflammation, mucosal desiccation and reduced ciliary function result when humidification is inadequate. The presence of an artificial airway increases respiratory secretions, decreases the effectiveness of cough, and hampers effective swallowing predisposing to aspiration of oropharyngeal secretions.

Resistance is directly proportional to tube length and inversely proportional to tube radius raised to the fourth power for laminar flow and to the fifth power for turbulent flow. Therefore, large increases in resistance derive from small reductions in tube radius. Turbulent flow occurs when flow rates are high, when secretions adhere to the inside of the tube, and because of tube curvature. Assuming equivalent internal diameter, the shorter length of the tracheostomy tube should decrease resistance compared to the endotracheal tube. In addition, tracheostomy tubes are more rigid, less likely to be deformed in the upper airway (by being placed below the vocal cords and the rigid structures of the subglottic region), and are easier to keep clean (they more effectively facilitate airway suctioning and removal of secretions) [3]. Although dead space is also lower with tracheostomy the magnitude is quite small. Tracheostomy tubes can also reduce the elastic work of breathing because, with less airways resistance, expiratory flow improves and the tendency to dynamic hyperinflation is reduced. The latter physiologic benefits may explain the improvement in patient ventilator synchrony seen by some investigators [4].

Taken together studies demonstrate modest reductions in work of breathing when the endotracheal tube is removed and replaced by a tracheostomy tube [3, 4]. In patients with marginal respiratory reserve this modest reduction may be clinically relevant and allow for successful liberation from the ventilator. That said, to date no study convincingly demonstrates improved success in difficult to wean patients when comparing tracheostomy to endotracheal tubes [5]. Nevertheless, anecdotally many experts can cite examples of patients who appeared to make sudden weaning progress after placement of a tracheostomy tube. Indeed, in one long-term weaning unit 30% of patients transferred as unweanable were successfully liberated within 48 hours of arrival [6]. Whether this weaning success results from the physiologic benefits described above or is the result of other benefits of tracheostomy is unknown (Table 3.7.2).

There is observational evidence that translaryngeal intubation is an uncomfortable procedure. Maintenance of the translaryngeal airway usually necessitates pharmacologic sedation and analgesia, often delivered continuously and intravenously.

Table 3.7.2   Purported benefits of tracheostomy tubes compared to endotracheal tubes.

- Physiologic
    - $\downarrow$ airways resistance
    - $\downarrow$ work of breathing (resistive and elastic)
    - $\uparrow$ expiratory flow, $\downarrow$ dynamic hyperinflation
    - Improved patient ventilator interaction
- Improved oral care and decreased injury to oral structures (e.g., teeth, tongue)
- Improved airway suctioning
- Improved comfort
- Improved communication (facilitates lip reading or placement of speaking valve)
- $\downarrow$ need for sedation
- More secure airway ($\downarrow$ unplanned or accidental airway removal)
    - Allows for increased patient mobility
    - Allows for earlier and safer transfer out of acute care ICU

The issue is of considerable clinical significance because excessive sedation may delay or limit successful liberation from mechanical ventilation. Indeed, excessive (continuous) intravenous sedation has been associated with prolonged mechanical ventilation and increased length of ICU and hospital stay [7]. In turn, strategies designed to reduce the use of intravenous sedation, employing either a sedation protocol or a strategy of once-daily cessation of sedation, lead to reductions in the duration of mechanical ventilation, length of stay, need for tracheostomy, and complications [8, 9].

Some experts recommend tracheostomy when the discomfort associated with translaryngeal intubation appears to contribute to the need for excess sedation [10]. In one investigation, patients undergoing percutaneous dilational tracheostomy required less intravenous sedative and narcotic administration after the procedure [11]. In contrast, a large single center retrospective study found no such benefit [12]. It is not known if sedation requirements change after surgical tracheostomy.

When the patient tolerates periods of spontaneous breathing enhanced communication becomes possible. Deflating the tracheostomy cuff and placing a one-way valve on the proximal end of the tube facilitates speech. The patient inspires through the tube but during expiration the valve closes forcing air across the vocal cords. Failure to tolerate this procedure often indicates the presence of upper airway obstruction.

3.7.4   Timing of tracheostomy

The optimal timing of tracheostomy is controversial and the standard of care has shifted over the years. Initially, tracheostomy tubes were usually considered once a patient required 21 days of translaryngeal intubation. Subsequently, an anticipatory approach was recommended where a key assessment occurred at Day 7 of mechanical ventilation [10]. In patients likely to be liberated within the next week, continued endotracheal intubation was recommended. If more than one week of additional mechanical ventilation was anticipated then tracheostomy was recommended.

Over the last decade retrospective, prospective observational, and randomized controlled trials have suggested benefit to early tracheostomy [13]. This literature must be interpreted cautiously; the definition of early timing has ranged from <48 hours to 10 days and the studies are impossible to blind. It has also proved difficult to predict who will need more prolonged mechanical ventilation (some patients randomized to "late" tracheostomy are successfully liberated or die before a tube can be placed). Shock and a high APACHE II score at admission (>25) identify a cohort likely to require prolonged mechanical ventilation [1]. In trauma patients the need for prolonged mechanical ventilation is suggested by a low Glasgow Coma Scale score (<9) and an increased Injury Severity Score (>24) [14].

A Cochrane meta-analysis of five randomized controlled trial comparing early versus late tracheostomy found the early procedure to be associated with fewer days on mechanical ventilation and a shorter length of stay in the ICU [15]. Unfortunately, no difference in risk for hospital-acquired pneumonia or mortality was noted. Therefore, the best strategy may be to combine the anticipatory approach while also using predictors of the need for prolonged mechanical ventilation to identify a cohort for earlier tracheostomy. Patients identified as being highly likely to require prolonged mechanical ventilation should be considered for early tracheostomy. All others are assessed at Day 7 using the approach outlined above. Using this strategy a recent analysis suggested consideration for early tracheostomy if any of the following were present: upper airway obstruction, Glasgow Coma Score ≤6 on Day 4, spinal cord injury at C4 or above, acute neuromuscular disease with autonomic dysfunction or underlying lung disease, acute respiratory distress syndrome (ARDS) score ≥2.5 on Day 7, and in burn patients with significant full-thickness burns or active infection [1].

3.7.5 Tracheostomy techniques

Open surgical tracheostomy can be performed in the operating room or at the bedside in the critical care unit. An incision is made in the anterior neck (between the suprasternal notch and cricoid cartilage) and retracting the overlying muscles and thyroid isthmus exposes the tracheal rings. A tracheal ring (often the third) is divided to create a cartilaginous flap that is reflected forward and sutured to the skin of the anterior neck creating a path from skin to trachea. Alternatively, the anterior portion of a ring is removed to create a tracheal stoma. With this approach, sutures run from the tracheal stoma to the opening in the neck to facilitate identification of the tracheal stoma if early emergency replacement of the tube is required [16].

Percutaneous dilational tracheostomy (PDT) is a procedure performed at the bedside [17]. A small incision is made over the upper tracheal rings, a needle is inserted between the rings to access the trachea, and a guide wire is passed through the needle. A series of dilators or a single tapered dilator is used to widen the opening from skin to trachea and then a tracheostomy tube is placed using the guide wire. Fiber optic bronchoscopy through the existing endotracheal tube (which has been withdrawn proximally) can be used to avoid injury to the posterior tracheal wall and ensure proper positioning. When compared to surgical tracheostomy, PDT takes less time to perform, can be scheduled with less delay (no operating room needed), and is less costly, though this may not be the case if surgical tracheostomy is performed at the bedside. A meta-analysis of 17 randomized controlled studies found no difference in bleeding, major perioperative or long-term complications, or mortality when comparing PDT to all surgical tracheostomies [18]. PDT was associated with fewer wound infections. When comparing PDT to surgical tracheostomy performed in the operating room the latter is associated with increased bleeding and death. One advantage of PDT is that it can be performed in a timely fashion by properly trained critical care physicians at the bedside, reducing the delay that may result from awaiting consultation with a surgeon and an anesthesiologist and the availability of an operating room.

3.7.6   Decannulation

Weaning from ventilatory support in a patient with a tracheostomy tube is similar to that for the intubated patient. In contrast, removal of an endotracheal tube (extubation) typically follows tolerance for a two-hour spontaneous breathing trial while decannulation (tracheostomy tube removal) is only considered after 24–48 hours off of ventilatory support. Several techniques have been described for facilitating decannulation [19]. The first entails placing a fenestrated tracheostomy tube (with one or more openings above the cuff). During ventilatory support an inner cannula occludes the fenestration to ensure that machine delivered tidal volume flows into the patient. When the inner cannula is removed the fenestrations provide another route for the flow of gas in and out of the patient. By deflating the tube cuff and occluding the proximal end with a cap the patient breathes through the native airway. The patient then undergoes capping trials of increasing duration until 24–48 hours can be tolerated without significant respiratory distress. At that point the tracheostomy tube is removed as long as the patient is deemed capable of protecting the airway and managing respiratory secretions. Another approach consists of progressively downsizing the tracheostomy tube. Tolerance for a very narrow tube signals readiness for decannulation. For patients who tolerate either technique but concern remains for the ability to clear secretions, the stoma can be maintained by using a tracheostomy plug or button. Patients intolerant of capping or tube downsizing should undergo bronchoscopy to identify the source of upper airway obstruction and determine the best therapeutic approach.

3.7.7 Complications

Surgical and percutaneous tracheostomy are safe procedures though early and late complications have been reported (Table 3.7.3) [20, 21]. In general, tracheostomy tubes are much more secure than translaryngeal endotracheal tubes [22]. Early accidental tube removal can be life threatening as replacement is challenging if the skin to trachea track has not fully matured. Under these circumstances the tube may be inadvertently placed in the pretracheal space, indicated by continuing respiratory distress, difficulty bagging the patient, or the development of neck subcutaneous emphysema. If tube replacement proves difficult the patient should undergo immediate translaryngeal intubation.

Late complications can be directly related to placement of the tube, leaving the tube in for a prolonged period, or abnormal healing at the site of injured tracheal mucosa. As with a translaryngeal endotracheal tube, complications may be related to the inflated cuff of the tracheostomy tube or the tip of the tube, especially when it impinges on the posterior tracheal wall. In contrast, the tracheostomy stoma leads to a unique set of airway complications. The most frequent late complication is the development of granulation tissue, a complication that can be subclinical or may present as failure to wean from the ventilator, failure to decannulate, or may manifest as upper airway obstruction with respiratory failure after decannulation. Granulation tissue may contribute to airway occlusion or contribute to airway stenosis [21].

Tracheal stenosis, an abnormal narrowing of the tracheal lumen, can occur at different sites: suprastomal, stomal, or infrastomal. Common to all sites is tracheal injury followed by abnormal healing with granulation tissue. Granulation tissue may obstruct the airway and cause difficulty in replacing the tracheostomy tube if accidental decannulation occurs. The vascular nature of granulation tissue increases the risk for bleeding during tube placement. Stomal and suprastomal granulation

Table 3.7.3 Early and late complications of tracheostomy.

Early
  Loss of airway with inability to correctly replace the tube
  Bleeding
  Stomal infection
  Pneumothorax
  Subcutaneous emphysema
  Tracheal ring rupture

Late
  Tracheal stenosis
  Tracheomalacia
  Tracheoinnominate fistula
  Tracheoesophageal fistula
  Aspiration

tissue can occlude tracheostomy tube fenestrations, preventing successful decan-nulation. Over time granulation tissue matures becoming fibrous and causing airway circumferential narrowing or stenosis [21].

Stenosis can also occur at the site of tracheal tube cuff related ischemic injury to the tracheal mucosa. This occurs when cuff pressure exceeds the perfusion pres-sure of the capillaries of the tracheal wall. Although the incidence of cuff stenosis has fallen with the change to high volume, low pressure cuffs, over-inflation can lead to ischemic airway injury [21]. The latter can be decreased by monitoring cuff pressure and removing air, as needed, to keep pressure below 25 mm Hg. In general, cuff pressures below 18 mm Hg are associated with aspiration of fluid around the tube and air leaks.

Up to 5% of patients with a tracheostomy may fail to wean secondary to tracheal stenosis or obstruction from granulation tissue [23]. Clinical clues to tracheal obstruction include the presence of elevated peak airway pressures, difficulty in passing a suction catheter, or intolerance for tube capping. Patients may also present as failure to decannulate. Bronchoscopic evaluation of the trachea is indicated to define the exact site of stenosis, the cause, and the length of the involved trachea. Therapeutic approaches include placement of a longer tube (bypassing the area of narrowing) or tracheal stenting if significant stenosis is detected. Granulation tissue can be removed bronchoscopically or by excision using a carbon dioxide or neodymium-yttrium-aluminum-garnet (Nd:YAG) laser. For other patients, exer-tional dyspnea, dyspnea at rest or stridor occurs weeks to months after decannula-tion. Some of these patients require surgical repair (tracheal sleeve resection) consisting of excision of the stenotic area followed be reanastomosis of the remain-ing elements of the trachea [21].

Tracheomalacia, or a weakening of the tracheal wall, results from ischemic injury and subsequent destruction and necrosis of supporting tracheal cartilage. The tra-cheal airway collapses during expiration resulting in expiratory airflow limitation, air trapping, and less effective removal of respiratory secretions. Tracheomalacia may also present as failure to wean. Bronchoscopy or chest CT will reveal exces-sive expiratory collapse of the trachea, using forced exhalation or cough. Tracheomalcia is defined as a 50% or greater narrowing of the tracheal lumen during the expiratory maneuver. Expiratory touching of the anterior and posterior tracheal walls indicates severe tracheomalacia. Therapeutic strategies include place-ment of a longer tracheostomy tube (to bypass the region of expiratory collapse) or a tracheal stent. Surgical options include tracheal resection or tracheoplasty (repair using cartilage or a graft) [21].

Tracheoinnominate artery fistula is a rare but life threatening complication. If the tracheostomy tube is placed to low, below the third tracheal ring, the inferior concave surface of the cannula may erode into the artery. An overinflated trache-ostomy cuff balloon or the tip of the tracheostomy tube can severely damage the tracheal mucosa, leading to necrosis and eventual erosion into the innominate artery. This complication typically occurs within 3–4 weeks of the tracheostomy and most commonly manifests as bleeding around the tracheostomy tube or massive hemoptysis. Treatment of active bleeding entails emergent digital or tube cuff compression of the fistula to achieve hemostasis as the patient is emergently transported to the operating room for surgical interruption of the artery [21].

Tracheoesophageal fistula resulting from injury to the posterior tracheal wall occurs in less than 1% of patients. Posterior tracheal wall injury can occur during PDT placement or secondary to excessive cuff pressure or the tip of the tracheostomy tube. Clinical features include copious production of secretions, recurrent aspiration of food, increasing dyspnea, persistent cuff leak, or severe gastric distension (as air moves from the respiratory side to the stomach via the fistula). Barium esophagography or CT scan of the mediastinum can help make the diagnosis. Treatment includes surgical repair or placement of a double stent (in the esophagus and trachea) in patients unable to undergo surgery [21].

Placement of a tracheostomy tube disrupts swallowing and increases the risk for aspiration. Based on the high prevalence of swallowing disorders, frequently clinically silent, it is recommended that a formal swallowing evaluation be conducted in all patients with a tracheostomy in whom oral nutrition is contemplated. Despite numerous studies it remains unclear whether tracheostomy decreases ventilator-associated pneumonia rates compared to intubation [1].

3.7.8   Illustrative case continued

Based on the diagnosis of critical illness neuromyopathy, the team predicted difficulty liberating the patient from mechanical ventilation. On Day 11 a percutaneous tracheostomy tube was placed in the ICU, the patient tolerated the procedure well. On Day 14 she remained stable and was transferred to the hospital's 10-bed long-term weaning unit. Over the next six weeks she continued to recover, demonstrating improvement in peripheral motor strength and a NIF of $-40\,cm$ H_2O. During this time she tolerated spontaneous breathing trials, of increasing duration, conducted on 30% oxygen delivered through the tracheostomy tub. She eventually tolerated 24 hours off of mechanical ventilatory support. At that time an attempt to deflate the tracheostomy cuff and cap the tube led to significant respiratory distress. Fiber optic bronchoscopy disclosed subglottic granulation tissue arising from the anterior tracheal window obstructing 80% of the tracheal lumen. The patient underwent successful laser resection of the granulation tissue with significant improvement. She subsequently tolerated capping of the tube and cuff deflation without distress. The tracheostomy tube was removed after she tolerated 48 hours of having the tube capped.

References

1. King, C. and Moores, L.K. (2008) Controversies in mechanical ventilation: when should a tracheotomy be placed? *Clin. Chest Med.*, **29**, 253–263.
2. Epstein, S.K. (2005) Anatomy and physiology of tracheostomy. *Respir. Care*, **50**, 476–482.

3. Davis, K., Jr., Campbell, R.S., Johannigman, J.A. *et al.* (1999) Changes in respiratory mechanics after tracheostomy. *Arch. Surg.*, **134**, 59–62.
4. Diehl, J.L., El Atrous, S., Touchard, D. *et al.* (1999) Changes in the work of breathing induced by tracheotomy in ventilator-dependent patients. *Am. J. Respir. Crit. Care Med.*, **159**, 383–388.
5. Pierson, D.J. (2005) Tracheostomy and weaning. *Respir. Care*, **50**, 526–533.
6. Vitacca, M., Vianello, A., Colombo, D. *et al.* (2001) Comparison of two methods for weaning patients with chronic obstructive pulmonary disease requiring mechanical ventilation for more than 15 days. *Am. J. Respir. Crit. Care Med.*, **164**, 225–230.
7. Kollef, M.H., Levy, N.T., Ahrens, T.S. *et al.* (1998) The use of continuous i.v. sedation is associated with prolongation of mechanical ventilation. *Chest*, **114**, 541–548.
8. Brook, A.D., Ahrens, T.S., Schaiff, R. *et al.* (1999) Effect of a nursing-implemented sedation protocol on the duration of mechanical ventilation. *Crit. Care Med.*, **27**, 2609–2615.
9. Kress, J.P., Pohlman, A.S., O'Connor, M.F. *et al.* (2000) Daily interruption of sedative infusions in critically ill patients undergoing mechanical ventilation. *N. Engl. J. Med.*, **342**, 1471–1477.
10. Heffner, J.E. (2003) Tracheotomy application and timing. *Clin. Chest Med.*, **24**, 389–398.
11. Nieszkowska, A., Combes, A., Luyt, C.E. *et al.* (2005) Impact of tracheotomy on sedative administration, sedation level, and comfort of mechanically ventilated intensive care unit patients. *Crit. Care Med.*, **33**, 2527–2533.
12. Veelo, D.P., Dongelmans, D.A., Binnekade, J.M. *et al.* (2006) Tracheotomy does not affect reducing sedation requirements of patients in intensive care–a retrospective study. *Crit. Care*, **10**, R99.
13. Groves, D.S. and Durbin, C.G., Jr (2007) Tracheostomy in the critically ill: indications, timing and techniques. *Curr. Opin. Crit. Care*, **13**, 90–97.
14. Durbin, C.G., Jr (2005) Indications for and timing of tracheostomy. *Respir. Care*, **50**, 483–487.
15. Griffiths, J., Barber, V.S., Morgan, L. *et al.* (2005) Systematic review and meta-analysis of studies of the timing of tracheostomy in adult patients undergoing artificial ventilation. *BMJ*, **330**, 1243.
16. Durbin, C.G., Jr (2005) Techniques for performing tracheostomy. *Respir. Care*, **50**, 488–496.
17. Rana, S., Pendem, S., Pogodzinski, M.S. *et al.* (2005) Tracheostomy in critically ill patients. *Mayo Clin. Proc.*, **80**, 1632–1638.
18. Delaney, A., Bagshaw, S.M. and Nalos, M. (2006) Percutaneous dilatational tracheostomy versus surgical tracheostomy in critically ill patients: a systematic review and meta-analysis. *Crit. Care*, **10**, R55.
19. Christopher, K.L. (2005) Tracheostomy decannulation. *Respir. Care*, **50**, 538–541.
20. Durbin, C.G., Jr. (2005) Early complications of tracheostomy. *Respir. Care*, **50**, 511–515.
21. Epstein, S.K. (2005) Late complications of tracheostomy. *Respir. Care*, **50**, 542–549.
22. Goldenberg, D., Ari, E.G., Golz, A. *et al.* (2000) Tracheotomy complications: a retrospective study of 1130 cases. *Otolaryngol. Head Neck Surg.*, **123**, 495–500.
23. Rumbak, M.J., Walsh, F.W., Anderson, W.M. *et al.* (1999) Significant tracheal obstruction causing failure to wean in patients requiring prolonged mechanical ventilation: a forgotten complication of long-term mechanical ventilation. *Chest*, **115**, 1092–1095.

3.8 Putting it all together: protocols and algorithms

Scott K. Epstein[1] and Maged A. Tanios[2]

[1] *Office of Educational Affairs, Tufts University School of Medicine, Boston, MA, USA*
[2] *Intensive Care Unit, St Mary Medical Center, Long Beach, CA, USA*

3.8.1 Illustrative case

A 56-year-old man was intubated four days ago for severe community acquired pneumonia. Upon admission an order was written to initiate the intensive care unit (ICU) weaning protocol by screening the patient each morning to determine readiness for spontaneous breathing trials. The patient has been ventilated using volume assist control with a respiratory rate of 16, tidal volume 500 ml, and PEEP 5 cm H_2O. Until yesterday he was requiring a FiO_2 of 0.50–0.60 and had been maintained on dopamine at 8 mcg/kg/min to keep the mean arterial pressure $\geq$65 mm Hg. Over the last 24 hours the patient has improved significantly. He was screened at 6 a.m. this morning by a respiratory therapist who noted: FiO_2 of 0.40, PEEP of 5 cm H_2O, PaO_2 of 80 mm Hg (yielding a PaO_2/FiO_2 of 200), respiratory rate 18 (machine back-up rate 14), and blood pressure of 130/70 (off of dopamine).

Following the ICU protocol, the respiratory therapist placed the patient on CPAP 5 cm H_2O (FiO_2 0.40), a spontaneous breathing trial. The ICU nurse carefully observed the patient during the trial, which lasted 120 minutes. The patient appeared comfortable throughout the trial, without significant change in vital signs or oxygen saturation level. The patient was then placed back on assist control and the ICU team, which was rounding in another part of the unit, was notified. The ICU team came to the patient's bedside and noted the patient to be awake and alert, with

A Practical Guide to Mechanical Ventilation, First Edition.
Edited by Jonathon D. Truwit and Scott K. Epstein.
© 2011 John Wiley & Sons, Ltd. Published 2011 by John Wiley & Sons, Ltd.

minimal respiratory secretions (last needing airway suctioning four hours previously), and a good cough. The ICU team proceeded with extubation at 10:15 a.m. and the patient did well.

3.8.2 Introduction

The preceding chapters have reviewed the essential elements to be addressed as the clinician seeks to discontinue mechanical ventilation and successfully extubate the patient (Figure 3.8.1). The process begins with recognition that sufficient recovery has occurred for the patient to undertake spontaneous breathing trials (SBTs). This decision is aided by the application of objective parameters indicating readiness for SBTs. A trial of spontaneous breathing is then conducted on no or minimal ventilatory support. Rigorous criteria are applied during the SBT to determine if the patient is tolerating the trial. If the trial is tolerated, the clinician applies objective parameters to determine whether the patient can be extubated. If the patients does not satisfy readiness criteria for an SBT or fails the SBT, the patient is ventilated on full support. The clinician then launches into a detailed investigation to identify treatable barriers to discontinuation from mechanical ventilation. Depending on the results of this evaluation, screening will be repeated the next day and the process repeated.

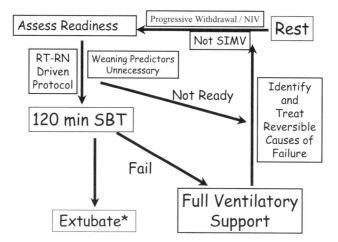

Figure 3.8.1 Overview of process of discontinuation from mechanical ventilation and extubation. RT = respiratory therapist; RN = ICU nurse; NIV = noninvasive ventilation; SIMV = synchronized intermittent mandatory ventilation. *Extubate if adequate cough, minimal respiratory secretions (airway suctioning needed no more than every two hours), and adequate mental status (awake or easily arousable).

Clinicians with substantial expertise in mechanical ventilation implicitly use this approach every day at the bedside. Unfortunately, the expertise of clinicians and the time they can spend at the bedside may vary considerably. This is especially true in an ICU with an open structure. Such ICUs may not have dedicated intensivists or the involvement of intensivists in any given case may depend on formal consultation. Under these circumstances an organized approach to weaning making use of the skills of critical care nurses and respiratory therapists can improve the outcome of mechanical ventilation. By using a protocol, variations in care can be reduced and the process of care can continue even if the ICU physician is not physically present at the patient's bedside. Although protocols bring standardization to the process of weaning, their use runs the risk of applying a general algorithm to a group of complex patients who display considerable physiologic variability (e.g., one size does not fit all). The best protocol is one that applies an algorithm that has been rigorously studied (ideally in randomized controlled trials) in a patient population similar to that in which it will be applied (the protocol has external validity). Protocols best serve as guidelines or defaults to initiate the process. They may be particularly effective in identifying a patient whose readiness for spontaneous breathing was not otherwise evident. The most effect protocols allow the clinician the power to override the algorithm to take into account individual patient characteristics (e.g., protocols must be flexible). Indeed, ICU physicians should adapt validated protocols to their particular ICU environment or distinctive patient population. Ideally this modified protocol would be rigorously tested at the institution, but this rarely happens. At a minimum, the outcomes resulting from protocol use should be periodically analyzed providing a feedback loop for continuous quality improvement.

3.8.3   Protocols for weaning

Uncontrolled investigations and randomized controlled trials (RCTs) demonstrate improved outcome with weaning driven by a protocol and implemented by physicians or by respiratory care practitioners and ICU nurses (Table 3.8.1). Protocols can be used to perform a daily screen to determine readiness for an SBT, to determine the pace of weaning using methods of progressive withdrawal, or to direct a search for treatable causes for weaning failure. Of these three applications, the first is more important than the second; the third application is likely to be very important but unfortunately has yet to be fully investigated.

3.8.3.1 Randomized controlled trials

The landmark study of a screening protocol randomized 300 mechanically ventilated medical patients to either standard care or an intervention strategy that combined readiness testing with a daily screen [1]. To pass the daily screen the patient had to satisfy *all* of the following criteria: $PaO_2/FiO_2 \geq 200$ (on PEEP ≤ 5 cm

Table 3.8.1   Application of weaning protocols to facilitate liberation from mechanical ventilation.

Weaning issue	Supporting evidence
A protocol, driven by respiratory care practitioners and ICU nurses, should be used to assess daily readiness (and monitor) for spontaneous breathing trials and to direct the weaning process.	High quality; based on RCTs.
A protocol combining daily awakening trials with daily spontaneous breathing trials is superior to using the SBT alone.	High quality, based on a single RCT.
Protocols have not proven superior to usual care in the Neurologic ICU, the Pediatric ICU, and in a Medical ICU managed by a highly experienced core of faculty and fellows.	High quality; based on multiple RCTs

H_2O), hemodynamically stable; adequate cough, no intravenous sedation, and f/$V_T \leq 105$ breaths/l/min. Control patients were screened but care was not influenced by the testing. In contrast, intervention patients passing the daily screen underwent a two-hour SBT (T-piece or CPAP) with a prompt for extubation if the trial was tolerated. The intervention strategy resulted in significant reductions in weaning time, duration of mechanical ventilation, complication rate, and ICU costs; no differences were noted in length of ICU or hospital stay, hospital costs, or mortality. In a follow-up analysis the authors noted that 30% of patients who never passed the daily screen could still be ultimately liberated from the ventilator (in 40% of these cases the f/V_T criteria was never satisfied). This raises two important points. Firstly, if the protocol was rigidly adhered to, 30% of patients would have been inappropriately maintained on mechanical ventilation. Therefore, protocols should be viewed as guidelines or starting points in the weaning process. Secondly, the study raised the issue about which components of the daily screen were essential to the process. This author's group conducted a randomized controlled trial of 304 patients in which all patients were screened but in only one group was the weaning predictor (f/V_T) used for weaning decision making (Figure 3.8.2) [2]. Using the f/V_T did not shorten the duration of mechanical ventilation or reduce length of stay. These two studies both included screening parameters that recent work indicates are more appropriately used as predictors of extubation rather than weaning outcome [3]. These parameters include cough, secretions (frequency of suctioning) and mental status. Indeed, the multisociety Task Force on Discontinuation from Mechanical Ventilation only recommended the PaO_2/FiO_2 ratio (≥ 150) and hemodynamic stability as routinely determined screening parameters to assess readiness for spontaneous breathing trials [4].

Another key feature of these two studies is that both used non-physician health care personnel to implement the protocol. For example, in the study by Tanios *et al.*, respiratory therapists conducted the daily screen and initiated the SBTs if the screen was passed. ICU nurses monitored patients during the SBT to determine whether they were tolerating the trial. Two additional randomized controlled trials

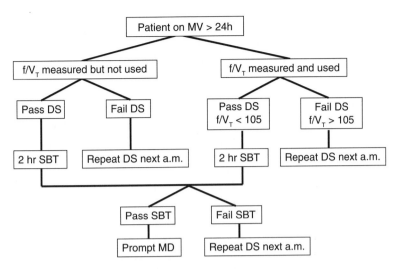

Figure 3.8.2 Flow diagram of randomized controlled trial comparing two daily screens (DSs) to determine readiness for SBTs. To pass the daily screen all criteria must be satisfied: $PaO_2/FiO_2 \geq 150$ or $SpO_2 \geq 90\%$ on $FiO_2 \leq 0.4$ and $PEEP \leq 5\,cm\ H_2O$; mean arterial pressure $\geq 60\,mm\,Hg$ without vasopressors or only requiring low dose vasopressors; awake or easily arousable; adequate cough during suctioning and suctioning required less often than every 2 h. f/V_T is the frequency tidal volume ratio determined by dividing the respiratory rate (breaths/min) by tidal volume (liters) [2].

in medical and surgical ICUs also found that protocols directed by a respiratory care practitioner-ICU nurse shortened mechanical ventilation duration [5, 6]. Another RCT found that a protocol combining a spontaneous awakening trial (SAT) with a SBT was superior to one using the SBT alone [7].

As noted earlier, it is essential that protocols be adapted to the local ICU environment and modified for application to unique patient populations. For example, subsequent studies performed in a neurosurgical ICU [8], a pediatric ICU [9] and in a medical ICU at a leading academic medical center with particular expertise in mechanical ventilation found no advantage to a protocol-led approach [10]. Though a protocol may serve as the default approach to weaning, flexibility and clinical judgment are highly recommended, as too rigid an approach needlessly prolongs weaning and extubation.

3.8.3.2 *Initiating and maintaining protocols*

Protocols have been successfully implemented in many aspects of medicine. Nevertheless, many physicians see protocol-led care as a threat to their clinical decision making autonomy. Given the complexity of individual patient characteristics physicians often rail against what may be perceived as "cookbook" medicine.

As noted above, considerable research supports the use of a protocol-led approach to weaning in certain settings. Despite high quality evidence some physicians are reluctant to alter their practice and management styles. Therefore, an essential element for successful implementation is getting "buy in" from physicians who practice in the ICU [11].

The process begins with institutional commitment to improving outcomes and provision of sufficient resources necessary for implementation. For example, the successful implementation of protocols requires adequate non-physician staffing, both ICU nurses and respiratory therapists. Indeed, when the number of nurses is reduced below a certain threshold the duration of mechanical ventilation increases [12]. The influence and leadership of respected local opinion leaders and experts in mechanical ventilation is an indispensable component of this process. The protocol should be based on evidence-based data, modified to meet the local environment. Once a specific protocol is designed, it is essential to assemble a multidisciplinary team (physicians, respiratory care therapists, ICU nurses, administrators, etc.) that will be charged with protocol roll-out and maintenance. The team should then craft a staged implementation process. Members of the team will be responsible for coordinating and providing education to all personnel who will participate in protocol implementation. During the education period, or before, it is useful to collect baseline data on mechanical ventilation outcomes (weaning success rate, duration of mechanical ventilation, length of ICU stay, etc.) that can serve for future comparison with outcomes observed after initiating the protocol.

With initiation of the protocol the emphasis switches to maintenance. This entails monitoring both compliance with the protocol and the resulting outcomes. A process of continuous quality improvement should be implemented so the protocol can evolve along with other changes in the ICU environment or in the patient population encountered. Educational efforts must be ongoing to educate new members of the team and to provide refreshers for continuing team members. Lastly, it must be re-emphasized that overly rigid following of protocol rules may delay the process of liberation from mechanical ventilation for some patients. Flexibility and the opportunity for using clinical judgment must not be forsaken [11].

3.8.4   A practical approach

Based on the considerations detailed in the last eight chapters, this author's institution has adopted a rigorous organized approach to discontinuation and extubation. Within 24 hours of admission to the ICU an order is written to initiate the protocol and conduct daily screening for readiness for spontaneous breathing trials (Figure 3.8.3). When writing the order the ICU physician also specifies how the spontaneous breathing trial will be conducted and what the duration should be. The ICU

MICU Weaning Protocol Orders

Patient:
Medical Record #:
Diagnosis:
Date intubated:

Institute MICU Weaning Protocol (patient to be screened every 8 am)

Method of Spontaneous Breathing Trial (SBT):

PSV _____ cm H_2O + PEEP _____ cm H_2O

CPAP _____ cm H_2O

Duration of Spontaneous Breathing Trial (SBT):

30, 60, 120 minutes (circle one)

MD signature:

Figure 3.8.3 Example of pre-printed order sheet allowing ICU nurses and respiratory therapists to initiate a process of daily screening followed automatically by SBTs if the screen is positive.

nurse screens the patient each day using a written protocol (Figure 3.8.4). Results of the daily screen are recorded on a separate bedside form to foster communication between ICU nurse, respiratory therapists, and ICU physicians. Previous work demonstrates that outcome improves when a bedside weaning board and flow sheet is used to enhance communication between critical care practitioners [13].

When patients undergo a spontaneous breathing trial the ICU nurse and ICU physician use a rigorous set of criteria to determine tolerance for the SBT (Figure 3.8.5). Vital signs (and blood gases if applicable) are carefully recorded every 15 minutes during the trial. If the SBT is not tolerated the reason is recorded (Figure 3.8.5), the patient is returned to full ventilatory support and an immediate investigation into the cause for failure is launched. The goal of the investigation is to detect potential reversible barriers to weaning success.

The author's protocol makes use of daily spontaneous breathing trials, returning the patient who fails to full ventilatory support. At any time the ICU physician is permitted to opt out of the approach and change to a strategy that employs a slow reduction in ventilator support using either pressure support ventilation, T-piece or constant positive airway pressure (CPAP) trials of increasing duration, or a combination of synchronized IMV (SIMV) and pressure support as outlined in Chapter 3.4. Daily spontaneous breathing trials may be combined with any of these techniques.

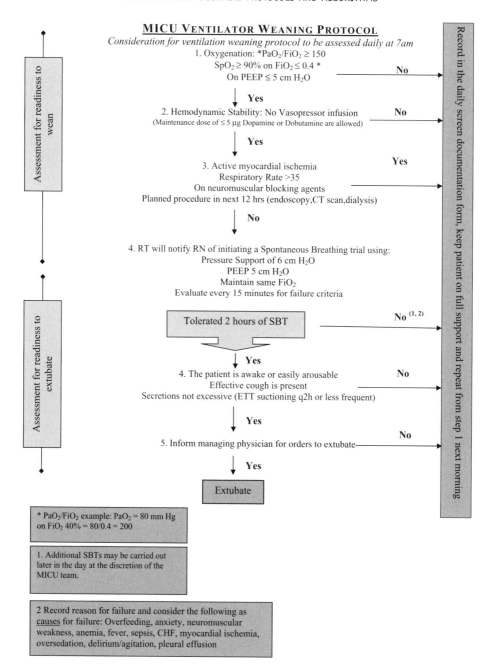

Figure 3.8.4 Weaning and Extubation protocol used in the author's Medical Intensive Care Unit (MICU). RT = respiratory therapist; RN = ICU nurse; ETT = endotracheal tube.

Daily Screen Protocol Documentation Form

Patient's name: _____ Medical Record Number: _____

Date:	/ /	/ /	/ /	/ /	/ /	/ /

Readiness to wean parameters	Yes	No	Yes	No	Yes	No	Yes	No	Yes	No	Yes	No
PaO2 / FiO2 (≥ 150 = pass)												
PEEP (≤ 5 = pass)												
Intravenous pressor (no = pass) (≤5µg Dopamine or Dobutamine is allowed)												
Passes Screen?												
SBT performed? If no, explain												

Criteria for failure of SBT:
1. Diaphoresis, agitation or dyspnea.
2. Signs of increased work of breathing* for >15 minutes.
3. Hypoxemia: PaO2 decreased to < 60 or SaO2 < 90%.
4. Hypercapnia: Increase PaCO2 > 10mmHg from pre-weaning.
5. Increased respiratory rate to >35 bpm for >10minutes.
6. Tachycardia HR > 140, or bradycardia HR < 50
7. Hypotension: Systolic blood pressure < 80 mmHg, or drop by > 20%.
8. Hypertension: Increase in systolic blood pressure > 20%.

Tolerated the 2-hour SBT?	Yes	No	Yes	No	Yes	No	Yes	No	Yes	No	Yes	No

If the answer is "Yes" in the previous
section, proceed to the next section.

Readiness to extubate parameters	Yes	No	Yes	No	Yes	No	Yes	No	Yes	No	Yes	No
Awake or easily arousable (yes = pass)												
Effective cough present (yes = pass)												
Requires suctioning more frequently than q2 hours (no = pass)												
Passes Screen?												
Orders to extubate obtained?												
Extubated?												
Date Extubated												

Date/Time	Comments	Initials

*Signs of increased work of breathing such as thoraco-abdominal paradox or the use of accessory muscles for breathing

Figure 3.8.5 Bedside flow sheet for recording results of daily screen for spontaneous breathing trials, tolerance for SBTs, and readiness for extubation.

References

1. Ely, E.W., Baker, A.M., Dunagan, D.P. *et al.* (1996) Effect on the duration of mechanical ventilation of identifying patients capable of breathing spontaneously. *N. Engl. J. Med.*, **335** (25), 1864–1869.
2. Tanios, M.A., Nevins, M.L., Hendra, K.P. *et al.* (2006) A randomized, controlled trial of the role of weaning predictors in clinical decision making. *Crit. Care Med.*, **34** (10), 2530–2535.
3. Epstein, S.K. (2002) Decision to extubate. *Intensive Care Med.*, **28** (5), 535–546.
4. MacIntyre, N.R., Cook, D.J., Ely, E.W., Jr. *et al.* (2001) Evidence-based guidelines for weaning and discontinuing ventilatory support: a collective task force facilitated by the American College of Chest Physicians; the American Association for Respiratory Care; and the American College of Critical Care Medicine. *Chest*, **120** (6 Suppl.), 375S–395S.
5. Kollef, M.H., Shapiro, S.D., Silver, P. *et al.* (1997) A randomized, controlled trial of protocol-directed versus physician-directed weaning from mechanical ventilation. *Crit. Care Med.*, **25** (4), 567–574.
6. Marelich, G.P., Murin, S., Battistella, F. *et al.* (2000) Protocol weaning of mechanical ventilation in medical and surgical patients by respiratory care practitioners and nurses: effect on weaning time and incidence of ventilator-associated pneumonia. *Chest*, **118** (2), 459–467.
7. Girard, T.D., Kress, J.P., Fuchs, B.D. *et al.* (2008) Efficacy and safety of a paired sedation and ventilator weaning protocol for mechanically ventilated patients in intensive care (Awakening and Breathing Controlled trial): a randomised controlled trial. *Lancet*, **371** (9607), 126–134.
8. Namen, A.M., Ely, E.W., Tatter, S.B. *et al.* (2001) Predictors of successful extubation in neurosurgical patients. *Am. J. Respir. Crit. Care Med.*, **163** (3 Pt 1), 658–664.
9. Randolph, A.G., Wypij, D., Venkataraman, S.T. *et al.* (2002) Effect of mechanical ventilator weaning protocols on respiratory outcomes in infants and children: a randomized controlled trial. *JAMA*, **288** (20), 2561–2568.
10. Krishnan, J.A., Moore, D., Robeson, C. *et al.* (2004) A prospective, controlled trial of a protocol-based strategy to discontinue mechanical ventilation. *Am. J. Respir. Crit. Care Med.*, **169** (6), 673–678.
11. Ely, E.W., Meade, M.O., Haponik, E.F. *et al.* (2001) Mechanical ventilator weaning protocols driven by nonphysician health-care professionals: evidence-based clinical practice guidelines. *Chest*, **120** (6 Suppl.), 454S–463S.
12. Thorens, J.B., Kaelin, R.M., Jolliet, P. *et al.* (1995) Influence of the quality of nursing on the duration of weaning from mechanical ventilation in patients with chronic obstructive pulmonary disease. *Crit. Care Med.*, **23** (11), 1807–1815.
13. Henneman, E., Dracup, K., Ganz, T. *et al.* (2001) Effect of a collaborative weaning plan on patient outcome in the critical care setting. *Crit. Care Med.*, **29** (2), 297–303.

Index

3-CPO trial 45–6
ABC *see* airway, breathing, and circulation
abdominal distension 264–7, 327
accessory muscles 32–4, 64–9, 83, 199–202, 289–90, 301–2, 337
achondroplasia 108–9
acidosis 163, 211, 216–17, 230, 264–6, 268, 290, 294, 301–2
acute CHF, noninvasive ventilation 41–8, 52, 85–7
acute lung injury (ALI) 56, 151–60, 166–70, 173–92, 221–3, 241–2, 244, 270, 277, 286
acute myeloid leukemia (AML) 51
acute pulmonary edema 5, 96–8, 168–70, 174–92, 241–2, 244, 250–1, 264, 270, 289
acute respiratory distress syndrome (ARDS) 52, 56–9, 85–90, 96–8, 151–60, 165–71, 174–92, 195, 205–12, 216–18, 220–3, 307–15, 323
   noninvasive ventilation 52, 56–9, 85–90
   outcomes 216–18, 220–3
   statistics 96, 216–18, 220–3
acute respiratory failure (ARF)
   causes 51–60, 250–1
   CRF contrasts 99–100

invasive mechanical ventilation 96–100, 141–2, 205–12, 246, 250–1, 319–27
non-CHF/COPD causes 51–60
noninvasive ventilation 3–4, 10, 17–27, 31–8, 51–60, 72, 83, 85–90, 100, 223–9
patient–ventilator interactions 18–21, 139, 145–53
acute respiratory failure from COPD 3–4, 10, 17–27, 31–8, 51–2, 72, 83, 85–90, 99–100, 223–4, 285–6, 301–2, 305, 315
adaptive support ventilation (ASV) 143–56
adjuncts to facilitate weaning 305–15
advanced cardiac life support (ACLS) 108–9
aerosolized medications 138, 201–2, 209–12, 289–90
age factors, outcomes 216–17, 219–21, 229–30, 260, 291–302
"air trapping" 158, 167–71, 186, 196–202
airway, breathing, and circulation (ABC) 103–8
Airway Care Score 88
airway management 3, 6, 18, 21–7, 33–8, 52, 56–60, 88–90, 103–31, 170–1, 200–2, 209–12, 241–2, 265–6, 293–8, 299–300
   see also invasive mechanical ventilation
bag-valve-mask (BVM) assisted ventilation 103–9, 120–5, 299–300

A Practical Guide to Mechanical Ventilation, First Edition.
Edited by Jonathon D. Truwit and Scott K. Epstein.
© 2011 John Wiley & Sons, Ltd. Published 2011 by John Wiley & Sons, Ltd.

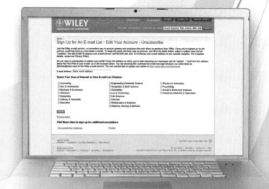
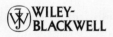